Mental Illnesses: Basic Concepts and Etiology

Mental Illnesses:
Basic Concepts and Etiology

Edited by **John Dalvi**

New Jersey

Published by Foster Academics,
61 Van Reypen Street,
Jersey City, NJ 07306, USA
www.fosteracademics.com

Mental Illnesses: Basic Concepts and Etiology
Edited by John Dalvi

International Standard Book Number: 978-1-63242-274-3 (Hardback)

Printed in the United States of America.

Contents

Preface

In my initial years as a student, I used to run to the library at every possible instance to grab a book and learn something new. Books were my primary source of knowledge and I would not have come such a long way without all that I learnt from them. Thus, when I was approached to edit this book; I became understandably nostalgic. It was an absolute honor to be considered worthy of guiding the current generation as well as those to come. I put all my knowledge and hard work into making this book most beneficial for its readers.

Major concepts and discoveries in the treatment of mental illnesses are discussed in this book. In this book, the main focus is on the various background factors that govern the understanding of public attitudes, immigration, stigma, and competencies surrounding mental illness. Many etiological and pathogenic factors, commencing from adhesion molecules on one side, and concluding with abuse and maltreatment in children and youth on the other, are linked with mental illnesses, inclusive of personality disorders that lie between mental health and illness. The book makes an attempt to integrate theory and research data in understanding particular ways to deal with mental illness.

I wish to thank my publisher for supporting me at every step. I would also like to thank all the authors who have contributed their researches in this book. I hope this book will be a valuable contribution to the progress of the field.

Editor

Part 1

Introduction – General Background

Stigma and Mental Disorders

Vesna Švab
University Ljubljana
Slovenia

1. Introduction

Stigma is recognised as a major obstacle to recovery and integration of people with mental health problems. In this chapter the definitions of cognitive, emotional and social aspects of stigma will be presented, as well as origins, main representations and coping strategies. The research on stigma is presented, beginning with Gofmann's work (Chapter History) and followed by contemporary research and critical overview. This work follows the International Study of Discrimination and Stigma Outcomes (INDIGO) led by professor Graham Thornicroft (UK), which was a cross-sectional survey in 27 countries, in centres affiliated to the INDIGO Research Network, by use of face-to-face interviews with 732 participants with schizophrenia. This research was followed by the creation of Antistigma European Network, with further research goals and a strong mission to overcome or at least reduce the consequences of mental disorder stigma in Europe. Each country participated in this projects produced additionally locally specific answers and solutions. Some of them are listed below-these are comments on stigma made by patients with schizophrenia in Slovenia. Each country involved in these research projects also produced locally specific answers and solutions to the stigmatization and particularly to discrimination problems.

The intent of this publication is, besides giving an overview of stigma research, to provide some additional insight into real life experience of people with severe mental illness.

2. Definitions

2.1 Stigma

Stigma is a term that applies to labelling certain people as different and inferior. It is a mark of shame, a sign of worthlessness applied to the stigmatized. Its consequence is avoidance and even expulsion from society. It can be described as a form of social monitoring or omission of minorities from certain competitive areas, working as a form of intangible control over groups of people with mental disorders (Goffman, 1963).

Its influence is in proportion to social, economic and political forces that make possible the creation of stereotypes, destruction of reputation, and other forms of discrimination (Link & Phelan, 2001). Stigma is obviously a wide concept, one that binds aspects of labelling, stereotyping, cognitive rejection, emotional reactions and discrimination - therefore, it has cognitive, emotional and social components, whose final result is the loss of social status for the person affected. Social status here refers to an individual's position in society and to an individual's reputation and influence. A high social status guarantees material goods, freedom, space, comfort, time and the feeling that one is appreciated. The fight for status is a fight to expose our inner wealth.

2.2 Stereotypes

Stereotypes are knowledge acquired by the majority of a social group so that knowledge of other social groups can be categorized. A stereotype is a collective agreement, needed for quick orientation as far as expectations and impressions are concerned. They are dynamic constructs, dependent on social judgment. Having a stereotypical opinion of a patient with metal health disorder would be thinking of him as dangerous and severely behaviourally disturbed. These stereotypes do not fit the facts. A typical patient lives in the community, his behaviour socially managed. A typical person with mental disorder has far less trouble in social adaptation than the usual hospitalised patient. Patients who must be treated regularly throughout their lives are a minority in the mentally ill fringe group. They function according to the severity of the illness, associated disabilities, the level and quality of available support and treatment capabilities. Patients who have recovered are usually invisible to professionals and public, as they generally hide their illness from others, because of stigma. They avoid institutions and social services so that they can pursue their careers, education or other personal goals. A diagnosis only describes the part of a person that the symptoms fit. A person with schizophrenic symptoms is not a schizophrenic, as these symptoms are only a part of his personality at the moment of diagnosis. A diagnosis is used to set treatment goals and methods and to estimate the illness' course. It is only to be referenced correctly in medical classification and professional assessment. Any other use of a psychiatrist's diagnostic terminology is considered to be stereotyping, aimed at discriminating against people with mental health disorders. Psychiatric diagnoses are often carelessly used to discredit political or other opponents, which is hurtful to people who have been diagnosed and have to live with illness and disability.

People do not always agree with stereotypes. Belief in them forms prejudice.

2.3 Prejudice

Prejudice is a wrong conviction, an ideological construct based on stereotyping and oversimplification. It motivates an authoritative bearing, hate and exclusion. In Nastran Ule's (1999) opinion, prejudice is simply a set of evaluations passed by privileged groups. Their main trait is helping repression. She defines repression as dominion of the strong over the weak, with the strong never allowing the weak to question the fairness of this arrangement. People are always very interested in learning how to have more power than others. If prejudice is collective, as those surrounding people with mental disorders are, people adapt to it. The general opinion is that people with mental disorders are less capable and that they require constant monitoring and care, which is followed by disdain and patronizing.

Almost every paper on stigmatization mentions prejudice as hard to change, relatively stable and spontaneous, affecting us no matter our will. This thesis introduced a certain amount of pessimism in all attempts to reduce stigmatization and rationalised poor results of anti-stigmatization campaigns. Social and psychological research, on the other hand, refuses this conclusion and proves that stigmatization is easily manipulated and very changeable in nature, as seen in Jew and women discrimination history (Henriquez et al., 1984) and the quick minimalisation of racial prejudice in the last few decades. It therefore follows historical experience that prejudice can be changed swiftly and successfully, if appropriate social circumstance and political goodwill exist. Politics can achieve position changes and improve tolerance through media access. But prejudice can not be created or stopped only with conviction. A complex social movement is required, one that provides both moral and financial consequences for those that break the rules. It has been proven repeatedly that the behaviour of people with mental illness even when completely normal is considered »weird« because of prejudice (Link & Cullen, 1986; Link et al., 1987, Link et al., 1999). Their behaviour is not incorrectly interpreted only by the general public, but also by professionals. In 1974 Langer and Abelson made an experiment in which two groups of analytic psychotherapists were shown s video interview with a young man. One group was told that this was a job interview, whereas the other was told that the man was a psychiatric patient. Despite watching the same tape the second group described his behaviour as abnormal, whereas those in the first group didn't see many problems at all (in Corrigan, 2005).

Prejudice means a poor life quality for the affected. It generates strong emotional responses, of which fear is the most important.

2.4 Fear

Most people are afraid of people suffering from mental illness. They fear »infection« despite it being general knowledge that mental illness can't be transmitted. For example, a common effect of fear are complaints from mental health staff about how hard it is to work with psychiatric patients, not because of the workload, but rather because they fear projective identification that could influence a staff member's mental health. This fear originates in prejudice of danger and unpredictability. People with mental health disorders may be dangerous, but only very rarely and always under foreseeable circumstances. Studies show that the percentage of patients with an affinity for violence is less than 10% in men and significantly less among women. Even this small percentage is not dangerous constantly, but only when they're under influence of psychoactive substances like alcohol and alternatively, when their psychotic symptoms are left untreated or poorly treated. Less severe mental disorders like depression and anxiety are not connected to violent behaviour. Research shows that 75% of the population believes that the mentally ill are dangerous, the number of people with this belief doubling over the last 40 years (Corrigan, 2005: 165). The rise of the danger myth can be explained by deinstitutionalization, meaning less access to hospitals and other social institutions; and primarily by media reports (Wahl, 1995). There was a series of papers published in the USA that "proved" psychiatric patients were dangerous. This research is methodologically dubious and its results were interpreted haphazardly at best. It was best refuted by the following statement: Mental illness has little connection to violence. This connection is used for discrimination of people with mental disorders and their families. People with mental disorders must be guaranteed quality treatment. The occurrence rate of criminal acts done with full awareness is much higher than of those who are motivated by illness.

Today, 6% to 15% of the American prison population are people with mental disorders. This number saw a 150% increase over the last 10 years. The reasons for this fact can be found in poor service accessibility, public fear, legislation that prevents hospitalization and lack of education. In the USA, officers of the law seem to have a role of doormen to the medical system, for which they are not educated. Furthermore, in the US, the number of psychiatric hospital beds is evidently over reduced.

Any behaviour that is caused by prejudice is discrimination (Corrigan & Watson, 2002, Corrigan et al., 2003).

2.5 Discrimination

The behavioural manifestation of "applied prejudice" is discrimination. Affected people are discriminated against by being marginalised, avoided and being victims of violence. Even though discrimination can be an upfront protest against the mentally ill, it more often takes the form of avoidance. Openly ridiculing patients is no longer acceptable due to rising awareness. Hostility or (at least) ambivalence is nowadays expressed more subtly.

But, many patients report feeling lonely, losing friends, not being in contact with their families, losing their jobs and being delegated to lower positions in their workplace. Discrimination is not authoritarian and directly aggressive anymore (Corrigan et al., 2001), most likely due to anti-stigmatization movements, which managed to influence the way discrimination is exhibited, but not what it's about. An Australian study researching nurses' relationships with their patients (Happel et al., 2002) showed that most of nurses agree with anti-stigmatization programs, yet wouldn't allow a mentally ill individual to be part of a job screening procedure in their workplace. 40% of them were found to believe that even though a users' view on mental illness is important, lectures on this topics should be given by nurses.

Social distance raises the levels of disability amongst the mentally ill and significantly worsens the illness. Stereotyping, prejudice and discrimination can thus stop people from realising their ambitions and life goals.

3. History of stigma

Any discussion of mental illness is accompanied by strong emotion. Psychiatrists are still considered to be modern witches, capable of both help and harm. The general population's view of psychiatry and psychiatrists is coloured by emotions such as fear, shame, guilt, hostility, admiration and ultimately, confusion. It is for this reason that most mental health disorders are only discussed and treated in a close circle of friends, family and acquaintances and professional help only being sought in extreme circumstances.

Throughout history, society constantly changed its treatment of people with mental disorders. Rejection, punishment and avoidance was replaced, in certain times, by relative tolerance and attempts at integration, but this trend was never exclusive, as different viewpoints coexisted, sometimes obviously in mutual opposition. The general consensus is that the more the group was removed into specific institutions and the edge of society, the more negative society's attitudes were. In Europe, the relationship between marginalised groups and public opinion had been primarily defined by the church, its own attitudes subject to change from acceptance to rejection. For instance, when the predominant belief was that people with mental disorders were possessed by demons, they were either jailed or banished from society, whereas when mental illness was seen as a gift from god, they were protected and respected. In 1486, the book Malleus Maleficarum (The hammer of the witches) was published, ushering in 150 years of persecution of people with mental illness. Women with hysterical or psychotic symptoms were labelled as witches and torture was used for making them admit their guilt. The subsequent executions and other extreme violence were not put to a stop until 1656, when, under the influence of more tolerant ideas, asylums were first opened in the French monarchy. During the next century, people with mental illness were joined in these buildings by orphans, prostitutes, homosexuals, the chronically ill and the elderly. The same century saw the first attempts to classify mental illnesses and understand them as medical disorders. There were attempts to improve the quality of care by the reformists Vincenzo Chiarugi (1759-1820) in Firenze, William Tuke (1732-1822) in York, and finally Jean Baptiste Pussin (1745-1826) and Philippe Pinel (1745-1826) in France. The removal of shackles from the Parisian hospital Bicètre marks the start of moral treatment. Pinel classified mental illnesses as being melancholy, mania, idiocy or dementia and claimed they were caused by both environmental and hereditary factors. He used education and persuasion as his methods and provided a comfortable environment for patients to heal in, but it wasn't until the 19th century that psychiatry became a branch of medicine, which brought about significant advances. In England, Tuke influenced the removal of restraints from hospitals. America saw a reform of psychiatric institutions, initiated by Benjamin Rush. The Kraepelin classification of mental disorders provided an accurate enough description of psychiatric symptoms. In 1920 electroconvulsive therapy was introduced.

Sigmund Freud (1856-1939), the founder of psychological interpretation of mental disorders, initiated the development of psychotherapeutic treatment through his personality, dream interpretation, sexuality and other theories. Social psychiatry began to evolve, using as it's tools both clinical and social theory knowledge. It dealt with the problems of poverty, racial prejudice, war and mass migration, even if it was apparent that no profession can solve them. The anti-psychiatry movement originated within social psychiatry, explaining mental disorders through social and family influences.

From 1954 to 1956, Ervin Goffman, the author of the famous Asylums(1961), was doing research in psychiatric hospitals and other institutions, precisely describing life in these »total institutions« (hospitals, prisons, homes for the elderly etc.) meant to hold patients away from society. He reasoned that any »total institution« has the same characteristics: the presence of a large number of people, group management and a clear structure of activities meant to institutionalise. In its essence a »total institution« was about controlling a large population with a bureaucratic institutional organisation, in which obedience was expected from both the population and the staff that oversaw it. A rift between the staff managing the asylum and the patients using it became apparent. The social distance between the superior, displeased staff and the weak, inferior patients was immense, with most of the staff's energy being directed at stopping patient to doctor (or any other staff member with more responsibility) communication. The simple effect of this was that patients were excluded from deciding their own fate. The secondary effects ranged from extreme boredom, the cause of which was that the patients were not trusted with anything, to post-treatment social exclusion. Upon leaving the hospital most patients had no established contacts with the outside world, as being institutionalized severed their bonds with the world. The mere entry into a psychiatric hospital was highly indicative of permanent loss: washing, disinfection, hair cut off, a personal search, listing of personal belongings and receiving instructions. In this way, a patient's life story became nothing more than property of a group of experts treating him, his actions only seen and evaluated through his diagnosis. The whole admission process could, in this light, be termed »programming« for an institutionalised life. A patient thus had no right to personal possessions and could have no space that could not be searched by anyone. Electroshocks were administered to patients in plain view of the rest of the patient population. Patients were only allowed spoons to eat their meals with. One way of ensuring obedience in the patient population was to demand humility, in any way deemed important by the staff, mainly by acknowledging the staff's superiority. The patients were talked about in their presence, and constantly asked to participate in sessions that forced them to acknowledge that their situation was their fault. These »mea culpa« sessions were but one form of mental torture, another example being that they were forced to discuss the conflicts within the patient population. In the name of behavioural therapy, patients were accorded material possessions that were part of normal life in the outside world: clothes, cigarettes, etc. Physical examinations were performed in common rooms, forcing the patients to be exposed to everyone. The hygienic standards were non-existent. Any and every action that was not in accordance with hospital regime was strictly sanctioned, no matter the triviality. Patients lived in a state of constant fear, starting to accept their "moral" careers as psychiatric patients, living their role as social outcasts.

The year 1952 brought about the first antipsychotic medication, which made a significant difference in severe mental disorder prognosis. Public opinion shifted, and under its influence many hospitals were closed. The deinstitutionalisation process and anti-psychiatrist movement were present in every country that had some form of institutional care, leading to thousands of patients ending up on the streets.

There is no clear answer to the question of choosing institutional or not-institutional care. Should the patients be treated in institutions or outside is not even a valid question, as they need versatile care. There seem to be two prevailing types of public opinion concerning this - the public should be protected from the mentally ill and on the other hand, they need to be liberated of any institutional control. Both viewpoints are stigmatizing as they take away both the power to decide one's own treatment and disregard the patient's specific needs. We need to note, however, that Goffman's Asylums and the subsequent debates about stigma brought about significant changes in psychiatry. Hospitals were renovated, the number of the personnel employed increased and their education was improved. Patient's human rights are now vigorously protected, through legislation, certain in-hospital rules and advocates and lawyers who take part in the treatment process.

The World Health Organisation and the World Psychiatric Association began a far reaching public campaign in 1996 aimed at reducing stigmatization. Interest in stigmatization prevention reached it's zenith in 2001 when the media actively advertised stopping any kind of biased behaviour toward the mentally ill. This message appeared in every important document in the international mental health community. Yet, the perceivable effect was low. There is no evident decrease of stigmatization of people with mental disorders. The prejudice against people with severe mental illness can even be, according to some authors, proven to be rising, mostly because of mass media (Stier & Hinshaw, 2007).

4. Causes of stigma

Stigmatization is grounded in a narcissistic emotional satisfaction that crosses the boundaries of rational self-criticism. One who stigmatizes others finds validation in discrediting another. This discreditation enables him to join the majority; he finds himself stronger and agreed with. Regardless of whether this is the real majority or simply a privileged group, the stigmatised represent a "problem" which needs to be solved. For Jews, this was the »final solution of the Jewish question«, for African Americans it was open disdain and disrespect of their basic human rights. The mentally ill face the same sort of persecution, in the form of avoidance and isolation. In the 1950's, Adorno's study showed that any kind of hate directed towards the different is rooted in early childhood repression and loss, which is directed towards others in later life. These others are selected by criteria of social acceptability, meaning that those whom society shuns will be selected most often. Understanding the problem of discrimination, does not, however, help in moderating it.

Social categorization plays a great part in the formation of prejudice, social categorization here meaning simply dividing people into two classes - us and them. Revulsion and violence directed toward stigmatized groups is only possible when personal prejudice finds either political or ideological backing (Nastran Ule, 1999: 305). Being affiliated with a certain group incites favouritism for that group, as is evident in families and work environments. A positive group identity is the motive for stereotyping others, which leads to a better self-image. Stereotypes are thus born from negative self-image, or rather a person's inability to create one. Identity is built on being accepted as separate from »the others«. For the stigmatizing, this is a natural and effective means of countering a potential threat. For the stigmatized it is simply suffering (Yang et al., 2007).

Negative attitude towards the mentally ill is being taught to people from their birth to their deathbed. The place we go to gather information is, for most of us, the media. Information is a market commodity and is being treated as such by the media, which consequently tailors the information to generate income. Reports from many different countries show that any event connected with mental illness is prone to be reported in manner that exaggerates danger and unpredictability of the mentally ill and shows specific behaviour as bizarre and incompetent. The mentally ill are often presented as unpredictable murderers, women with split personalities or homeless people having conversations with themselves. Anyone with a mental disorder is 10 times as likely to be labelled dangerous; additionally, three quarters of such reports graded this danger as extreme. Only six percent of TV shows discussing mental illness included mentally ill people or recovered patients in their panels. Those included were commented on in a stigmatizing fashion (Wahl., 1999; Wahl et al., 2002). These representations have little in common with objective reality.

These claims hold true for American and British media especially. There are few reports of negative media coverage from other countries, with the exception of Australia. Public disdain and branding not only significantly affect ill individuals, but also the services provided to them, which is the reason for numerous educational programs aimed at

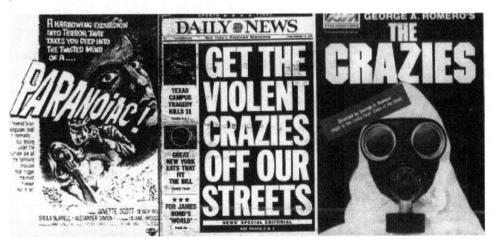

Newspaper headings in US journals

reporters. One of them was an international warrant for stigmatizing media reports (http://www.mentalhealthstigma.com/cinemania.html), aimed at identifying stereotype and media violence.

A close examination of media responses shows that there was no significant change in less stigmatizing way (Wahl et al., 2002).

Media, however, is the most important tool in fighting discrimination and stigmatization, which was proven in several countries, i.e. Australia, Slovenia etc.

5. Signs of stigma

A significant change can be observed in how prejudice shows itself. It is not shown aggressively and openly, but rather as exclusion in the form of avoidance, passive refusal and ignoring. Fringe groups are not the focus of clear negative beliefs, be it to their advantage or not. Simply put, stigmatization is moving into the subconscious (Nastran Ule, 1998: 323).

Mental illness stigma is strongly linked with prejudice against patients with mental disorders: of danger, incompetence and irresponsibility. The World Health Organization (WHO), aware of this problem, issued a statement in 2001 that described the most common myths concerning mental illness and, of course, demystified them with scientific evidence, summarized below.

"Mental disorders are not imaginary, they are real diseases that cause suffering and reduce capabilities. It is not true that people with mental disorders or brain damage can not be helped. They can be treated and mental health can be restored, which is true of all mental disorders. Patients' suffering can be eased, their symptoms can be managed, and many make a complete recovery. Mental illness has nothing to do with a person's character, as it is always a consequence of biological, psychological and social causes. Furthermore, the correlation between genetics, lifestyle, environment and illness is as well established as with physical illness. Managing mental illness requires not only a serious effort on the patient's side, but also professional help. The WHO emphasized avoiding moralizing and projecting guilt onto patients and their families. People with mental health problems should not be treated exclusively in hospitals and asylums, as they have the same rights regarding special care and intimacy as other people do. They should be provided with specialized treatment plans and be treated at home, clinics and at psychiatric wards. Rehabilitation can be organised in housing communities, employment programs and in support groups. Only 20% of patients are unable to handle regular employment. "

Signs of stigma are myths. One of the most persistent myths concerning the mentally ill is the myth of danger. The WHO emphasized that the vast majority of patients with mental disorders is not in any way a danger to others. When a mentally ill person actually becomes dangerous it is mostly for the same reasons other people do, namely, drug and alcohol abuse. The risk that a mentally ill person could be dangerous is compounded if the person in question exhibited violent behaviour before the illness, if they have delusions and hallucinations, if their psychosis is left untreated and if they abuse alcohol and drugs. This was confirmed by numerous studies. These risk factors are moderate and comparable to risk factors in groups without mental disorders, such as those with a lower education, teenagers, those excluded on the grounds of gender and those who have previously exhibited violent behaviour (Corrigan, 2005). Moreover, this risk factor is significantly lowered by the fact that violent behaviour among the mentally ill is correlated with a specific set of psychotic symptoms which can be immediately recognised by a professional. Mentally ill people are two and a half times more likely to be victims of violence than other social groups (Chapple et al., 2004).

People with mental disorders are employable and they do the same work as others. Any conviction to the contrary is simply wrong. Their career potential is the same as with others, dependent entirely on their talents, capabilities, cleverness, experience, motivation and health. Any myth about mental disorders decreases the life quality of the stigmatized and significantly hampers their treatment and recovery.

6. Types of discrimination

6.1 Overprotection and patronizing
Feelings of anger, compassion, sadness and uncertainty often fortify discriminatory behaviour in families and experts. The most common defensive behaviour when having these feelings is patronizing. The term can be explained as behaviour that denies a person his remaining capabilities because of his mental wound. Patients often report patronizing language and feel as they are being talked to as if they were children instead of adults. Another common behaviour being the previous' opposite is that the illness and related problems are not talked about at all.

Discussing the disease with nothing but well-meant advice is considered patronizing, if there is no personal experience involved. On the other hand, not talking about the illness spawns feelings of isolation and loneliness, whereas talking about it too much leads to stress, one of the main causes of relapse. Patronizing is a sign of under appreciating the role of the patient in treating and coping with the illness. The main reasons for this type of behaviour amongst professionals are a lack of knowledge, apathy and inertia (Sartorius, 2002).

6.2 Violent behaviour toward the mentally ill
Despite the persistence of the myth that the mentally ill are dangerous, the fact is that they are far more likely to be on the receiving end of violent behaviour. This is supported by research that states, for instance, that 97% of homeless women in the USA have reported being victims of violent behaviour. Studies report that 16% of all psychiatric patients are victims of abuse (Walsh et al., 2003).

An Australian study (Chapple et al., 2004) reported that 18% of psychiatric patients had been abused in the year preceding the study, three times more than in any other population group. A Finnish study (Honokonen et. al., 2004) reported a lower percentage, yet the group researched was far less exposed to such behaviour. Still, it was felt that the number was too high and steps were taken in order to protect this vulnerable group of patients. The mentally ill are also far more likely to be victims of false promises and religious fraud. Their already poor resources are ruthlessly exploited by shamans, charlatans and nonprofessional psychotherapists (Goffman, 1963).

6.3 Courtesy stigma
Stigma spreads from the individual to his loved ones (Goffman, 1963) and to all people close to the stigmatized person. Goffman's term "courtesy stigma", i.e. stigma by association, applies to those who are in contact with mental illness but not ill themselves. Research

proves that it contributes to the low level of interest for psychiatry exhibited by medical students. Further examples include denying a psychiatrists' medical professionalism by other physicians and specialists and consequent neglect of physical illness in psychiatric patients. The most common effect of courtesy stigma is family burden because of prejudice and discrimination.

A family's reaction to mental illness, at least in the beginning, bears all the traits of loss and grief. Mental illness exceeds all normal deviant behaviour. Surprise and outrage of family members expresses itself first through denial, then through attempts at re-education of the affected family member and finally through anger and/or overprotection. The diagnosis itself provides some answers and solutions, but it is only the beginning of the process. Acceptance and the realization that life needs to adjust to these new circumstances are usually a long way off. We now know that professional help often comes too late on this path and that there is too little of it (Stier & Hinshaw, 2007). Numerous studies have shown that family care causes stress, financial difficulties and depression (Wancata et al., 2006). Families often feel that discrimination directed toward the patient is also directed at them (Gonzales Torres et al., 2007).

Most patients with mental illness receive as much care from their families as they can provide. The feelings of guilt that the family experiences are correlated to false beliefs which claim that the reason for mental illness is most often connected to the family or to psychological traits of the patient's parents. In the 20th century a prevailing belief amongst experts was that most psychological problems can be attributed to patients' family situations. These theories have been refuted, but they still caused damage that is very hard to repair. The damage is obvious in families that are unable to help patients due to feelings of guilt.

Families face objective burdens of responsibility and subjective feelings of social exclusion. They are embarrassed by how the affected individual behaves, are under continuous psychological and financial stress which affects their physical and mental health. Guilt can foster either overprotection or hatred, either denial or attempts at correcting »the mistake«. This, of course, leads to stress in a patient's life and can jeopardize treatment and recovery. Families often try to hide that their loved ones got ill. Research reports that the family of a patient with a severe mental disorder often experience the same social exclusion and loss of their social network as the patient does. There is proof to the fact that relatives of these patients experience physical illness, depression, anxiety and other consequences of prolonged stress (Awad & Voruganti, 2008).

Relatives find it hardest to accept structural stigma, namely unfair and unbalanced treatment and rehabilitation in medical and social services, inadequate legislation and thoughtless political decisions that lead to financial crisis and family deprivation. Their most often voiced complaint is poor care quality. They describe being left on their own as far as patient care is concerned and being sent from one institution to another without any apparent concern for their problems. A lack of cooperation between institutions and exclusion of families from the treatment process seem to be two of the more pressing issues (Angermayer et al., 2003). Legislation that protects patients' rights often stops relatives from being informed, even though they need to be. Information can only be distributed by the doctor and only if the patient agrees to it, which can be a problem where mental problems are concerned. Most families try to get the necessary professional help as soon as possible and adjust their lifestyle so that symptoms and disability can be managed.

- My mom was very concerned about my education, she wondered if I'll manage when I grow up.
- I live with my parents; they tolerate much more from me than they did before the disease. They don't bother me with their problems.
- My family supported me all the way.
- No one in the family treated me differently. Not my parents, not my husband. There was no pity.

Mental illness scares the family, leading to overprotection, which hampers the patient's self-reliance. Before the patient's family reaches a balances that allows adequate help, too much time passes.

- When I got sick, my family really just didn't understand it at first. They didn't treat me as an equal. It's better now.
- Too much care seriously hampers treatment and rehabilitation. It leads to prejudice and hostility.
- They treat me differently now. I can't go out Friday and Saturday night, my parents think something'll happen. I'm not allowed to drink or use any drugs...not that I would, but still.
- My parents don't think I can take care of myself.
- They were embarrassed at first, that I was in the hospital. Mom wouldn't tell her friends or our neighbours. My parents had a lot of trouble accepting things.
- My sisters think that I can't be a good parent, so they interfere all the time.

Families can be counselled and helped to reduce the feelings of exclusion and helplessness. Educating the family on how to manage the illness in family groups which share experience and help each other is an invaluable tool in combating stigma. Patients' relatives organised on national and international levels wield considerable political power that is used in creating, developing and overseeing different mental health services, including psychiatry.

6.4 Self respect damage, self-discrimination, internalised stigma
A person's lack of success is considered to be his own fault. Victims of prejudice are forced to hide their disabilities, or at least act in a way that enables them to stay in contact with the dominant culture - one that reinforces the fantasy of a strong, unbreakable self that holds dominion over itself and others (Goffman, 1963, Nastran Ule, 1999).

6.4.1 Hiding the illness
The act of hiding a mental disorder strengthens the vicious circle of prejudice. Psychiatric patients most often choose not to talk about their disorder or diagnosis since they are subject to strong feelings of guilt and shame due to the aforementioned prejudice. They lead a double life in fear of exposing themselves, which leads to avoiding other people, as they are a direct threat to their exposure. They become lonely and, in turn, feel insecure, constantly threatened and inferior. Withdrawing from society, fearing ridicule, the stigmatized become more and more alone (Goffman, 1963). Despite the above stated, patients admitting their disease actually severely limits their chances of being a member of any privileged social groups. Most often admittance means a membership in the vast group of second class citizens and losing the battle for status (Thesen, 2001). Attempts to hide and obscure their condition are a source of continuous stress, which forces patients to expend enormous amounts of energy on their disguises. When it was suggested by professionals that psychiatric hospitals should be established in city and town centres, the patients' wish to be

unrecognized was overlooked. Being in the centre is not the interest of the majority of them. The following statements were made by patients who feel that this is the case.

- *I really want people not to know that I've been diagnosed. When somebody asks me how I'm doing, I never tell the truth- that I'm ill and I'm not doing well. Most wouldn't even understand, if I told them that I have schizophrenia.*
- *I don't say to people: I'm sick. I don't say that I'm going to the hospital. It seems smarter to not say anything.*
- *He asked me if I was in the hospital. So I lied.*
- *I'm ashamed of my diagnosis. I must keep it to myself. If it's important I tell people, but not all the time. It's better to stay quiet.*
- *I don't advertise that I'm being treated.*
- *I can't tell people that I've been diagnosed.*
- *When I meet somebody new, I don't say a thing.*
- *I only go to the library, but they noticed and now they look at me different.*
- *I'm not sick, but those who think that I am, avoid me.*

Despite everything, some have decided to admit their illness and risk unforeseeable consequences:

- *My friend said that I'm living in my own world, one that others can't understand. But I think that she's the sick one - always nervous and stressed. On the other hand, my friends at college don't even understand why I've been sent to the hospital. It depends on the person, I guess.*
- *When I was first in the hospital I felt stigmatized, but only because my mom told me all about that. I had trouble fitting in. I noticed later that people don't care much about whether you're in the hospital or not. I told my classmates that I'm being treated. The more you hide it, the harder it gets. It just gets to be another burden. I now tell everyone, because if I don't, I keep having to think about what I told to who. I have lots of friends, so now it's not a problem anymore.*

6.4.2 Anticipated discrimination
What they have been taught in their childhood and adult lives makes many patients with mental disorders expect discrimination. The general belief, that the mentally ill are dangerous and incompetent, turns on a patient in the moment of his diagnosis. Becoming a part of an inferior group makes him expect discrimination which leads to demoralization.

Negative cultural concepts start to be felt on a personal level. Prejudice works as a self-fulfilling prophecy, which means that expectations of discrimination come true sooner or later. The actual identity of an individual is replaced by a »virtual« social identity, one defined by others through stereotyping (Goffman, 1963).

The general social opinion of the mentally ill is largely created by the media. In movies and reports, a negative outcome of treatment, low quality of life and dangerous and incompetent behaviour are attributed to the mentally ill. These myths endanger self-respect and demoralize patients to an extent that doesn't allow them to fight for a better life. The affected individual is taught society's expectations of him and re-identifies himself; starts controlling his own expectations and avoids any confrontation, thus missing almost every opportunity (Angermeyer et al., 2004). Their social networks shrink, leading to poverty and unemployment, which in turn leads to social exclusion (Kroska & Harkness, 2006). Oversensitvity to any communication involving stigma emerges, presenting itself as embarrassment on both sides, meaning not only with those who expect to be stigmatized but also those who try to cover up their worry for the affected.

- *The opinion of others affects me a lot. I can't talk about that.*
- *Sometimes people say that I would be better if I don't get married and have kids. I agree with them now.*
- *I don't try to make friends.*

Patients believe that expected discrimination is far worse than the smaller number of options they actually have. Still, some do not allow themselves to expect discrimination.

- *I went back to work and back to school. It was a little uncomfortable at first, but now it's OK, I almost never feel that way. I still have trouble meeting people, but I don't give up. Sometimes it works out, sometimes it doesn't.*
- *People had trouble accepting me, but it wasn't me who had a problem, it was them.*
- *I never went back to my old job. My doctor advised me against continuing in this profession, so I changed careers and finished a course. I didn't want to retire.*

6.4.3 Self-stigma
The psychological cause for self-loathing is internalization of prejudice. Some people accept disdain to be justified and legitimate. They start to act passively, dependently and helplessly as is expected of them. A social quarantine devoid of encouragement and responsibility is formed around the individual. Expectations are reduced (Lysaker et al., 2007). One withdraws and gives up hope and wishes, making himself less emotionally dependent and less likely to speak out – which are all recognised as »negative« symptoms of mental illness. It was proven that people, who identified themselves as being stigmatized, compare poorly to others, who do not feel stigmatized regarding their intellectual capacity. This means that a stigmatized social group actually functions below their intellectual potential, stigma being the reason for their impairment and not only their illness. They feel incapable of functioning as rational, competent and functional individuals, have lower self-esteem and are often depressed, anxious and hostile (Quinn et al., 2004).
Being a part of a stigmatized group is a barrier to one's success and often means a loss of life opportunities. People with mental disorders are often isolated, unemployed, poor, single and alone (Thessen, 2001). Recognising their situation many in turn disdain and even hate their fellow patients - a group of people with mental illness. They may exhibit the same or even worse stigmatizing behaviour as those outside of the group towards their fellow, more stigmatized patients (Zalar, Strbad & Švab, 2007). The individual does not want to be a part of the disadvantaged group (Goffman, 1963).
The anger and outrage directed towards the barriers keeping them out of social life is turned on themselves. Self-stigma is exhibited in feelings of shame, exclusion and loss of importance. Still, the consequences of self loathing do not stop there. Patients in its grasp do not argue their rights or interests, thus maintaining the vicious circle of stigma and legitimizing the fact that non-stigmatized people avoid and exclude them (Goffman, 1963).
It must be noted at this point that mental illness does not necessarily mean a loss in effectiveness and self-esteem. People react differently to disease and possible disability. Some fight discrimination and abuse and some are indifferent, depending on an individual's personality and the situation. People who refuse to accept the stereotype feel angry and

strong, and justifiably so. Sometimes, as members of a marginalized group which has been wronged, they feel even stronger and more assertive than before. Similar to the reaction of the Afro-American culture, they say that anger is the fair response to stigma. This expression of just anger is more likely to happen if the stigmatized individuals connect in a group focusing on improving the situation. People who fail to identify with a group more often treat discriminatory practices with indifference, regardless of their personal experience (Corrigan, 2005).

The only way to resist self loathing is to stand up to discrimination and resist abuse.

- *They avoid me a lot. I don't care. There is difference between being stupid and mad. I don't think I'm stupid.*
- *I broke it off with some of my friends. Not just because of the diagnosis. Though I'm ok with those that I kept being friends with. If I manage to sort myself out, find a job and my family is fine, then nobody can say I'm schizophrenic, I know that.*
- *I think of being diagnosed as an advantage. Me and my family figured it out, what being ill means and we know exactly what to do when I start acting differently, it is the illness that gets worse.*

6.5 Structural discrimination

Structural discrimination happens on a systematic level, in a way that automatically stops any attempts to acquire a different social status. The mentally ill are pushed to the edge of society, drastically reducing their life options. Being of the edge of society means that any group can be forced into humility, anonymity and silence. Any discussion of equal rights, respecting diversity and understanding is futile if discrimination is built by the general society and the state itself as the ultimate defence against intrusion of marginalized groups, dreamers and the unadjusted into any decision making system. Some countries include special mental illness clauses in their visa application forms. There are countries or states that deny their mentally ill citizens the right to vote, not considering if an individual can manage the illness or not. But the most generally present effect of structural stigma is poor quality of mental health services and their inaccessibility (Angermeyer et al., 2003), basically denying patients their right to treatment and care in an apparently accidental way. The reasons for this can be found in social service management, political decisions and poor legislation. In a cultural environment with strong values on work and income, a patient is stigmatized and cornered. He is unemployed because of not being able to reach the required production norms. As unemployed individual he is labelled twice: being mentally ill and unproductive or even lazy, unable to achieve the socially required criteria to be considered a productive member of the community. The only possible way out of this situation is belonging to a wider community of people who also feel wronged by the prejudice directed towards the mentally ill. Patients who are able to find a way to belong to such a group and identify with it have more self-esteem and are significantly stronger (Corrigan et al., 1999, 2004).

Stronger individuals report better recovery (Anthony, 2000). Those who are politically connected influence the quality of mental health services.

Poor care for the patients' physical health is one of the more serious problems that mental health care faces. People with mental disorders have the same somatic diseases as other people do, yet the standard for hospital care drops severely whenever a mental problem appears. The risk for physical problems such as diabetes, high blood pressure and cardiovascular disease is far greater amongst people with mental disorders than in other groups. Cardiovascular disease is the main cause of death in this group. The paradox here is that with severe physical health problem good mental health is not possible. All physical illness is strongly connected with depression, anxiety and other mental health problems. It follows logically that every physician should be trained in identifying and treating mental health problems, yet psychiatry is mostly treated as unimportant at most medical schools, by the teaching staff and students alike. The average medical student is likely to have the same opinion of mental health problems as the general public. They mostly feel that psychiatry as a branch of medical science is ineffective and unscientific (Feldmann, 2005).

The basis for improving the life and treatment quality of patients with mental disorders is improving the education on all levels of the educational system, including lessons on needs, rights and the reality of life in fringe groups.

7. Areas of discrimination

7.1 Friendship

Compared to others, people with mental disorders have scarce social networks and are more strongly linked to their families and more dependent on them (Thornicroft, 2006:27). A small social network can be a consequence of stigmatization and the mental disorder itself. Loneliness is a risk factor for poor recovery. Most patients try to hide their illness from their friends, as they believe hiding is essential for their social survival. They believe that mental illness makes them social lepers and rarely see it as an opportunity to improve on the quality of their existing relationships and, perhaps, finding new ones.

- *True friends stay by your side. You can check who your friends really are and start all over again, or even improve them.*
- *We're better friends than before I got ill.*
- *My friends listen more, stand by my side and encourage me.*
- *My friends stuck around, mostly. Those who didn't, weren't my friends, were they?*
- *I didn't exactly have a lot of friends. I met new people when I was admitted to the hospital. They're my friends now.*

But there seems to be much more negative experience. Friends disappear, flat out decline to see the patient and avoid him. Every friendship lost strengthens feelings of loneliness and despair.

- *I had one friend. I went to visit him once. He told me to leave. He avoided me after that, so I did the same.*
- *When they say: »she's the crazy one«, I know they're making fun of me. Nobody can stop it from happening.*
- *Some of my friends, when I told them I was in, didn't come to see me. I don't trust them anymore.*
- *I feel distant. People don't know what to say when I'm around.*
- *People that know treat me differently. If they don't, everything is much easier.*
- *I didn't make any new friends after I was admitted.*
- *I feel they don't want to be around me. It takes a lot of time for anyone to get through to me, I know that.*
- *Nobody ever comes to visit, nobody ever calls me.*
- *I called my friend and wished her happy holidays, She said she'd come, but she didn't. I think her husband doesn't let her.*

- When I still had a job, I lost my best friend when he found out. He never called me again, so I didn't want to call him.
- My childhood friend was shocked, when she found out. She was scared of visiting me, so she never did. I'm sad because I lost my best friend.
- They think they're better than me.
- My friends were shocked. They avoided me.

7.2 Partnership

People with mental disorders are much less likely to be in a committed relationship. There are many reasons for this, the most common being low self-esteem and lack of opportunities. Many existing relationships are discontinued due to the severity of the disease, stigma and financial difficulties. On the other hand many couples manage the illness and find new challenges and qualities in their relationships.

- For me, it's an advantage. She's great.

Divorce is one of the most stressful events in an average person's life. Most people need to be helped when faced with divorce, the mentally ill especially so. Several cases of patient's being used and manipulated during the separation process have been reported.

- My boyfriend dumped me the second I was admitted to hospital. He didn't want to be with me anymore.
- I was married. My husband left me when I got ill. I had no relationships since.
- My husband left me because of my diagnosis.
- Once people know you're ill, it's hard to find somebody who's willing to share your life. You can't have kids when you're taking medication.
- My husband isn't understating. He had all the power so he had me hospitalized.
- He met somebody else, fell in love and that was that.
- Nobody wants to have a physical relationship with you once they know you're ill. People are afraid.
- Who am I going to get? People see a cripple when they look at me.
- When I went to see my girlfriend her mother wouldn't leave us alone. She couldn't trust someone who was in the hospital.

7.3 Parenting

Nurturing and caring for a child after giving birth is one of the hardest physical and mental tests for mothers. Sleeplessness, hormonal imbalance, physical stress, financial difficulties, breastfeeding and relationship difficulties can shake even the strongest of women. Those who are sensitive to psychiatric disorders often experience a relapse in the year following birth. Admitting this, there is little evidence to suggest that schizophrenic mothers are unable to take care of their children. Women with mental disorders often lose their children, despite all the facts. This can be attributed to not receiving any assistance when it is most needed. Mothers don't have access to counselling, education or family therapy (Thornicroft, 2006: 38).

Most parents who have some form of mental disorder provide excellent care to their children and are considered good parents, if sufficient support is provided for possible overloads.

- When I was hospitalised, I was handicapped, had no energy. When I went to pick my son up from kindergarten everybody was very correct. I didn't have any bad experiences, none good too; they just treated me like everyone else.
- There was some doubt at home, but I went through with it anyway. I'm really happy I had a baby.
- My ex-husband tells me I'm not strict enough when the kids are with me. I don't think so, I think he's too strict and they have to let of some steam when they're with me. It's a very small flat and there are five of us when they come over, but they like being here.

People with severe mental disorders like schizophrenia want children the same as everybody else.

- We tried to adopt a child with my wife, but we couldn't.

7.4 Sexuality
People with mental health disorders often exhibit radical sexual behaviour, the outstanding group being those with mania. Women with mental health disorders are far more likely to be sexually abused. Research states that there are a lot of cases when a patient should be treated both for sexual abuse and illness (Thornicroft, 2006).
Several drugs used in psychiatric treatment have a negative effect on libido, erection and ejaculation, which is one of the leading reasons for avoiding use.

- I have no libido…It's just gone.
- It's true I don't have any desire to be sexually active since it got sick.
- I can't get a woman pregnant. The medicine would harm the kid.
- When I got ill, I couldn't perform. My wife cheated on me a lot, she wasn't happy with me.
- Sexual disorders are another cause of slow self-esteem.

Intercourse is, because of the above mentioned, less likely to happen in psychiatric institution than in other institutions, but it does occur and not rarely. Prohibiting sexual activity is discrimination, yet it must be implemented sometimes in order to stop people acting on basis of their reduced reasoning because of the illness. People with low self-esteem who agree to intercourse they would otherwise reject also need to be protected. Effects of these dilemmas presented themselves through hospital management decisions conflicting over gender separation. In the name of normalization, England implemented mixed wards for a couple of decades, which are being separated again. The reasons for this are numerous reports of abuse and women's dissatisfaction due to a lack of privacy. Closed wards fared the worst in this experiment of gender mixing, as the patients there have a problem controlling their behaviour. Women who experienced abuse before admission often demand their right for privacy very strictly The number of women being treated because of traumatic sexual experiences in psychiatric hospitals is not low (Thornicroft, 2006).
A patient's right to sexual expression needs to be balanced with the reasonable demand for protection. In clinical practice, this means that in closed wards sexual intercourse is usually prohibited, even though it is a breach of their basic human rights.

7.5 Employment
Employment discrimination is one of the most often encountered forms of stigma.

- I rarely got a reply to my work applications and I was never accepted. I wrote about my diagnosis in these applications.

Work is known to improve mental health, helps manage an individual's life and makes a person feel appreciated. Unemployment deprives people of social interaction, reduces their self-esteem, intensifies feelings of incompetence and pushes people into poverty. Research proves that most people with mental disorders   possess work capabilities and desire to employ them (Brohan &Thornicroft, 2010). The low employment rate of people with mental disorders can be blamed on discrimination.

- I want to work, but I am locked up at home. I have nothing to do
- They told me to find another job, when they found about my medication.

Employers expect mentally ill workers to be unproductive and frequently absent. They fear unpredictability and damage to the workplace or the company. Physically disabled people are twice as likely to be employed compared to the mentally disabled. If people with mental disorders get employed, they can expect a lower and less lucrative position, their experience and education not taken into account.

- This is a big obstacle and big stress. Employer looks at me very carefully, what I speak and what I do.
- I was moved to a lower paid work position, and then finally to some unimportant office. Then I quit.
- From team leader to worker and finally a cleaner.

Given time, a lot of them give up on finding employment and accept their social status (Wahl, 1999; Link, 1982). Half of available and appropriate positions are terminated or changed to the mentally ill worker's disadvantage because of poor workplace relations (Becker et al., 1998). The most commonly asked question when discussing possible employment with a patient is whether the individual should reveal his diagnosis to his employer. There is no simple answer to that question. It depends on the employer's prejudice and on whether the position is more or less stressful. Hiding the diagnosis might lead to difficulties. If the individual can not perform set tasks or can not handle the stress, the most common response is inefficiency.

- There was too much overload, I collapsed and had to go away.

Honesty, on the other hand, might expose the individual to rejection and victimisation.

- Nobody said I won't get the job because I was sick, they never say "You are schyzophrenic and we don't want you", but it's obvious.

The most common solution seems to be denying the illness and covering up problems (Stuart, 2004).
Experts who try to lower their patients' or clients' expectations and try to get them to accept social aids or pensions are also an issue.
Adjusting the work to the needs of people with mental health disorders improves their job performance (Waghorn, 2011). This means making the workplace a little more serene, employing people to work from their homes, adjusting the work hours or just making sure

that individuals work in a tolerant environment where they are entitled to support when needed. There are clear guidelines how to organize work for people with mental health disabilities (Corrigan & McCracken, 2005). People with mental disorders need adjusted work hours and support at the work place (Crowther et al., 2001). An organizational culture which respects mental health, diversity and offers support is therefore necessary, as job performance can be significantly improved even with the most severe mental disorders (Thornicroft & Brohan, 2008). Legislation can speed up the process of employing people with mental disorders, but only slightly as employers still see them as a threat, despite the financial stimulation the government offers for their employment. Productivity is the cornerstone of respect in many cultural environments. To get and keep a job is the best path to recovery, on walked also by many people with severe mental illness. There are many examples of people who received enough support to recover in this way.

7.6 Education
A student with a mental disorder can experience significant difficulties. Their reduced capabilities show themselves as problems with studying, communicating, memory, thinking and sleep which significantly affects their studies. Such students are hard to recognise as most student difficulties are attributed to a lack of motivation and poor working habits. Research of their special needs is very scarce. The astounding diversity of mental disorders and their varied symptoms further complicate the problem. Student may suffer from depression, anxiety, addiction, psychotic disorders or personality disorders. Each and every of these problems requires a different treatment and different types of support. The diagnosis, however, should not be the reason for program adjustment, it should rather be the reduced capabilities caused by the illness and its other effects - including stigmatization. Obstacles that prevent the student from reaching optimal results need to be removed. Specific social skills, for example, in obtaining information can be improved upon by an appropriate mentor. Additional rights can be provided for a student who just finished recovering from a mental illness, such as additional timelines, additional flexibility, adjustment of class attendance requirements, providing additional mentors and tutors, additional lectures arranged for specific problem areas and the option of at-home studying. Counselling, stress control classes, study planning classes and social skill classes should also be considered. Adjusting the study process should not jeopardise its quality, only change its difficulty. It is not expensive to adjust educational programs, the difficulty lies in combating discrimination against the mentally ill in all stages of the educational system (Rickerson et al., 2004). Rights and needs awareness need to be raised among the staff working in education.
Students who have received sufficient support have proved that education can help control a mental disorder.

- *Learning helps me get through the day.*

Students with mental disorders have reported that some teachers try to help them manage their duties, which depends on the sensibility of the teachers themselves, not on school rules.

- *In college my professors became lenient when they found out about my illness, with homework or even tests. One even gave me a solved test and just told me to copy it.*
- *I got special treatment in high school.*

They frequently experience discrimination and avoidance.

- When I was doing my requalification everybody looked at me funny.
- Teachers, professors-they all underestimated me.

Some further guidelines for educational adjustment can be found here:
(http://www.bu.edu/cpr/jobschool).

7.7 Accommodation, communities
Different social and cultural environments mean different types of care for people with mental disorders. The Slovenian social environment, for instance, sees most patients living in primary families, similar to the Mediterranean countries. In northern and western countries, most patients live on their own (Thornicroft, 2006).
Today numerous patients live in sheltered living arrangements. This form of accommodation offers diverse levels of care and is an alternative to living with relatives. Patients mostly choose to live in such a community when their domestic situation offers no advantage to recovery, when they feel they have no chance of living on their own and when they require help with everyday obligations. These alternative living choices can only work when competent staff is available, one that can recognise and answer the many different needs that people in such a community have. In Slovenia, social institutions are still one of the most common types of long-term accommodation, and however far they are developed, they still seem to face the same problems - an often reported high risk of neglect and inadequate treatment.

- Looking for an apartment when mentally ill isn't easy. When I did it, I never told anyone I was ill. People don't like people who are...different. It's best to stay unnoticed.

- My landlord knows that I'm ill, she's a bit more careful now. I think it's because I didn't tell her much, but she still tries to make conversation and understand me. I know it's a bit awkward for the both of us, but I fell it's ok, it's her house.

- My parents think I'm not mature enough to have my own flat, even though I have one. I can cook for myself. Ironing and washing up are still problems, but I'll get help from a therapist so I can look after myself after I'm discharged.

7.8 Social relations, finances, civil rights
A person's social life outside the bonds of family and the workplace depend on his social skills, opportunities, rights, resources and his perceived worth in society. The mentally ill can be discriminated against by having no means for day to day recreation, quality time and simple pleasures. The most common reason for this is financial deprivation, usually caused by unemployment and poor pension or social aid, sufficient only for the bare necessities. Most patients desire employment that would improve their financial status. Even if they do manage to find some form of employment they have to deal with management that s not always tolerant. Furthermore, they are most often not sufficiently informed of their rights and subsequently do not enforce them. Others do not want to enforce their rights because they want to enter any relationship on equal grounds. Some accept their inferior status because of their low expectations.

People with severe mental disorders are poorer than the general population and suffer from disrespectful behaviour, sometimes physical violence and underestimation. It should be noted however, that there are numerous reports of tolerance, cooperation and equal treatment.

- They encouraged me. In the library, the staff knew what I'm interested in and they helped me.

7.9 Neighbours

Reports from Great Britain and the US claim that people with severe mental disorders are being avoided and excluded by in their communities. When the non-government organization ŠENT in Slovenia was establishing group homes, we believed that people who were living in the neighbourhood should not be given prior information concerning the possible (absence of) danger to help them accept the newcomers. We have firmly stated, however, that any event out of the ordinary, even if it's just an unscheduled visit by an ambulance, should be explained to everyone affected. The recommendation (Thornicroft, 2006: 15) that in the earliest stage of creating the community, residents should be notified carries weight, which might be relativised by the right to confidentiality and the fact that half of the world's adult population will be affected by a mental disorder at some point in their life and that three quarters of this population know somebody who suffers from one. Reports given by interviewed people with schizophrenia in INIGO differ significantly. Often the neighbours are those who notice that an individual requires help. The individual affected may perceive this as an intrusion into his autonomy that damages his self-respect.

- Of course, my neighbours called the ambulance. It's annoying if your neighbours know they can out you away. They just call the ambulance and tell them to take me. When I bought this flat, my own little place, I locked myself in for 14 days straight - I wanted to put it in order. It was my first apartment! In the ghetto, really small, doesn't matter. Then suddenly, cops came to take me away. And I was so happy to get my own flat. It's unpleasant to say the least, when somebody can send you to the hospital anonymously. They just come, handcuff me and take me away.
- The neighbours know when I'm in the hospital. My blinds are down. It bothers me, a little.
- I live in a small village; my mom-she's the village gossip. She always cares most about what the neighbours will say. I think that's the source of a lot of problems. If I lived alone, there would be none of that. People in my village are always watching me.

People in a community most often help one another.

- I was elected house president twice. I told nobody in the building that I was in the hospital. That's why they listened to me.
- My neighbours didn't know I was ill for a long time. They know now, they understand.

7.10 Professionals

Patients with mental disorders are most stigmatized by professionals (Lauber et al., 2006, Nordt et al., 2006). Stigma in professional services is one of the main causes of treatment discontinuation amongst patients (Tehrani et al., 1996). Professionals stigmatize the mentally ill for the following reasons. They are pessimistic about their recovery, despite all the scientific evidence to the contrary. The prognosis for most mental disorders is far better than for most recurring physical illnesses. Experts rarely meet recovered patients, only those in grave need of assistance. Another reason is the need for distance and superiority, in short, power, which can be easily satisfied in any type of institution. Most professionals claim that they do not stigmatize, that problems arise from patients' oversensitivity to what they say. This anticipated discrimination contributes to patient stress. Stigma directed against the professionals themselves is also very much a reality- people often perceive professionals as arrogant and uncomprehending and therefore don't trust. This leads to procrastination in seeking assistance. Research shows that most people with mental disorders never seek treatment (Wittchen et al., 2005). The most stigmatized diagnoses are alcohol addiction, eating disorders, personality disorders, self-harm and schizophrenia. The most stigmatized patient groups are men with financial problems and the homeless. Discriminatory behaviour of staff increases in case it is decided that he mental problem is the patient's own fault, if the patient is admitted frequently, if violent or criminal behaviour is assumed, if it is believed the patient has little chance of recovery or, finally, if the patient is believed to be dishonest. Besides patronizing, double standards are a common type of stigmatization - every act is judged according to the patient's diagnosis even when there is no objective reason to do so. For example, a patient being upset with the quality of his treatment could be interpreted as agitated because of the illness, even if his complaints are legitimate. People with mental disorders encounter the same discrimination in every institution, not just the hospital. Professionals' attitude towards the mentally ill has a large influence on others' behaviour. Psychiatrists and nurses who see their profession as stressful, hard and unsatisfying lead the public to see apathy, ignorance and poor patient treatment as the way to behave toward people with mental disorders. On the other hand, committed experts who appreciate their choice of profession set an example of respect, hope and the need to cooperate.

- *Social services are like that: they decide instead of you, they treat you differently.*
- *The court doesn't take me seriously. He raped me long ago, I was in the hospital and I am still here, and he, the criminal, is out.*
- *I feel the gap between staff and patients, between "healthy" and "mad". Outside the hospital, I'm worried my professors will find out about me, because we are a very small study group.*
- *My tooth was extracted in spite of my resistance to do that. The dentist just did it. I'm not in control of my life.*
- *They didn't tell me about the effects and side effects of drugs, an also about the length of my hospitalization. They didn't tell me anything.*

Others don't experience such problems.

- *My gynecologist knew about my illness, but she didn't treat me diferently.She encourages me to have children, but we decided against it, with my husband, since it's a genetic disease.*

7.11 Privacy
New legislation demands that a patient be accorded his right to privacy. This can not always be done due to current hospital conditions. Living conditions depend on many factors, chief amongst them the budget available and the level of structural stigmatization. Respect for the right to privacy depends on the staff also - some might see the patients'need to be alone as important, others not. Obviously, a closed ward is needed for patients who need to be observed for their and others' safety.

- There is no privacy in the hospital. For any of us, none has it better.
- It's hard to say. There's not a lot of freedom, but they expect you to cooperate with everyone, the doctors, parents. No inner peace.
- Patients in psychiatric hospitals don't have privacy. You can't do anything on your own, just what they tell you.
- I had to sleep on a „temp", in the living room. People were coming to look at me all night long, made noise. I cried all night.
- They were always ok with it, when I wanted to be alone.

8. Coping with stigma

8.1 Protest
Protest is the most used strategy to fight injustice, as unsuccessful as it is. People who discriminate are prone to responding with more discrimination when subject to outrage and opposition. They are less likely to cease their behaviour when other opinions are forced on them. Protest can only positively affect media coverage, specifically those reporters who have failed to form a clear opinion on the matter at hand. Protest is a reactive strategy; it attempts to diminish negative attitudes about mental illness, but fails to promote more positive attitudes that are supported by facts (Corrigan & Watson, 2002).

8.2 Education
The belief that prejudice is irrational inevitably leads to the logical conclusion that it can be fought with reason. If we were only able to understand the whole truth of mental disorders, the people it affects and ourselves we would be able to overcome prejudice and weaken their connection with our emotions easily. This thesis is the ground on which all anti-stigmatization educational programs are founded, including those that promote meetings between the non-discriminated and the discriminated. Promoting mental illness awareness is by far the most accepted method of combating stigmatization and discrimination. The same method was used in intercultural dialogue campaigns, aimed at reducing racism and homophobia. It was assumed that people could rationally »delete« their prejudice. It was proven that although short educational programs improve relationships and awareness (Roman & Floyd, 1981, Link et al, 1987, Brockington et al., 1993), they only have short-term effects. Their effect on discriminatory behaviour is unproven and there is some doubt as to whether they influence the behaviour itself or merely change the understanding of a problem (Corrigan et al., 2005, Pinfold et al., 2005, Shulze et al., 2003). People understanding more about mental disorders, however, doesn't mean much to stigmatized individuals. The main problem of educational programs seems to be that discussion is always focused on the stigmatized group, not on the group that stigmatizes. Instead of paying attention to prejudiced individuals, objects of their prejudice are being focused on, as Henriques noted in 1984 in his book »Changing the subject«. Following years showed that more than convictions, actual discriminatory behaviour needed to be stopped, which required knowledge of history, institutions, legislation and the cultural traits of the affected environment (Gonzales Torres et al., 2007).

8.3 Contact
Establishing direct contact with those who recovered from mental illness is another way to educate. Stories and reports by empowered individuals are a strong weapon against

stigmatization. (Brockington et al., 1993; Wolf et al., 1996, Corrigan et al., 2001; Happpel et al., 2002, Pinfold et al., 2005). They were proven more successful than educational campaigns, especially in combating fear (Angemayer et al., 2003), yet even these programs only managed to fight stereotyping (Wolf et al, 1996; Thompson et al., 2002), not social distance. Relating to an individual with mental disorder experience does not affect the social nature of stigma. But, even direct contact effects can be relativised, as individuals can consider the one they are talking to, an exception. An informed and competent individual does not affect the reputation of his whole group, except when he is a recognised representative (Oakes et al., 1994). People with mental health problem experience know where to expect stigma in day to day life. Professional representatives of the mentally ill that give speeches at conventions and seminars aren't typical representatives of the group. Similar to professionals, they require frequent public appearances to maintain their status. Their posture is consequently militant, disdainful and they are constantly trying to find mistakes in their healthy colleagues' communication. They demand »appropriate« behaviour, in keeping with the marginalised group's code. Their expectations differ significantly from the bulk of the population's, who try to be polite and careful in order not to jeopardize their position. Most individuals with mental disorders try to demonstrate that they are well adjusted, behaving similar to others. At the same time, they try to convey that they are not the same; that they are at a disadvantage that needs to be accepted as a fact (Goffman, 1963). Most of the discriminated have developed careful and artful forms of communication, which enables them to be at least partially accepted and prevents severe problems.

9. Research on stigma

Already in 1999 US research on stigma argued that socio-psychological research of ethnic minorities and other group stereotypes should be considered when implementing anti-stigma strategies. It indicates that (a) attempts to suppress stereotypes through protest can result in a rebound effect; (b) education programs may have limited effectiveness because many stereotypes are resilient to change; (c) contact is enhanced by a variety of factors, including equal status, cooperative interaction, and institutional support (Corrigan & Penn, 1999).

In 2004, Link and others identified a variety of mechanisms allowing observation and measurements of key components present in a stigmatization process. These are: labelling, stereotyping, cognitive separating, emotional reactions, status loss, discrimination experiences and discrimination expectations, structural discrimination and behavioural responses to stigma. Structural discrimination was found not to be adequately researched. Strong proof of prevalence of expected discrimination over actual, experienced discrimination was found. Most studies show that older people, individuals with a relatively poor education and persons who have never known anyone with a mental illness are more likely to desire social distance than their younger, more educated counterparts who have had more contact with the mentally ill. The main limitation of majority of research by then was found to be social desirability bias. People do not want to state openly that they are reluctant to accept people with mental disorders. Opinion measuring scales and Community Attitudes Toward the Mentally ill scales showed major improvement after contact with people with mental disorders (Crisp et al., 2005), which produced incentive to further anti-stigma strategies. The positive influence of contact was also proved by measuring emotional reactions to people with mental disorders (Angermeyer & Matschinger, 1996) and opened a path to research on stigmatizers.

The stigmatized were, from 1987 onward, repeatedly assessed on rejection, perceived rejection and anticipation. Some measures on coping orientations were taken as well. The stigma on the affected' carers and relatives was measured with different scales from the one of the last developed in Germay (Wancata et al., 2006).

The biggest stigmatization control project was »Open the Doors«, a study and a campaign under the World Psychiatric Association, which got underway in 1996 in 20 different countries around the globe (Thompson et al., 2002; Sartorius & Schulze, 2005). It was meant to combat prejudice and discrimination against schyzophrenia. The first phase consisted of public polls in 6 different countries, the second a wave of social service public education programs. The project enjoyed some success, achieving, for example, a reduction in social exclusion in Germany (Gaebel, 2004). The following years showed that more than convictions, actual discriminatory behaviour needed to be stopped, which required knowledge of history, institutions, legislation and the cultural traits of the affected environment (Gonzales Torres in dr., 2007). One of the larger anti-stigmatization campaigns »Moving People« proved this as during the campaign, from 2002 to 2005, of 30 milion British reached, 17% more started believing that mental illness and violence are correlated, whereas in Scotland the exact opposite was true- the number of people convinced that the mentally ill are prone to violence dropped by 17% . Before the campaign started 40% more people in Scotland believed in this stereotype than in Wales and England. This result proves that campaigns need to be adjusted to social and cultural environments.

The media research gaps were identified by Stout and others (2004). It was nevertheless clear that those who watch a lot of television hold more negative views of individuals with mental illness than those who watch it less (Granello & Pauley2000). Most of the articles on media influence on stigma share the same conclusion - this is outrage on media reports. A lack of differentiation among different media channels and the scarcity of research on children perception is nevertheless obvious. Additional problems include non-representative results – the people studied are primarily college students. A link between media depiction and individuals' perceptions is thus still theoretical at this point. Replication and expansion of research in this area is required, and particular emphasis should be given to identifying links between exposure to media images and subsequent perception impact. Simply stated, more precise research is needed.

A major improvement in research was applying qualitative methods , being essential for appreciating the subtle, damaging effects of stigma, for example structural discrimination. The Goffman work described above was the first and still most influential qualitative research on stigma. Major gaps in stigma research still remained: lack of results on structural discrimination, emotional responses of patients and cross cultural approaches.

The importance of understanding the social context of the stigma is presented in research about attitudinal and structural barriers that prevent people with mental disabilities from becoming active participants in the competitive labour market (Stuart, 2006).

The connection between mental disorder and physical illness researched proved that the increased frequency of physical diseases in schizophrenia might be on account of factors related to schizophrenia and its treatment, but undoubtedly also results from the unsatisfactory organization of health services, from the attitudes of medical doctors, and the social stigma ascribed to the schizophrenic patients (Leucht et al., 2007). One of the major approaches to overcome low service use, poor adherence rates, and stigma was defining mental disorders as neurobiological medical disease. The 10-year comparison of public endorsement of treatment and prejudice proved that this approach translates into support for services but not into a decrease in stigma. Reconfiguring stigma reduction strategies may require providers and advocates to shift to an emphasis on competence and inclusion of patients with mental disorders (Pescosolido et al., 2010).

In Pinfold et al. a review (2005) of relevant literature and the results of the recent Mental Health Awareness in Action (MHAA) programme in England was published to discuss the current evidence base on the active ingredients in effective anti-stigma interventions in mental health. The key active ingredient identified by all intervention groups and workshop facilitators were the testimonies of service users. The statements of service users (consumers) about their experience of mental health problems and of their contact with a range of services had the greatest and most lasting impact on the target audiences in terms of reducing mental health stigma.

Research on stigma and mental disorders has faced several problems: it has made few connections with clinical practice or health policy (for example in relation to help-seeking and access to care); it has been largely descriptive in its use of public attitude surveys or portrayal of mental illness and violence by the media. Few systematic assessments of user experience have been made. The research has been focused on hypothetical rather than real situations, out of context, addressed stigma indirectly rather than directly and has not provided a clear answer on how to intervene to reduce social rejection (Thornicroft et al., 2009). The review of self-stigma research shows lack of longitudinal research in this area and the need for greater attention on disentangling the true nature of the relationship between internalized stigma and other psychosocial variables (Livingston & Boyd, 2010). Public campaigns' efforts to reduce stigma have not been convincing and the field suffers from a lack of applicable solutions (Thornicroft, 2006; Angermeyer et al. 2009; Gaebel et al., 2008)]. The process of destigmatization appears to be a slow one. Data on the economic impact of anti-stigma campaigns is scarce and evaluation is intrinsically difficult (Sharac et al., 2010).

The overall conclusion of research gave some premises that the best course of action to support people with mental illness is empowerment, including a connection with supported employment and job coaching, national policy changes, development of quality services and anti-stigma education of mental health workers. The strongest evidence at present for active ingredients to reduce stigma pertains to direct social contact with people with mental illness and social marketing on the population level (Thornicroft & Brohan, 2008). The research should focus on measures directed at personal stigma of mental illness as it is increasingly being used as a key factor in anti-stigma interventions.

The need to schedule research from public to the affected persons was followed with the introduction of the INDIGO study aimed to describe the nature, direction, and severity of anticipated and experienced discrimination reported by people with schizophrenia. A cross-sectional survey in 27 countries was made, in centres affiliated to the INDIGO Research Network, by use of face-to-face interviews with 732 participants with schizophrenia. Discrimination was measured with the newly validated discrimination and stigma scale (DISC), which produces three subscores: positive experienced discrimination; negative experienced discrimination and anticipated discrimination. Rates of both anticipated and experienced discrimination were found to be consistently high among people with schizophrenia, mostly in establishing and keeping friendship, in family relationships and in work places. Almost three thirds of the participants were found to want to conceal their diagnosis (Thornicroft et al., 2009). The theory that contact with mentally ill people reduces stigma and discrimination is not fully supported by latest qualitative INDIGO results (Rose et al., 2011).

The INDIGO study is followed by the ASPEN project which is currently underway (2009-11) in 27 countries of the EU. It's goals are ambitious and include the creation of stigma and discrimination assessment scales, creation of detailed analytical European profile of stigma and discrimination as experienced by young people and adults with depression, including both anticipated and expected discrimination and self-stigma. The focus groups research, literature search and interviews were applied to identify best-practice, relevant problems in local environments and presentations of structural stigma and social exclusion (ASPEN, retrieved 7.7.2011on webpage http://mdac.info/aspen).

INDIGO and ASPEN projects are seen as a step forward towards improvement of research on attitudes, systems, personal testimonies and discriminative behaviours.

10. Conclusion

Prejudice can be fought by associating it with the political and social environment. Stigma can not be removed by open protest, explanations or examples - the only solution is a complex social movement aimed toward the better investment in the position of the mentally ill. All stigma reducing interventions need to be adjusted according to local experience and founded on daily observation of problems individuals face. Prejudice that affects the areas of life important to the affected individual needs to be determined (Yang et al., 2007). A set of social and institutional measures needs to be taken, one that encourages tolerance of illness, patients, treatment and symptoms. The anti-stigma movement should be connected with big mental service planning issues- those of psychiatric rehabilitation and community mental health that give some promise to improve the social position and access to care and treatment of people with mental disorders. Community care for people with mental disorders is important, since it provides multi-sectoral programmes of action to promote the social inclusion of people with mental illness.

The only way we as individuals can affect stigma is by leading by example, openly opposing derogatory terms and stereotypes. In basic education, schools and teachers should provide also mental health education, care for mental health and wellbeing of pupils and teachers alike. An inclusive school, promoted, can foster tolerance and make possible early recognition of mental disorders. Every educational level needs to prohibit derogatory language directed at the people with mental disorders and consistently view them as individuals, not diagnoses. Changes in educational curricula should include involving mental health service users and their carers at all educational levels as experts and teachers in mental health issues.

11. Acknowledgment

This work is published with the support of the national association for Mental Health ŠENT, Slovenia.
Translation: Gregor Cotič.

12. References

Adorno, T. W. (1950). *The Authoritarian Personality*. Harper and Row, 0393311120, New York
Angermeyer, M. C. & Matschinger, H. (1996). Relatives' beliefs about causes of schizophrenia. *Acta Psychiatrica Scandinavica*, Vol. 93, No. 3, (march 1996), pp.199–204, 16000447

Angermeyer, M.C., Shultze, B. & Dietrich, S. (2003). Courtesy Stigma. *Soc Psychiatry Psychiat Epidemiology*, Vol. 38, No. 10, (april 2003), pp. 593-602, 14564387

Angermeyer, M. C., Matschinger, H., Corrigan, P.W. (2004). Familiarity with mental illness and social distance from people with schizophrenia and major depression. *Schizophr Res.*, Vol. 69, No. 2-3, (august 2004), pp. 175-182, 10474548

Angermeyer, M. C., Holzinger, A. & Matschinger, H. (2009). Mental health literacy and attitude towards people with mental illness: a trend analysis based on population surveys in the eastern part of Germany. *Eur Psychiatry*, Vol. 24, No. 4 (may 2009), 225-232, 19361961

Anthony, W.A. (2000). A recovery oriented service system: Setting some system level standards. *Psychiatric Rehabilitation Journal*, Vol. 24, No. 2 (fall 2000), 159-168, 1095158X

Awad, A. G., & Voruganti, L. N. (2008). The burden of schizophrenia on caregivers: a review. *Pharmacoeconomics*, Vol. 26, No. 2, (january 2008), pp. 149-162, 18198934

Becker, D.R., Drake, R.E., Bond, G.R., Xie, H., Dain, B. J. & Harrison, K. (1998). Job terminations among persons with severe mental illness participating in supported employment. *Community Ment Health J*, Vol. 34, (februar 1998), pp. 71-82, 00103853

Brockington, I. F., Hall, P., Levings, J. & Murphy, C. (1993). The community's tolerance of the mentally ill. *The British Journal of Psychiatry*, No. 162, (january 1993), pp. 93-99, 14721465

Brohan, E. & Thornicroft, G. (2010). Stigma and discrimination of mental health problems: workplace implication. *Occup Med*, Vol. 60, No.6, (september 2010), pp. 414 - 415, 14718405

Chapple, B., Chant, D., Nolan, P., Cardy, S., Whiteford, H., & McGrath, J. (2004). Correlates of victimisation amongst people with psychosis. *Soc Psychiatry Psychiatr Epidemiology*, Vol. 39, No. 10, (october 2004), pp. 836 - 840, 15669665

Corrigan, P.W., Faber D., Rashid, F. & Leary, M. (1999). The construct validity of empowerment among consumers of mental health services. *Schizophrenia Research*, Vol. 38, No.1, (July 1999), pp. 77-84, 10427613

Corrigan, P.W. & Penn, D. L. (1999). Lessons from social psychology on discrediting psychiatric stigma. *Am Psychol.* Vol. 54, No. 9, (september 1999), pp. 765-776, 10510666

Corrigan, P. W., Backs Edwards A, Green A, Lickey Diwan S, Penn DL. (2001). Prejudice, Social Distance and Familiarity with Mental Illness. *Shizophrenia Bulletin,*Vol. 27, No. 2, pp. 219-225.

Corrigan, P.W., Watson, A. C. (2002). Understanding the impact of stigma on people with mental illness. *World Psychiatry*, Vol. 1, No. 1(february 2002), pp. 16–20, 1489832

Corrigan, P. W., Watson, A. C., Ottati V. (2003). From whence comes mental illness stigma? *Int J Soc Psychiatry*, Vol. 49, No.2, (june 2003), pp. 142-157, 0020-7640

Corrigan, P. W., Markowitz, F. E., Watson, A. C. (2004). Structural levels of mental illness stigma. *Schizophrenia Bulletin*, Vol. 30, No. 3, pp. 481-491, 17451701

Corrigan, P.W. (ed.). (2005). *On The Stigma Of Mental Illness: Practical Strategies for Research and Social Change.* American Psychological Association, 9781591471899, Washington DC

Corrigan, P. W. & McCracken, S. G. (2005). Place first, then train: an alternative to the medical model of psychiatric rehabilitation. *Social Work*, Vol. 50, No.1, (january 2005), pp. 31-39, 00378046

Crisp, A., Gelder, M., Goddard, E., Meltzer, H. (2005). Stigmatization of people with mental illnesses: a follow-up study within the Changing Minds Campaign of the Royal College of Psychiatrists. *World Psychiatry*, Vol. 4, No. 2, (june 2005), pp. 106–113, 16633526

Crowther, R.E., Marchall, M., Bond, G.R. & Huxley P. (2001). Helping people with severe mental illness to obtain work: systematic review. *BMJ*, Vol. 322, No.7280 ,(january 2001), 204-208, 11159616

Feldmann, T., B.(2005). Medical Students' Attitudes Toward Psychiatry and Mental Disorders. *Acad Psychiatry*, Vol. 29, No. 4, (october 2005), pp.354 - 356, 16223897

Gaebel, W., Zäske, H., Baumann, A. E., Klosterkötter, J., Maier, W., Decker, P. & Möller, H. J. (2008). Evaluation of the German WPA "program against stigma and discrimination because of schizophrenia--Open the Doors": results from representative telephone surveys before and after three years of antistigma interventions. *Schizophr Res.*, Vol. 98, No.1-3, (january 2008), pp. 184-193, 17961985

Goffman, E. (1961). *Asylums. Essays on the Social Situation of Mental Patients and Other Inmates.* Doubleday Anchor, 0385000162, New York

Goffman, E. (1963). *Stigma: Notes On The Management Of Spoiled Identity.* Pelican Books, 0671622447, Harmondsworth

Gonzales Torres, M.A., Oraa, R., Arsegui, M., Fernandez-Rivas, A., & Guimon J. (2007). Stigma and discrimination towards people with schizophrenia and their family members. *Soc Psychiatry Psychiatr Epidemiol*, Vol. 42, No. 1, (january 2007), pp. 14-23, 17036263

Granello, D. H., Pauley, P. S. (2000). Television viewing habits and their relationship to tolerance toward people with mental illness. *Journal of Mental Health Counseling*, Vol. 22, No. 2, (april 2000), pp. 162-175, 10402861

Happell, B., Pinikahana, J., Roper, C. (2002). Attitudes of postgraduate nursing students towards consumer participation in mental health services and the role of the consumer academic. *International Journal of Mental Health Nursing*, Vol. 11, No. 4, (december 2002), pp. 240–250, 08839417

Henriquez, J., Holloway, W., Urwin, C., Venn, C. & Walkerdine, W. (1884). *Changing the Subject*, Methuen. In: Nastran Ule M.(ed). (1999). *Predsodki in diskriminacije (Prejudice and Discrimination)*. Znanstveno in publicistično središče, 9616294083, Ljubljana.

Honokonen, T., Henriksson, M., Koiviso, A. M., Stengard, E. & Salokangas, R. K. R. (2004).Violent victimization in schizophrenia. *Soc Psychiatry Psychiatr Epidemiol*, Vol. 39, No. 8, (august 2004), pp. 606-612, 14339285

Kroska, A. & Harkness, S. K. (2006). Stigma Sentiments and Self-Meanings: Exploring the Modified Labeling Theory of Mental Illness. *Social Psychology Quarterly*, Vol. 69, No. 4, (december 2006), pp.325-348, 1472-1465

Lauber, C., Nordt, C., Braunschweig, C. & Rössler, W. (2006). Do mental health professionals stigmatize their patients? *Acta Psychiatrica Scandinavica Suppl.*, No. 429, pp. 51-59, 16445483

Leucht, S., Burkard, T., Henderson, J., Maj, M. & Sartorius, N. (2007). Physical illness and schizophrenia: a review of the literature. *Acta Psychiatr Scand.*, Vol. 116, No. 5, (november 2007), pp. 317-333, 17919153

Link, B. G. (1982). Mental patient status, work, and income: an examination of the effects of a psychiatric label. *Am Sociol Rev.*, Vol. 47, No.2, (april1982), 202-215, 00031224

Link, B. G. & Cullen, F. T. (1986). Contact with the mentally ill and perceptions of how dangerous they are. *Journal of Health and Social Behaviour*, Vol. 27, No. 4 (december 1986), pp. 289-302, 21506000

Link, B.G., Cullen, F.T, Frank, J. & Wozniak, J. (1987). The social rejection of formal mental patients: Understanding why labels matter. *American Journal of Sociology*, Vol. 92, No. 6 (may 1987), pp. 1461-1500, 0001690X

Link, B. G. & Phelan, J. C. (2001). Conceptualizing Stigma. *Annu. Rev. Sociol.*, Vol. 27, pp. 363-385, 1526-5455.

Link, B. G., Yang, L. H., Phelan, J. C. & Collins , P. Y. (2004). Measuring mental illness stigma. *Schizophr Bull.*, Vol. 30, No. 3, pp. 511-541, 15631243

Livingston, J. D. & Boyd, J. E. (2010). Correlates and consequences of internalized stigma for people living with mental illness: a systematic review and meta-analysis. *Soc Sci Med.*, Vol. 71, No.12, (december 2010), pp. 2150-2161, 21051128

Lysaker, P. H., Roe, D., Yanos, P. T. (2007) Toward Understanding the Insight Paradox: Inetrnalized Stigma Moderates the Association Between Insight and Social Functioning, Hope and Self-esteem Among People with Schizophrenia Spectrum Disorders. *Schizophr Bull*, Vol. 33, No.1,(januray 2007), pp. 192-199, 16894025

Nastran Ule, M. (1999). *Predsodki in diskriminacije (Prejudice and Discrimination)*. Znanstveno in publicistično središče, 9616294083, Ljubljana

Nordt, C., Rössler, W. & Lauber, C. (2006). Attitudes of Mental Health Professionals Toward People With Schizophrenia and Major Depression. *Schizophrenia Bulletin*, Vol. 32, No. 4, (october 2006), pp. 709-714, 16510695

Oakes, P. J., Haslan, A. & Turner, J. C. (1994). *Stereotyping and social reality*, pp. 186-213, Blackwell Publishers, 063118872X, New York

Pescosolido, B. A., Martin, J. K., Long, J. S., Medina, T. R., Phelan, J. C. & Link, B.G. (2010). A disease like any other"? A decade of change in public reactions to schizophrenia, depression, and alcohol dependence. *Am J Psychiatry*, Vol.167, No.11, (november 2010), pp.1321-1330, 20843872

Pinfold, V., Thornicroft, G., Huxley, P., Farmer, P. (2005). Active ingredients in anti-stigma programmes in mental health, *Int Rev Psychiatry*, Vol. 17, No. 2, (april 2005), pp. 123-131, 16194782

Quinn, D. M., Kahng, S. K., Crocker, J. (2004). Discreditable: stigma effects of revealing a mental illness history on test performance, *Pers Soc Psychol Bull.*, Vol. 30, No.7,(july 2004), pp. 803-815, 15200689

Rose, D., Willis, R., Brohan, E., Sartorius, N., Villares, C., Wahlbeck, K., Thornicroft, G.& INDIGO Study Group. (2011). Reported stigma and discrimination by people with a diagnosis of schizophrenia.Epidemiol Psychiatr Sci., Vol. 29., No. 3, (june 2011), pp.193-204, 21714366

Rickerson, N., Souma, A., Burgstahler, C. (2004). *Psychiatric Disabilities in Postsecondary Education* , 1.7.2011, Available from http://www.ncset.hawaii.edu/institutes/mar2004/papers/pdf/Souma_revised.p df

Roman, P.M. & Floyd, H.H. (1981). Social acceptance of psychiatric illness and psychiatric treatment. *Social Psychiatry and Psychiatric Epidemiology*, Vol. 16, No. 1, pp. 21-29, 00207640

Sartorius, N.(2002). Iatrogenic stigma of mental illness. *BMJ*, Vol. 324, No. 7352, 1470-1471, 12077020.

Sartorius, N.& Schulze, H. (2005) *Reducing the stigma of mental illness: a report from a Global Programme of the World Psychiatric Association,* Cambridge University Press, 0521549434, Cambridge

Schulze, B. & Angermeyer, M.C. (2003). Subjective experiences of stigma. A focus group study of schizophrenic patients, their relatives and mental health professionals. *Social Science & Medicine*, Vol. 56, No.2, (february 2003), pp. 299-312, 17583217

Schulze, B., Richter-Werling, M., Matschinger, H., & Angermeyer, M. C. (2003). Crazy? So what!? Project weeks on mental health and illness. Their effect on secondary school students' attitudes towards people with schizophrenia. *Acta Psychiatrica Scandinavica*, Vol.107, No.2, (February 2003), pp. 142 -150, 15591255

Stier, A. & Hinshaw, S. (2007). Explicit and implicit stigma against individuals with mental illness. *Australian Psychologist*, Vol. 42, No.29, (august 2007), pp. 106-117, 17716044

Sharac, J., McCrone, P., Clement, S. & Thornicroft, G. (2010). The economic impact of mental health stigma and discrimination: a systematic review. *Epidemiol Psichiatr Soc.*, Vol. 19, No 3, (september 2010), pp.223-232, 21261218

Stout, P. A., ViUegas, J. & Jennings, N. A. (2004). Images of Mental Illness in the Media: Identifying Gaps in the Research *Schizophrenia Bulletin*, Vol. 30, No.3, (january 2004), pp. 543-561, 15631244

Stuart, H. (2004). Stigma and work. *Healthc Pap*, Vol.5, No. 5, No. 2, pp.100-111, 15829771

Stuart H. (2006). Mental illness and employment discrimination., *Curr Opin Psychiatry* ,Vol.19, No. 5, (september 2006), pp. 522-526, 16874128

Tehrani, E., Krussel, J., Borg, L., & Munk-Jorgensen, P.(1996). Dropping out of psychiatric treatment: A prospective study of a first-admission cohort. *Acta Psychiatrica Scandinavica*, Vol. 94, No.4,(october 1996), pp. 266–271, 16000447

Thessen, J. (2001). Being a psychiatric patient in the community – reclasified as the stigmatized »other«. *Scand J Public Health*, Vol 29, No.4, (december 2001), pp. 248-255, 11775780.

Thompson, A. H., Stuart, H., Bland, R. C., Arboleda Flores, J., Warner, R. & Dickson, R. A. (2002). Attitudes about schizophrenia from the pilot site of the WPA worldwide campaign against the stigma of schizophrenia. *Soc Psychiatry Psychiatr Epidemiology*. Vol. 37, No. 10, (october 2002), pp. 475-482, 02275910

Thornicroft, G. (2006). *Shunned: Discrimination against People with Mental Illness,* University Press, 00453102, Oxford

Thornicroft, G., Brohan, E. (2008). Reducing stigma and discrimination: Candidate interventions. *Int J Ment Health Syst.* Vol. 2, No.1,(april 2008), pp. 3, 18405393

Thornicroft, G., Brohan, E., Rose, D., Sartorius, N., Leese, M., for the INDIGO Study Group. (2009). Global pattern of experienced and anticipated discriminationagainst people with schizophrenia: a cross-sectional survey. *Lancet*, Vol. 373, No. 9661, (January 2009), pp. 408–415, 19162314

Waghorn, G. & Lloyd C. (2011). The employment of people with mental illness. *Advances in Mental Health.* Vol. 4, No. 2 , pp: 129 – 171, 18374905

Wahl, O.F. (1995). *Media Madness: Public images of mental illness,* Rutgers, 0813522137, New Brunswick

Wahl, O.F. (1999). Mental health consumers' experiences of stigma. *Schizophr Bull,* Vol.25, No.3, (march 1999), pp. 467-478, 17451701

Wahl, O. F., Wood, A., Richards , R. (2002). Newspaper Coverage of Mental Illness: Is It Changing? *American Journal of Psychiatric Rehabilitation,* Vol. 6, No. 1., pp. 9-31. 3387865

Walsh, E., Moran, P., Scott, C., McKenzie, K., Burns, T., Creed, F., Tyrer, P., Murray, R.M. & Fahy T. (2003). Prevalence of violent victimisation in severe mental illness. *Br J Psychiatry,* No. 183, (september 2003), pp. 233-238, 12948997

Wancata, J., Krautgartner, M., Berner, J., Scumaci, S., Freidl, M., Alexandrowicz, R., Rittmannsberger, H. (2006). The "Carers' needs assessment for Schizophrenia", *Soc Psychiatry Psychiatr Epidemiol,* Vol. 41, No.3, (january 2006), pp. 221-229, 16435078

Wittschen, H. U., Jacobi F.(2005). Size and burden of mental disorders in Europe – a critical review and appraisal of 27 studies. *European Neuropsychopharmacology.* Vol. 15, No. 4, (august 2005), pp. 357-376, 15961293

Wolf, G., Pathare, S., Craig, T. &, Leff, J. (1996). Public education for community care: A new approach. *Br. J. Psychiatry,* Vol. 168, pp. 441-447, 1472-1465

Yang, L. H., Kleinman, A., Link, B. G., Phelan, J. C., Lee, S. & Good, B. (2007). *Soc Sci Med.,* Vol. 4, No. 7, (april 2007), 1524-1535, 17188411

Zalar, B., Strbad, M. & Švab, V. (2007). Psychiatric education : does it affect stigma? *Acad. psychiatry,* Vol. 31, No. 3, (october 2007), pp. 245-246, 10429670

Public Attitudes, Lay Theories and Mental Health Literacy: The Understanding of Mental Health

Adrian Furnham and Kate Telford

Research Department of Clinical, Educational and Health Psychology
University College London,
UK

1. Introduction

There is a large body of research into public conceptions of mental illnesses and disorders going back over 50 years (Star, 1955). This chapter seeks to review the complex literature on this topic scattered over a wide range of disciplines including anthropology, psychology, psychiatry and sociology. The aim is to provide the researcher in social psychiatry and allied disciplines the opportunity to have a comprehensive and critical review.

Over the years there are *three* slightly different but overlapping research traditions with regard to this topic: public attitudes, lay theories and mental health literacy. The first concerns studies of *attitudes towards people with mental disorders* (Nunnally, 1961), that is, beliefs about what people with mental illness are like and also, how they should be treated. These studies may be about specific mental disorders, such as schizophrenia (Siegler & Osmond, 1966) and depression (Rippere, 1977, 1979) or more generally about mental illnesses. These are nearly always large survey based studies typical of market research or attitudinal studies. These studies are important as they can offer an explanation for negative and stigmatising attitudes towards mental disorder (e.g. Nunnally, 1961; Link, Phelan, Bresnahan, Stueve, & Pescosolido, 1999), and why so few of those diagnosed, seek help (Lin, Goering, Offord, Campbell & Boyle, 1996; Andrews, Hall, Teesson & Henderson, 1999).

Secondly, studies relating to *lay theories* of mental illness have been conducted primarily by Furnham and colleagues (i.e. Furnham & Lowick, 1984; Furnham & Manning, 1997; Furnham & Haraldsen, 1998), focusing specifically on the nature, causes, and treatments of disorders, such as heroin addiction (Furnham & Thompson, 1996), and schizophrenia (Furnham & Rees, 1988). These studies are concerned with the structure of beliefs about aetiology and cure and the relationship between them. They originate in social attribution theory in psychology and are concerned with the extent to which lay people endorse biological, psychological or sociological theories for the causes of various illnesses. They are also concerned with the extent to which there is a clear logical correlation between perceived cause and recommended cure for specific individual illnesses.

The third approach is the term *'mental health literacy'* introduced by Jorm and colleagues (Jorm, Korten, Jacomb, Christensen, Rodgers, et al., 1997b) to refer to public knowledge and more specifically recognition of mental disorders. This encompasses theories of mental disorders, as well as other important issues such as knowing how and where to seek help (i.e. pathways to professional help). There are now well over two dozen papers that fall into this field. Most (but not all) are based on large population surveys and the ability of people to identify mental illnesses specified in vignettes of hypothetical situations of people suffering from the mental illnesses.

This chapter will concentrate on the topic of lay theories of mental illness.

2. Lay theories of mental disorder

As Furnham and Cheng (2000) described, researchers have distinguished between three types of everyday theories that may be deployed to explain phenomena: *lay* theories which are thought of as personal and idiosyncratic; *folk* theories which are thought to be shared by certain subgroups; and *scientific* theories which are usually thought to be empirically and observationally derived and tested. Furnham (1988) noted that research about lay theories is usually concerned with one or more of six different issues:

1. *Aetiology* (How do these theories develop? What factors seem to lead to the development of particular ideas?);
2. *Structure* (What is the internal structure of these theories? How is the mental architecture arranged?);
3. *Relationships* (How are various theories about different topics grouped or linked? What is the underlying structure of lay theories in different areas: health, economics, education?);
4. *Function* (What function do theories hold for individuals themselves? What are the implications for change?);
5. *Stability* (Do these theories change over time? What influences them?);
6. *Behavioural Consequences* (How is social behaviour related to these different theories?)

Most lay theory studies adhere to the following methodology. Once a particular disorder is identified, be it ADHD, anorexia, autism or alcoholism to sexual disorders, schizophrenia or suicide, a questionnaire is constructed based on interviews with, and reports from non-experts. The questionnaire is usually structured around three issues: the cause of the problem; the behavioural manifestation of the complaint, and the optimal cure of the problem. The analysis usually follows a pattern: beginning with a multivariate analysis of the structure of the three parts of the questionnaire, followed by correlations between cause, manifestation and cure factors and then possibly regressions with the belief factors and the criterion variable and various individual variables (demography, personality, ideology) as the predictor variables.

Recent studies into lay theories have focused specifically on beliefs about the causes and treatments of mental disorders and the relationship between them (e.g. Furnham & Thompson, 1996; Furnham & Buck, 2003), in order to find possible links between negative attitudes and erroneous beliefs. These studies have produced a number of interesting findings. For example, lay theories are not arbitrary or incoherent, but can be classified into categories such as 'psychological' or 'social' in the same way as academic theories (Furnham & Rees, 1988; Furnham & Thompson, 1996). This suggests that lay persons have a basic, possibly implicit, understanding of the different levels of explanation for mental disorder. Studies have shown that the structure of the categories of lay and academic theories overlap to a certain extent, for example 'biological' and 'psychological'. However, some may differ. For example, 'external' which includes beliefs about the roles of luck and religion in the aetiology of mental illness (Furnham & Buck, 2003).

There are also differences between the content of lay theories and academic theories of mental disorders. The main finding is that lay people place more emphasis on psychological, social, and familial causal factors (Sarbin & Mancuso, 1972; Angermeyer & Matschinger, 1996; Furnham & Thompson, 1996), which can be compared to primarily biological and genetic academic theories. However, lay beliefs about causes vary depending on the disorder. For example Jorm and colleagues (1997a) found that schizophrenia was more likely to be attributed to genetic factors than depression, and autism was more likely to be biological than theories of obsessive-compulsive disorder, which were more likely to be psychodynamic (Furnham & Buck, 2003). It is therefore necessary to investigate the structure and content of lay theories of bipolar disorder, as previous studies show that it is difficult to generalise across disorders. Notably, the finding that lay theories are generally psychosocial, rather than biological, has been frequently replicated and can therefore be used to make predictions about lay theories of bipolar disorder.

Lay theories about the treatment of mental disorders show marked differences from current practices in the mental health service, which involve drug treatment for mental disorders and/or psychotherapies such as Cognitive Behavioural Therapy (CBT). It has been found that lay people generally prefer psychotherapy to drug treatment (Angermeyer & Matschinger, 1996; Angermeyer & Dietrich, 2006) due to the perceived side effects (Angermeyer, Daumer, & Matschinger, 1993; Priest, Vize, Roberts, Roberts & Tylee, 1996; Fischer, Goerg, Zbinden, & Guimon, 1999). There is also a common lay belief that 'will power' can effectively facilitate recovery from mental disorders (Knapp & Delprato, 1980), such as agoraphobia and anorexia nervosa (Furnham & Henley, 1988). However, medication is believed to be the most effective treatment for disorders with a higher perceived severity (Furnham & Rees, 1988; Furnham & Bower, 1992), thus showing that lay and academic theories of treatment overlap to an extent. It is unclear how these findings may relate to bipolar disorder, especially since the perceived severity of the disorder is not known. However, it is predicted that psychotherapies will be preferred to drug treatment.

Other studies have focused on assessing whether there is a logical relationship between lay theories of cause and treatment. For example, it is expected that if cause is attributed to biological factors, medication should be endorsed as treatment. This has been found in a number of studies which show a strong relationship between similar cause and treatment theories (Furnham & Buck, 2003), and those which are "sensibly" linked (Furnham & Haraldsen, 1998, pp. 696). However these findings are not always replicated. To demonstrate, medication was the preferred treatment for schizophrenia, despite participants attributing the cause to psychosocial factors (Furnham & Bower, 1992; Furnham & Rees, 1988). However, in this case it is predicted that there will be a coherent relationship between theories of causes and treatments of bipolar disorder due to the predominant findings of previous literature.

Two general models of lay beliefs have been proposed. The 'medical' model (Rabkin, 1974), which suggests that mental disorders are like any other illness with symptoms caused by an underlying biological pathology and a treatment which addresses this. This has positive implications as it suggests that people with mental disorders should not be viewed differently than those with a physical illness. The second model is the 'psychosocial' model (Sarbin & Mancuso, 1972), which suggests that causes of mental disorder are psychological and environmental. This has positive implications for treatment as it advocates social and community support rather than hospitalisation. However, it has been found that people with beliefs which correspond to this model are less trusting of ex-psychiatric patients than ex-medical patients (Sarbin & Mancuso, 1972). These models can therefore be used to classify lay theories and have wide implications for attitudes towards those with mental illnesses, causal beliefs and treatment preferences.

3. Determinants of lay theories and mental health literacy

Attempts have been made to determine why particular theories are endorsed more than others. A number of studies have found that lay theories are predicted by demographic variables. Specifically, studies show that both younger and more educated people have more informed beliefs about mental disorders (Shurka, 1983; Hasin & Link, 1988; Yoder, Shute & Tryban, 1990; Fisher & Goldney, 2003). Significant effects of gender (Furnham & Manning, 1997), political persuasion (Furnham & Thompson, 1996), and religiousness (Furnham & Haraldsen, 1998) have also been found. This suggests that demographic variables may have some value in predicting many lay theories.

In relation to familiarity with, and knowledge about, mental disorders, it has been found that participants with less knowledge of autism endorse external theories of cause, such as luck and religion, rather than academic theories (Furnham & Buck, 2003), whereas correct recognition of schizophrenia predicts more informed causal beliefs (Jorm et al., 1997a). A large increase in recognition of mental disorders has also been found for mental health professionals compared to the general public (Jorm, Korten, Rodgers, Pollitt, Christensen et al., 1997d). These studies suggests that informed beliefs about the nature, causes and treatments of mental illness come from diverse reading, academic study and/or extensive contact with people affected by mental disorders. Therefore, these variables should have some predictive value for both recognition and theories of mental illness.

4. The studies

Table 1 summarises the results of two dozen studies on over a dozen mental illnesses. The table shows, in essence, the method and results of the studies which will not be repeated here. All were completed in western developed countries and participants were generally better educated and younger than the population as a whole. This would suggest that they probably have more sophisticated lay theories

Disorder	Authors	Study
Alcoholism	Furnham & Lowick (1984)	265 participants completed a questionnaire in which they rated 30 explanations for their importance in explaining the causes of alcoholism. • Findings indicated a gender effect: females, more than males, believed alcoholics to be socially inadequate and anxious and held the belief that there is too much social pressure and not enough prohibitions against drinking. • Furthermore, there was an age effect: middle aged rather than younger or older tended to explain alcoholism in terms of poor education, social and cultural pressures and biological and genetic mechanisms.

Disorder	Authors	Study
		Factor analysis revealed six factors: psychological stress, personal and social problems, psychoanalytic theories, socio-cultural explanations, biological or genetic explanations and social desirability or pressure.
Anorexia Nervosa	Furnham & Hume-Wright (1992)	168 participants completed a 105-item questionnaire which explored their beliefs regarding the cause, correlates and cures of anorexia nervosa. • Findings suggested lay people hold elaborate, consensual and moderately accurate (parallel to clinical theories) beliefs about the description, cause and cures of anorexia nervosa. • Sex, personal experience of eating disorders and being acquainted with an anorexic were significant correlates of a number of factors. • Factor analysis identified clusters of responses that showed underlying factors of family, stress of change, conflict in contradictory social roles, goals and demands, rebellion and security.
	Furnham & Manning (1997)	147 participants completed a 108-item questionnaire, based on Furnham & Hume Wright (1992). The four parts of the questionnaire were individually factor analysed and an interpretable factor structure emerged for each. • Results indicate young people (16-19 year olds) hold moderately accurate beliefs about the causes and cures of both anorexia nervosa and obesity. • Participants seemed to see social pressure affecting the development of anorexia as most important; and self-worth as most important for cures. • Sex, actual body size, estimated body size and having experience with an eating disorder were found to correlate significantly with a number of factors. • Factors of cause and cure were not correlated regarding anorexia but were for obesity.
	Benveniste, Lecouteur & Hepworth (1999)	Lay theories of anorexia nervosa using critical psychology perspective (Discourse Analysis) were investigated through 10 semi-structured interviews with 5 women and 5 men aged 15-25. • Three discourses emerged: Socio-cultural, Individual and Femininity. • It is concluded that lay theories of anorexia nervosa were structured through these key discourses which maintain separation between socio-cultural and individual psychology in relation to anorexia nervosa. • This reinforces the concept that anorexia is a form of psychopathology.

Disorder	Authors	Study
Autism and obsessive compulsive disorder	Furnham & Buck (2003)	A total of 92 participants were involved in the two studies. In study 1 parental interviews of sufferers were conducted and revealed that, as hypothesised, parents hold predominantly biomedical views regarding autism. • Participants then completed the questionnaire with varied levels of experience of autism (no experience-relatives of sufferers) which involved rating a range of theories of aetiology and treatment approaches for each disorder. • Statistical analysis confirmed that lay beliefs about autism were primarily biomedical and beliefs about OCD were primarily psychological. • Multiple regression analyses indicated that a range of individual difference factors (i.e. religiousness and age) predicted beliefs about the importance of the factors derived from factor analysis of the belief statements.
Depression	Furnham & Kuyken (1991)	After a pilot study asking people to list the causes of depression, 201 participants completed a questionnaire which involved rating 32 explanations and 5 current theories of depression. • Results indicated reasonable agreement in ratings of importance of causal attributions and with current theories of depression • Factor analysis revealed 6 interpretable factors; social deprivation, interpersonal difficulties, traumatic experiences, affective deprivations, negative self-image and interpersonal loss. • Overall lay people believe experience of loss was the major cause of depression, which is not consistent with clinical theories. • Demographic correlates were present but only accounted for between 10-12 percent of variance.
	Lauber, Falcato, Nordt & Rossler (2003)	Data was collected from 873 interviews from a representative telephone survey. A vignette depicting a man with depression satisfying the Diagnostic Statistical Manual (DSM) III-R criteria was presented. • For more than half of respondents (56.6%) difficulties within the family or the partnership are causal for depression. Occupational stress being the second most mentioned (32.7%). • Few correlations were found between causal attributions, labelling and demographic factors. • Attributions are shaped primarily by psychosocial ideas about aetiology; however one third of the sample held biological or disease-related beliefs about the causes of depression.

Disorder	Authors	Study
	Heim, Smallwood & Davies (2005)	128 Students were presented with vignettes describing individuals with symptoms of depression based on the DSM-IV to investigate lay perceptions of depression in terms of perceived severity. Descriptions varied in terms of gender, social status and a self-referent manner of communicating depressive symptomology. • When asked to rate on a likert-type scale the degree to which vignette characters were thought to be depressed, a non-self referent style of communicating symptoms of depression, by female vignette characters, was seen as an indication of elevated levels of depression.
	Çirakoğlu, Kökdemir & Demirutku (2003)	The study reports university students' attributions for the causes of and cures for depression in Turkey. • Results indicated 6 components for causes: trauma, job-related problems, loss, disposition, intimacy, and isolation. • Seven components were found for cures: hobby, sensation seeking, avoidance, professional help, religious practices, esteem and spiritual activities. • Men rated religious practices as more useful than women did. • No other gender differences were found.
	Budd, James & Hughes (2008)	The study aimed to develop a robust factor structure of lay theories of depression, while more adequately sampling from the full range of hypothesised causes of depression. • The reasons rated most important for depression were related to recent bereavement, imbalance in brain chemistry and suffering sexual abuse or assault. • The data was best described by a 2-factor solution, the first representing stress and the second depressogenic beliefs.
Anxiety & Depression	Kinnier, Hofsess, Pongratz & Lambert (2009)	In the study, 3 expert populations were consulted: popular self-help literature (10 books), well-respected therapists (17) and individuals who believe that they have successfully recovered from either anxiety or depression (18) for their recommendations to those suffering from anxiety or depression. • Content analysis and descriptive statistics indicated recommendations were for anxious and depressed individuals to actively seek help from multiple people and interventions, as well as to being open to innovative self-tailored interventions. • Affirmations relating to 'not being crazy' in relation to anxiety and that the depression will subside in time were deemed most helpful for recovery.

Disorder	Authors	Study
Gender Identity Disorder (GID)	Furnham and Sen (in press)	124 participants completed a questionnaire based on previous interviews regarding views on possible causes and cures of GID. <ul><li>As hypothesised, participants believed most in biomedical causes and cures of GID.</li><li>Factor analysis identified four factors in relation to causes of GID: upbringing and personal, pregnancy and brain abnormalities, environmental, biomedical causes.</li><li>Five factors identified in relation to cure were: psychological assistance and personal, extreme medical and behavioural changes, alternative therapies and external factors and medical treatments.</li><li>Results indicated participants were unclear of the causes and cures of GID but these beliefs were logically related.</li></ul>
Heroin Addiction	Furnham & Thompson (1996)	144 participants completed a questionnaire examining the structure and determinants of lay people's implicit theories of heroin addiction. They had to rate 105 statements about the causes, correlates and cures of heroin addiction. <ul><li>Factors seemed similar to explicit academic theories; except beliefs about cure which did not show support for most clinical models.</li><li>When a higher order factor analysis was performed, four factors emerged: moralistic, psychosocial, socio-cultural and drug treatment which reflect coherent views on the nature of heroin addiction.</li><li>The strongest demographic determinant of lay beliefs in these factors was political beliefs. Right wing voters emphasised moralistic and individualistic theory and left-wing voters supporting the psychological and societal ideas.</li></ul>
Neurosis	Furnham (1984)	Three experiments aimed to investigate various determinants of the common-sense conception of neuroticism. In the first experiment subjects completed various standardized psychological tests measuring neuroticism and anxiety, while also estimating the extent of their own anxiety and neuroticism. In the second experiment subjects attempted to detect items measuring neuroticism in a standard personality questionnaire and secondly estimate the extent of their own and the 'average' person's neuroticism. Finally, in the third experiment subjects rated the typicality of various neurotic traits and behaviour which had been supplied by subjects in the previous two experiments. <ul><li>Findings demonstrated some similarities in expert explicit theories and lay-person implicit theories, though there appeared systematic biases in subject's perception of their own neuroticism.</li></ul>

Disorder	Authors	Study
Paraphilia	Furnham & Haraldsen (1998)	The paper examined four types of Paraphilia: fetishism, paedophilia, sexual sadism, and voyeurism. 105 participants completed a four part questionnaire divided into: demographic details, perceptions of etiology, ratings of cure for each Paraphilia and the Eysenck Personality Questionnaire. • Factor analysis revealed a clear and logical factor structure for etiology and cure items. • Further, etiology and cure items correlated strongly with each other but only moderately with demographic and personality differences.
Phobia	Furnham (1995)	150 people completed a two-part questionnaire that investigates beliefs about the nature and cure of phobia. Five factors emerged from the 23-item attitude section: • The ideas that: certain personality factors related to phobia, there are physical correlates of phobia, observational learning causes phobia, phobias are caused by behavioural pairing, and Freudian ideas of unconscious association. The 13-item treatment section showed four factors: • Alternative medical practices, psycho-analytic practices, desensitisation and flooding. • There was a clear and logical relationship between perceptions of the causes and treatment of phobia demonstrating that lay people have coherent theories of the etiology and cure of phobia.
Schizo-phrenia	Furnham & Rees (1988)	Subjects completed two brief questionnaires, one concerning the description of, and attitudes towards schizophrenia and schizophrenics and the second on the possible cause of schizophrenia. Beliefs about the conceptions of mental illness suggested four factors labelled dangerous, amoral, egocentric and vagrant. The items on the causes factored into five factors labelled stress and pressure, biological, genetic, backward and brain damage.
	Furnham & Bower (1992)	106 Lay respondents (students, nurses, employed and unemployed) aged 18-60 answered a questionnaire examining five identified main academic theories of schizophrenia (medical, moral-behavioural, social, psychoanalytic and conspirational) along various dimensions (e.g. aetiology, behaviour, treatment). • No single model was favoured exclusively but seemed to point to a synthesis of several academic theories. Lay subjects stressed the importance of patient environment in the aetiology of schizophrenia rather than a physiological malfunction, but tended to stress the personal rights of the schizophrenic.

Disorder	Authors	Study
	Angermeyer & Matschinger (1994)	Results were obtained from a population survey of 2118 in Germany. Interviews revealed participants showed: • A strong trend to revert to social and individual psychological concepts in the search for a reason for the occurrence of schizophrenic disorders; in particular, stress. An unmistakable preference for psychotherapy as opposed to treatment with psychotropic drugs
	Jorm, Korten, Jacomb, Christensen, Rodgers & Pollitt (1997a)	Data from a national household survey of the beliefs of 2031 Australian adults about causes and risk factors for mental disorders was collected. • Results indicated that for schizophrenia, social environmental factors (day-to-day problems, traumatic events) were often seen as causes which are a contrast to the weak epidemiological evidence for such a role. • Genetic factors attracted more attention as a cause of Schizophrenia than Depression. Of notable concern was the popular belief (over half) of respondents that weakness of character was a likely cause of both depression and schizophrenia, implying a negative evaluation of the sufferer as a person.
	Furnham & Wong (2007)	The study investigated 200 (101 female, 99 male) British (100) and Chinese (100) participants' beliefs about the causes, behaviour, manifestations and treatments of schizophrenia. Results confirmed the three hypotheses that: 1. Chinese would hold more superstitious and religious beliefs towards the causation and treatment of schizophrenia and would prefer the use of alternative medicine. 2. The British emphasised more on internal (biological and psychological) and external (sociological) beliefs for the causes and treatments. 3. Chinese participants held more negative attitudes and beliefs about the behaviour manifestations of schizophrenia than the British.
	Furnham, Raja & Khan (2008)	A total of 305 British, British Pakistani and Native Pakistani medical students completed a questionnaire on general beliefs about people with schizophrenia, causal explanations concerning aetiology and the role of hospitals and society in treating people with schizophrenia. • There was strong evidence to suggest Pakistanis possessed more negative beliefs and attitudes about people with schizophrenia, but no evidence to suggest Pakistanis believed more in superstitious causal explanations.

Disorder	Authors	Study
		• Pakistanis were more likely to consider seeking help from faith healers, but not God, compared with the British Pakistani and British participants.
		• Results confirm cultural (European-Asian) difference in the understanding of the cause, manifestation and cure of schizophrenia.
Suicide	Knight, Furnham & Lester (2000)	Attitudes toward suicide were explored in 150 young people.
		• The strongest correlate of these attitudes was psychoticism scores, with the respondents with higher psychoticism scores viewing suicide more positively than those with lower scores.
	Walker, Lester & Joe (2006)	African Americans' lay beliefs and attributions towards suicide were examined in 251 undergraduate college students using the Attitudes Towards Suicide Scale, Life Ownership Orientation Questionnaire, Stigma Questionnaire and Suicide Ideation Questionnaire.
		• Beliefs about stigma were comparable across ethnic groups.
		• African American students were significantly less likely than European American students to attribute suicide to interpersonal problems and report the individual or government as responsible for life.
		• African American students were significantly more likely to report that God is responsible for life.

Table 1. Previous studies of lay theories of mental disorder

Table 2 shows the results of various studies concerned with lay theories of the process of psychotherapy. They are concerned with the perceptions of what occurs in a (typical) therapy session, the efficacy of different cures, the prognosis for different problems, and the differing perceptions of lay people and clinicians.

Author(s) "Title"	Study
Furnham & Wardley (1990) "Lay Theories of Psychotherapy I: Attitudes Toward, and Beliefs About, Psychotherapy and Therapists"	Two hundred people completed two questionnaires that concerned their beliefs about what psychotherapy clients experience and their attitudes toward psychotherapy.
	• Overall, the participants appeared to be very positive toward psychotherapy. They expected that psychotherapy clients receive considerable benefits from therapy.
	• They appeared to have a fairly realistic idea of what occurs in psychotherapy. They tended to

Author(s) "Title"	Study
	agree that psychotherapists aim to help clients achieve self-insight and express emotions. • The results of this study suggest that lay people have fairly complex, multi-faceted views of psychotherapy and the experience of psychotherapy clients. This was particularly the case with respect to beliefs about clients of psychotherapists' experiences. • There were no sex differences, but some age differences, which indicated that older people tended to be more sceptical, indeed even possibly cynical about the benefits of psychotherapy. • Education was related predictably to certain beliefs and showed that better-educated people tended to believe less than less-well-educated people in the whole process of psychotherapy. • The most powerful correlates of belief factors were actual psychological experience, exposure and knowledge. The most experienced participants tended to be less optimistic about progress in therapy and more aware that psychotherapy is not entirely about teaching new behaviours or dealing with conflict and emotions.
Furnham & Wardley (1991) "Lay Theories of Psychotherapy II: The Efficacy of Different Therapies and Prognosis for Different Problems"	Two hundred lay people completed two questionnaires, the first examining their perceptions of the efficacy of 22 different types of psychological treatment. The second questionnaire required them to rate the perceived prognosis for 36 different and relative common psychological problems derived from (with definition) the DSM III. • Participants perceived cognitive and group therapies as most effective and the physical and surgical therapies as least effective to "cure" a wide range of problems. They were most impressed by traditional psychotherapy but least impressed by primary scream or rebirth therapy. • The more experience participants had the less they believed in the efficacy of most therapies especially regressional techniques but also cognitive and psychodynamic therapies to "cure" a wide range of psychological problems.

Author(s) "Title"	Study
	• Overall, participants seemed moderately optimistic about the prognosis of certain neurotic disorders especially enuresis, insomnia and agoraphobia, while very pessimistic about the prognosis for epilepsy, dementia, and homosexuality.
	• The strongest correlate of the prognosis factor was psychological experience. The results tended to indicate that psychological experience tended to be associated with beliefs in the prognosis of problems concerned with general anxiety, but beliefs about the poor prognosis of problems associated with serious cognitive problems.
	• There seemed to be more belief in, perhaps as a consequence of understanding about, behaviourism and learning theory.
Furnham, Wardley, & Lillie (1992) "Lay Theories of Psychotherapy III: Comparing the Ratings of Lay Persons and Clinical Psychologists"	Approximately 200 lay people (working adults and students) and over 50 practicing psychologists completed a four-part questionnaire that examined attitude to psychotherapy, beliefs concerning what patients report during psychotherapy, the efficacy of quite different types of psychological treatment, and finally the prognosis for a wide range of psychological problems.
	• The results revealed numerous and consistent differences which showed that, compared to lay people, psychotherapists seemed more skeptical and pessimistic about the efficacy of therapy and the prognosis for various psychological illnesses.
	• Psychotherapists believed that clients in psychotherapy tended to report more positive, favourable reactions than lay adults and students.
	• Psychotherapists tended not to believe that therapists teach specific skills but rather that they provide some sort of social support and help vent fears and other negative emotions.
	• Therapists seem more skeptical in beliefs about the efficacy of different therapies and the prognosis of different problems. Therapists believe that different therapies are suitable for particular problems (and that some therapies are by-and-large fairly useless), while lay people believe therapies are suitable for a wide range of

Author(s) "Title"	Study
	psychological problems. • Lay people believe the prognosis for a wide range of psychological problems to be better than the therapists.
Wong (1994) "Lay Theories of Psychotherapy and Perceptions of Therapists: A Replication and Extension of Furnham and Wardley"	Two hundred and forty undergraduates and 43 non-faculty staff members at the University of Northern Iowa participated in the study. Each participant completed four questionnaires and read a vignette of a part of a psychotherapy session in order to examine the laypersons' perceptions of psychotherapy, the experience of psychotherapy clients, and therapist credibility. • The participants appeared to have realistic conceptions about what occurs in therapy and to be quite optimistic about treatment outcomes. Participants tended to disagree with most of the popular stereotypes about psychotherapy (e.g., most clients lie on a couch; women make better therapists than men) and to agree with the goals and techniques of most types of modern psychotherapy (e.g., therapists teach strategies to reduce conflict or frustration; psychotherapists encourage the expression of emotions). They also indicated that the therapeutic experiences and relationship lead to improvements for a variety of problems and client types. • They did endorse some common misconceptions about psychotherapy (e.g., most therapists ask about dreams, believe psychological problems start in childhood, or use personality questionnaires). They also responded neutrally to statements about some important aspects of therapy, such as the client-therapist relationship and the length of therapy. • Males, older individuals, and those with more psychological experience were less optimistic, but perhaps more realistic, about the potential benefits of therapy. However, the more experienced participants, surprisingly, did not differ from the less experienced ones in their beliefs about the experience of clients. As expected, when age, experience, and sex were controlled, the student and staff did not differ in their psychological experience or in their beliefs about psychotherapy.

Author(s) "Title"	Study
	• Neither participant's sex nor the amount of fee charge affected participants' perceptions. Also, treatment modality (client-centered vs. behaviour vs. rational-emotive) significantly affected ratings of overall, and each dimension of, therapist credibility. • Only a few beliefs about psychotherapy influenced perceptions of (only limited aspects of) therapist credibility.

Furnham, Pereira, & Rawles (2001) "Lay Theories of Psychotherapy: Perceptions of the Efficacy of Different 'Cures' for Specific Disorders"	Two hundred and seventeen participants completed a two-part questionnaire in order to study the structure and determinants of lay beliefs about psychotherapy in general and specifically the effectiveness of various therapies for four different disorders.
	• It was clear from the factor analysis of the ratings (across all four conditions) that participants did not distinguish between a range of talk therapies including psychoanalysis, gestalt and existentialist therapies, on the one hand, and group/marital therapies on the other, as well as more social-behavioural therapies like CBT, assertiveness and thought-stopping. To the participants they all appeared to involve talk which aims to change cognitions and emotions.
	• Participants clearly differentiated between the efficacies of the different therapies. Whether considered to be moderately efficacious (cognitive/talk therapies) or not, participants saw some as being significantly more appropriate than others.
	  • Cognition therapy was seen as efficacious for depression and delusional disorders.
	  • On the other hand, physical therapies were perceived moderately useful with anorexia but not at all for depression.

Furnham (2009) "Psychiatric and Psychotherapeutic Literacy: Attitudes to, and Knowledge of, Psychotherapy"	In total 185 British adults, recruited by a market research company, completed a four-part questionnaire, last about 20 minutes to study what lay people think happens during psychotherapy; what the processes and aims are; and the aetiology, treatment and prognosis for mood and psychotic (bipolar, schizophrenia) and two neurotic (depression, obsessive-compulsive) disorders.

Author(s) "Title"	Study
	• Participants saw psychotherapy as supportive, creating insight and improving coping skills. However, they do recognize that clients are occasionally required to confront uncomfortable and painful ideas and feelings.
	• Participants were generally very positive about psychotherapy believing the experience to be highly beneficial.
	• Schizophrenia was seen to have a biological basis; depression and bipolar disorder were perceived to have family, work and other stress-related causal issues.
	• Participants thought psychotherapy a very effective treatment but drug treatments more effective for schizophrenia and bipolar disorder.
	• 'Talking it over' was judged highly relevant, specifically to depression.
	• Participants believed that depression had a good chance of cure, and remission, but that neither schizophrenia nor bipolar disorder had much chance of an effective cure.

Table 2. Studies on lay theories of Psychotherapy

5. Limitations

The studies shown in Table 1 and Table 2 suffer various limitations. The first is *sampling*. Many studies have sampled relatively small, better educated, Western participants, often with disproportionate numbers of students. Far fewer have looked at the ideas of patients, their relatives or psychiatric staff. Further, very few studies have been conducted in third world or developing countries where it is known that people hold very different lay theories. Ideal studies would use large, representative samples. The second is *method*. Most studies have been questionnaire based after initial testing with interviews. All methods have limitations, and it would be most desirable to use multiple methods to investigate lay theories. It would also be most beneficial to trace theories over time, particularly if some attempts were made to change them via an intervention like mental health education. The third is *topic*. It is clear from Table 1 that only a small number of disorders have been investigated. They are however not arbitrary as the topics covered are often the more common mental illnesses (i.e. depression), as well as those most discussed by the public.

6. Conclusion

It is plausible to draw five conclusions from the scattered literature on lay theories of mental illness. *First,* as many have noted, knowledge of the various mental illnesses is both patchy and highly varied. Whereas lay people seem relatively well informed about some, like depression, they are surprising ignorant about others, like schizophrenia. This seems to be related to the prevalence of the illness in the population as well as media coverage of the problem, particularly celebrities admitting to being "sufferers". Many hold antiquated and unsubstantiated views on the nature or manifestation of mental illnesses that educators have been trying to correct for years.

Second, when thinking about the cause of mental illness it is common to find five types of explanations: psychological; sociological; biological/genetics; psycho-analytic and moral/behavioural. Most people rate typical psychological explanations seeing the cause to be individual mal-functioning of some system. They are also happy to acknowledge group, societal and structural variables as contributing to illness. To a limited extent, and highly specifically with respect to particular illness, people rate biological (i.e. hormonal, brain damage) and genetic factors as a major causal role in the mental illness aetiology. There is also a surprising number of people who endorse classic Freudian explanations of dysfunctional early relationships with parents or others. For some mental illnesses lay people are happy to suggest the cause is "wickedness" of one sort or another: that is, that the cause is gross moral turpitude. For some people in third world countries the cause is seen to be spiritual: that is the intervention and possible punishment from a "higher force" or "pantheon of gods". The extent to which people appear to endorse one type of theoretical explanation over another is a function of the illness in question, as well as their education and ideological orientation.

Third, lay people seem less certain about cure/intervention/management than cause. Once again, various types of cures are seen to be, at least in part, relevant to many problems. For most problems, the favoured cure, in terms of perceived efficacy, is a variety of the "talking cures": that is, psychotherapy of one sort of another. Cures that are acknowledged, but rated as less appropriate and effective, are behavioural, pharmacological(drugs) or surgical. For some illnesses incarceration or some change in the way society operates is seen as effective.

Fourth, there is often a weak and not always coherent, relationship between perceived cause and the cure of a mental illness. Usually there is a weak positive correlation between psychological causes and cures, though it is recognized that although the cause may be psychological, the effective cure may be drug related. Certainly it does seem that people do not hold very coherent theories for the origin, progression, manifestation and alleviation of mental illnesses.

Fifth, studies that have attempted to identify the demographic and experiential correlates of mental health knowledge or literacy have shown some predictably and explanatory results. Thus, those that are younger, better educated people know more; those with training on psychology/psychiatry know more; and those with personal experience (self/relatives) are better informed. However, the significant effects are very weak.

7. Acknowledgement

We would like to acknowledge the help of Steven Richards for his work on this project.

8. References

Andrews, G., Hall, W., Teesson, M., & Henderson, S. (1999). *The Mental Health of Australians*. Canberra: Commonwealth Department of Health and Aged Care.

Angermeyer, M. C., Daumer, R., & Matschinger, H. (1993). Benefits and risks of psychotropic medication in the eyes of the general public: results of a survey in the Federal Republic of Germany. *Pharmacopsychiatry*, 26, 114–120.

Angermeyer, M.C. & Dietrich, S. (2006). Public beliefs about and attitudes towards people with mental illness: a review of population studies. *Acta Psychiatrica Scandinavica*, 113 (3) 163–179.

Angermeyer, M.C., & Matschinger, H. (1996). Public attitude towards psychiatric treatment. *Acta Psychiatrica Scandinavica*, 94, 326–336.

Angermeyer, M. C., & Matschinger H. (1994). Lay beliefs about schizophrenic disorder: the results of a population survey in Germany. *Acta Psychiatrica Scandinavica*, 89, 39–45.

Benveniste, J., Lecouter, A., & Hepworth, J. (1999). Lay Theories of Anorexia Nervosa: A discourse analytic study. *Journal of Health Psychology*, 4, 59-69.

Budd, R., James, D., & Hughes, I. (2008). Patients' Explanations for Depression: A Factor Analytic Study. *Clinical Psychology and Psychotherapy*, 15, 28-37.

Çirakoğlu, O., Kökdemir, D., & Demirutku, K. (2003). Lay Theories of causes and cures for depression in a turkish university sample. *Social Behaviour and Personality*, 31, 795-806.

Fischer, W., Goerg, D., Zbinden, E., & Guimon, J. (1999). Determining factors and the effects of attitudes towards psychotropic medication. In *The Image of Madness: The Public Facing Mental Illness and Psychiatric Treatment* (eds. J. Guimon, W. Fischer & N. Sartorius), pp. 162-186. Basel: Karger.

Fischer, L.J. & Goldney, R.D. (2003). Differences in community mental health literacy in older and younger Australians. *International Journal of Geriatric Psychiatry*, 18, 33– 40.

Furnham, A. (1984). Lay conceptions of neuroticism. *Personality and Individual Differences*, 5, 95-103.

Furnham, A. (1988). *Lay theories*. Oxford: Pergamon.

Furnham, A. (1995). Lay beliefs about phobia. *Journal of Clinical Psychology*, 51, (4), 518–525.

Furnham, A., (2009). Psychiatric and psychotherapeutic literacy. *International Journal of Social Psychiatry*, 55, 525-537,

Furnham, A. & Bower, P. (1992). A comparison of academic and lay theories of schizophrenia. *British Journal of Psychiatry*, 161, 201–210.

Furnham, A. & Buck, C. (2003). A comparison of lay-beliefs about autism and obsessive-compulsive disorder. *International Journal of Social Psychiatry*, 49, 287–307.

Furnham, A. & Chan, E. (2004). Lay theories of schizophrenia. A cross cultural comparison of British and Hong Kong Chinese attitudes, attributions and beliefs. *Social Psychiatry and Psychiatric Epidemiology*, 39, 543–552.

Furnham, A., & Cheng, H. (2000). Lay Theories of Happiness. *Journal of Happiness Studies*, 1, 227-246.

Furnham, A. & Haraldsen, E. (1998). Lay theories of etiology and "cure" for four types of paraphilia: Fetishism, pedophilia, sexual sadism, and voyeurism. *Journal of Clinical Psychology*, 54, (5), 689-700.

Furnham, A., & Henley, S. (1988). Lay beliefs about overcoming psychological problems. *Journal of Social and Clinical Psychology*, 26, 423–438.

Furnham, A. & Hume-Wright, A. (1992). Lay theories of anorexia nervosa. *Journal of Clinical Psychology*, 48, 20–37.

Furnham, A. & Kuyken, W. (1991). Lay theories of depression. *Journal of Social Behaviour and Personality*, 6, (2), 329–342.

Furnham, A. & Lowick, V. (1984). Lay theories of the causes of alcoholism. *British Journal of Medical Psychology*, 57, 319–322.

Furnham, A. & Manning, R. (1997). Young people's theories of anorexia nervosa and obesity. *Counseling Psychology Quarterly*, 10, (4), 389–415.

Furnham, A., Periera & Rawles, R. (2001) Lay theories of psychotherapy. *Psychology, Health and Medicine, 6,77-84*

Furnham, A., Raja, N., & Khan, U. (2008). A cross-cultural comparison of British and Pakistani medical students' understanding of schizophrenia. *Psychiatry Research*, 159, 308-319.

Furnham, A. & Rees, J. (1988). Lay theories of schizophrenia. *International Journal of Social Psychiatry*, 34, 212–220.

Furnham, A. & Thomson, L. (1996). Lay theories of heroin addiction. *Social Science and Medicine*, 43, 29–40.

Furnham, A., & Wardley, Z. (1990). Lay theories of psychotherapy I. *Journal of Clinical Psychology, 46,* 878-890.

Furnham, A., & Wardley, Z. (1991). Lay theories of psychotherapy II. *Human Relations*, 44, 1197-1211.

Furnham, A., Wardley, Z. & Lillie, F. (1992). Lay theories of psychotherapy III. *Human Relations, 45,* 839-858.

Furnham, A., & Wong, L. (2007). A cross-cultural comparison of British and Chinese beliefs about the causes, behaviour manifestations and treatment of schizophrenia. *Psychiatry Research*, 151, 123-138.

Hasin, D., & Link, B. (1988). Age and recognition of depression: implications for a cohort effect in major depression. *Psychological Medicine, 18,* 683-688.

Heim, D., Smallwood, J., & Davies, J. B. (2005). Variability in lay perceptions of depression: A vignette study. *Psychology and Psychotherapy: Theory, Research and Practice, 78,* 315-325.

Jorm, A., Korten, A., Jacomb, P., Christensen, H., Rodgers, B., & Pollitt, P. (1997a). Public beliefs about causes and risk factors for depression and schizophrenia. *Social Psychiatry and Psychiatric Epidemiology*, 32, 143–148.

Jorm, A., Korten, A., Jacomb, P., Christensen, H., Rodgers, B., & Pollitt, P. (1997b). "Mental health literacy": a survey of the public's ability to recognize mental disorders and their beliefs about the effectiveness of treatment. *Medical Journal of Australia*, 166, 182–186.

Jorm, A., Korten, A., Rodgers, B., Pollitt, H., Christensen, H., & Henderson, A. (1997d). Helpfulness of interventions for mental disorders: beliefs of health professionals compared to the general public. *British Journal of Psychiatry*, 171, 233–237.

Kinnier, R. T., Hofsess, C., Pongratz, R., & Lambert, C. (2009). Attributions and affirmations for overcoming anxiety and depression. *Psychology and Psychotherapy: Theory, Research and Practice, 82*, 153-169.

Knapp, J., & Delprato, D. (1980). Willpower, behavior therapy, and the public. *Psychological Record*, 30, 477–482.

Knight, M., Furnham, A., & Lester, D. (2000). Lay theories of suicide. *Personality and Individual Differences*, 29, 453-457.

Lauber, C., Falcato, L., Nordt, C. & Rossler, W. (2003). Lay beliefs about causes of depression. *Acta Psychiatrica Scandinavica*, 108, (suppl. 418), 96- 99.

Lin, E., Goering, P., Offord, D. R., Campbell, D., & Boyle, M.H. (1996). The use of mental health services in Ontario: epidemiologic findings. *Canadian Journal of Psychiatry*, 41, 572-577.

Link, B.G., Phelan, J.C., Bresnahan, M., Stueve, A., & Pescosolido, B.A. (1999). Public Conceptions of Mental Illness: Labels, Causes, Dangerousness, and Social Distance. *American Journal of Public Health*, 89, 1328-1333.

Matschinger, H., & Angermeyer, M. (1996). Lay beliefs about the causes of mental disorders: a new methodological approach. *Social Psychiatry and Psychiatric Epidemiology*, 31, 309-315.

Nunnally, J. (1961). *Popular Conceptions of Mental Health*. New York: Holt, Rinehart & Winston.

Priest, R. G., Vize, C., Roberts, A., Roberts, M., & Tylee, A. (1996). Lay people's attitudes to treatment of depression: results of opinion poll for Defeat Depression Campaign just before its launch. *British Medical Journal*, 313, 858-859.

Rabkin, J.G. (1974). Public attitudes toward mental illness: A review of the literature. *Psychological Bulletin*, 10, 9-33.

Rippere, V. (1977). Commonsense beliefs about depression and antidepressive behaviour. A study of social consensus. *Behaviour Research and Therapy*, 17, 465-473.

Rippere, V. (1979). Scaling the helpfulness of antidepressive activities. *Behaviour Research and Therapy*, 17, 439-449.

Rippere, V. (1981). How depressing: Another cognitive dimension of commonsense knowledge. *Behaviour Research and Therapy*, 19, 169-181.

Sarbin, T.R., & Mancuso, J.C. (1972). Paradigms and moral judgments: Improper conduct is not disease. *Journal of Consulting and Clinical Psychology*, 13, 6-8.

Shurka, E. (1983). Attitudes of Israeli Arabs towards the mentally ill. *International Journal of Social Psychiatry*, 29, 101-110.

Siegler, M. & Osmond, H. (1966). Models of madness. *British Journal of Psychiatry*, 112, 1193-1203.

Star, S. (1955). The public's ideas about mental illness. Paper presented at: Annual Meeting of the National Association for Mental Health; November 5, Indianapolis, Ind.

Walker, R., Lester, D., & Joe, S. (2006). Lay Theories of Suicide: An Examination of Culturally Relevant Suicide Beliefs and Attributions Among African Americans and European Americans. *Journal of Black Psychology*, 32, 320-334.

Wong, J. (1994) Lay theories of psychotherapy and perceptions of therapists. *Journal of Clinical Psychology*, 50, 624-632.

Yoder, C.Y., Shute, G.E., & Tryban, G.M. (1990). Community recognition of objective and subjective characteristics of depression. *American Journal of Community Psychology*, 18, 547-566.

3

The Psychology of Immigration, Relief or a Burden? Immigrant Need and Use of Psychiatric Care

John E. Berg
Oslo and Akershus University College, Oslo
Norway

1. Introduction

The diversity we meet both in the group of immigrants and in the recipient countries is bewildering. In areas, both in Europe and further away from Europe or North America, the emigration rates were higher from areas where the welfare of the individual's nuclear family was the deciding economic factor[1]. Such a decision was driven by a sense of hopelessness and lack of prospect of a better future. When the family no longer could feed all the members, there was an exodus in great numbers. This inability to concert activities beyond the immediate family may aptly be called amoral familism, which for instance in remote areas of Italy was produced by three factors. They were, acting in combination to achieve such a state: a high death rate, certain land tenure conditions, and the absence of the institution of the extended family. During much of the 19th century almost a million people emigrated from Norway to the US (similar numbers also for Ireland). A Norwegian psychiatrist investigated large groups of these emigrants, and found increased incidence of severe mental illness after some years, thus indicating that the emigration process had its costs [2].

The big colonial powers of the 19th and 20th century had rules giving citizens of the colonies easier access to the mother country. Great numbers of people from Surinam in the Netherlands, Indians in Great Britain and Algerians and people from colonies in Sub Saharan countries in France are examples of a special type of immigration. Psychiatric needs of these immigrants compared to other immigrants have not been studied. Today the big colonial powers have restricted the access of citizens from the colonies.

1.1 Conflicts within emigrating countries are chaperons after immigration

Scandinavians, Germans and Japanese immigrants to the US were mainly rural whereas Irish, Chinese and Italians were urban [3]. Immigrants to Western Europe today are similarly divided, and give rise to different challenges as most are settled in urban areas. This meant and means a change also for the people already present in the host country. During the 1820th immigration of German Ashkenazi Jews to the US changed the situation for the then settled Sephardic Jews. The newly arrived Ashkenazi did not accept the Sephardic synagogues and several new synagogues had to be built. Discrimination in home countries led to emigration, but when immigrated the new group maintained a discriminatory attitude towards others within the same faith. Coping skills including the necessity of discrimination were perpetuated in the new setting. German and Irish Catholics did not immediately commute with the American Catholic communities. Refugees from Viet Nam where divided between those who escaped because they had supported the Americans, and others because they had fought against the government in the south. Several groups of Muslims repeat the divides from their home countries by entering non-cooperating helping facilities representing their Muslim faith. Help with adaptation and your religious or ethnic compatriots may thus not be as straightforward as you would expect after exodus.

1.2 Multiculturalism as a solution?

Multiculturalism is one conceptualisation of society with many diverse ethnic groups. The recipient countries in the Western world differ greatly in this respect. Australia, Canada and the US are countries based on immigration from all over the world, to such an extent that the existing cultural rules are a mixture of all foreign influences. Canada seems to be the country where the immigration process has led to less criminality, less interracial conflicts and a great flexibility in accommodating new entrants. Countries as Finland and Norway are more homogenous societies with little influx of immigrants. They are met by publicly organized affluent facilities catering for housing, language skills and health care, but with a backdrop of xenophobia in the population. The double communication from the host country may be bewildering [4]. Present immigrants are starting to reshape the countries in a more accepting and multi-ethnic direction, although far-right ethnocentric groups exist and grow. Fear of foreigners (xenophobia) is greater in such countries and will drip down on the immigrants as part of their identity adjustment challenges. This is aptly described in immigrant novels covering the apparently contradictory impulses of class, privilege and standing [5].

2. Immigration as relief

Emigration from hardship, poverty and small prospects of change was a relief for groups leaving Europe from Ireland and Norway during the 19th century. Arriving in USA they were investigated thoroughly and only the "fit and able" were accepted. Though starting at bottom level, a majority managed to attain a level of living conditions exceeding the one they left. Emigrating persons from Turkey, South West Asia and India today may be of the same category, whereas immigrants of African or Roma decent have greater hardships after entering countries as Spain, Greece and Italy. Whether the last groups in the end feel that emigrating was a relief has not been studied yet.

2.1 Why do some refugees conquer extreme hardship with intact mental balance?

It is observed that the capacity of humans to adapt to new environments and rules is high. Sufficient clarifications of who will adapt are not given by observable characteristics of the persons as educational level, age and somatic and mental health status. The American sociologist Aaron Antonovsky developed a theory of salutogenesis after encounters with survivors of concentration camps during World War II. His point of departure was the observation that some people seemed to adapt well to life after the traumatising and death threatening experiences, often combined with loss of several members of own family. He wanted to advance the understanding of the relations between life stressors, coping and health[6]. An emphasis on pathogenic (disease giving) factors has been and is still in use to explain lack of health and behaviours in biomedical as well as social science disease research. Antonovsky's salutogenic model looks to find signs of adaptive coping. According to the model this is the secret of movement towards the healthy end of the sick – healthy continuum. People develop resistance resources, and this is a perfect frame to understand the process of the psychology of emigration. The resources were wealth, ego strength, cultural stability and social support [7]. After immigration many people have little wealth, cultural instability and lack the former, natural social support, even if they maintain ego strength. An example is the observation that immigrant minorities in New York in the US have higher cancer rates than the majority population [8]. The authors explain this by stating: "immigrants face cancer care and research access barriers, including economic, immigration status, cultural, and linguistic barriers".

Notwithstanding, some maintain that people emigrating often constitute a resource rich and rather healthy part of the population in the country they left. The poor and feeble do not have the strength or endurance to flee or move. Those who faired well after immigration or great trauma had according to Antonovsky the ability which he called Sense of coherence. The construct encompasses more than concepts as self-efficacy, internal locus of control, problem oriented coping, or the challenge component of hardiness. The sense of coherence concept has been shown to be less bound by particular subcultures, thus useful in an immigration context [7]. When sense of coherence is low, the future risk of morbidity and mortality in drug abusers increase [9] [10]. In order to counter the effect of low sense of coherence in immigrants German researchers advocate the establishment of a complementary system of health care in order to give a sustainable medical care for small migrant groups or not optimally integrated immigrant populations [11].

3. Immigration as a burden

Forced emigration during conflicts, either internally in own country or to a neighbour country is initially a burden. Depending on experiences before an emigration, during the flight and the reception in a new country, disease may develop and the immigration may pose grave problems in accommodating to a new life.

An Australian initiative organised multidisciplinary primary healthcare for newly arrived humanitarian entrants [12]. The clinic achieved to see and investigate the refugees within a median of five days. GPs were present at the clinic, but later transfer of the patients to outside GPs in the community remained problematic.

Goth et al studied whether the engagement of GPs is sufficient. She studied immigrants' use of primary health care in the form of contact with general practitioners or emergency services in two recent papers from Norway [13, 14]. Immigrants to Norway tend to use emergency primary health care services more than the registered GP, despite the fact that every citizen by law has a designated GP. There is lack of relevant information in several languages; immigrants use key informants from their own group to partly overcome this. There is also a reluctance to accept the democratic attitude of Norwegian GPs, who involve the patients in decisions of treatment, and even a lack of confidence in the quality of the doctor if he/she consults handbooks or colleagues. Her most striking finding is, however, that the group of immigrants is very diverse both in health literacy, attitude towards peers and language skills.

3.1 The different generations of immigrants

Several generations of a family may emigrate. Either at one time point, or as a result of family reunion some time after the immigration of a part of the family. There are often strong bonds between the generations and they depend on each other. Eventually the oldest generation needs more support from their children or grandchildren. The meaning of family support among older Chinese and Korean immigrants to Canada has been studied [15]. The authors found that the immigrants above 60 years had the following perspectives on the family life:

1. They had become more peripheral family members
2. Parents were no longer authority figures in the family
3. The older generation was more independent in the sense that they had a changed economic environment, were living alone and had a social network beyond the family

This all promoted a move to biculturalism. A statement of one of the participants underscores this: "I believe we should not depend on them...I suggest we should save enough money for our future when we are young...if you hade better apply for living in senior houses so that the children can drop by when they are free". Such a view is in contrast to what cultural obligations from the emigration country would prescribe. In another small study from Australia aging Chinese immigrants valued financial security and an active lifestyle as the most important aspect of getting old, whereas the Anglo-Australians regarded growing old gracefully and accepting the limitations of life as important aspects of successful aging [16].

Internet-usage of immigrants may enhance the intercultural adaptation when they accommodate to host country sites [17]. Thus it is important to guide immigrants to local sites where knowledge and understanding of the new host country may be established.

Immigrants from certain countries have a low acceptance rate for mental health problems. This is a cultural question, but also a question of possible access to mental health care. Number of psychiatrist per 100,000 inhabitants is for instance around 8 within the European Union, 35 in Norway, but only 0.3 in India. Integration of primary health care and psychiatry for immigrants may improve acceptability to receive mental health guidance and treatment, as shown by Yeung et al. in Boston [18]. They used a specially trained nurse to bridge the patients between primary care and the psychiatric services, thus increasing the number of patients turning up at the mental health clinic after referral.

One expression of felt strain in life may be suicidal ideation. This was studied in adolescents in the Netherlands [19]. Turkish adolescents had higher levels of suicidal ideation than both the majority and other minority group adolescents. Turks and Moroccans enjoyed being at home less than the Dutch. On the other hand, having a good relationship to mother and father had a protective effect against suicidal ideation. Many factors play a role here. The authors also concluded that discussing their problems at home increased suicidal ideation in Turkish adolescents, but had a protective effect in Dutch and Moroccan adolescents. Having a friend was a buffer. Different coping strategies in families may be the important factor, whether or not the family and its surroundings is of native or foreign descent.

4. Understanding illness behaviour in a new culture

Transcultural psychiatry is difficult. Understanding the verbal and social aspects of people in need of psychiatric care demands knowledge of aspects of culture, race, religion and expectations in both the caregivers and the recipients of care, as described in for instance

Fernando "Mental health, race and culture" [20]. The Western European psychiatric tradition in most countries receiving immigrants may be less understanding when exposed to spiritual healing, Chinese medicine and the use of the family group as a treatment arena.

4.1 Case

An Albanian woman from Macedonia was referred to the acute psychiatric facility with a diagnosis of psychosis. She told the doctor on duty that her aunt had put an evil spirit in her body, and she could not get rid of him. The psychiatrist in training categorized her notion of an evil spirit as a sign of a paranoid psychosis. Later it turned out that she only was in severe conflicts with her family members. Treating her with antipsychotic medication only made her very tired, her opinion of evil spirits did not subside.

Immigration is a risk factor for developing mental disorders. This risk can be viewed as a combination of a demographic divergence from the host population, increased psychosocial stress, and environmental factors as housing and cultural difficulties in giving a proper diagnosis to the patient. Torture survivors may be prone to post-traumatic stress disorder. Immigrants from Surinam and Morocco to the Netherlands were shown to have a fourfold relative risk of schizophrenia, purportedly due to the rapid change in lifestyle [21, 22]. On the other hand, immigrants seem to have a lower rate of substance abuse than the host population [23]. This was also corroborated in a cohort study from a Norwegian acute psychiatric facility [24].

4.2 Referrals of migrants to psychiatric acute resident care

Most immigrants, as most other inhabitants are not referred to acute psychiatric care. Acute onset of mental illness may illuminate special problems brought to an extreme level. Some aspects of extreme behaviour would be cultural, socioeconomic or religious in origin. By studying specifically referrals to acute care, many general aspects of differences between immigrants and native populations could be demonstrated. Two papers from Norway are described in the following in some detail.

All patients referred during a year were grouped as immigrants or native Norwegians [24]. There were more men among the immigrants (68.8% versus 43.3%), they were somewhat younger, but more referrals under compulsion (75.5% versus 51.9%) according to the Mental Health Act. Suicide attempts or suicidal ideation were equal between immigrants and native Norwegians. Multiple referrals were not different as shown in the table below.

Referrals in one year	Immigrants (N=80) Patients (% of 80)	Other referrals (N=335) Patients (% of 335)
2	12 (15.0%)	50 (14.9%)
3	4 (5.0%)	14 (4.2%)
4	1 (1.3%)	5 (1.5%)
5	1 (1.3%)	2 (0.6%)
6	0	4 (1.2&)
9	0	1 (0.3%)
Total	18	76

Table 1. Multiple referrals during a year of individual patients to an acute psychiatric facility in Oslo according to ethnicity

The clinicians had an impression that relatively more immigrants were referred. As shown in the table below this was not the case. The rate of referrals from the catchment area, three boroughs in the capital, was 0.0049 for immigrants and 0.0052 for native Norwegians (X2 = 0.1; p = 0.74), i.e. the same fraction of the immigrants and the native population were acutely referred to the hospital.

Borough	3	5	6
	Number (%)	Number (%)	Number (%)
Total population	28678	26857	25682
Non-Western immigrants	1993 (6.9)*	6144 (22.9)*	8038 (31.3)*
Other immigrants	1854 (6.5)	1442 (5.4)	1196 (4.7)

*) The material for the study was from three boroughs, where borough 3 was more affluent, and thus with a lower rate of immigrants.

Table 2. Population in the catchment area for an acute psychiatric facility in Oslo and number of immigrants according to borough

4.3 What may explain these findings?

Slightly more women than men are in general referred to acute psychiatric care and to ambulatory psychiatric treatment in Western societies. How come that more men were referred to the clinic in Oslo? There are several possible explanations to this. More men than women emigrate; men or young boys are the vanguards for later family reunion. Accept or even recognition of mental disorders is less among immigrant groups. Thus men, who are frequently the breadwinner in the family, must conform to the standards of working life in the host country, whereas the women, who stay at home, only are referred to psychiatric treatment when they cannot fulfil their homely tasks. The expression of severe mental illness is non-conform to the host culture, often with gesticulating and noisy or culturally awkward behaviour. That may be the reason for the clinicians' impression of more severe illness among immigrants.

Psychometric tests at entry to an acute facility may improve diagnosis and subsequent treatment [25]. Such tests are seldom employed in Norway, and even less so among immigrant patients, probably due to language barriers and culturally biased tests.

Immigrants have different expectations of the future depending on their status when emigrating; as asylum seeker, refugees or more or less a poverty-driven exodus [26]. A significantly higher proportion of asylum seekers than refugees had nightmares, feelings of guilt and feelings of hopelessness. Similarly asylum seekers had more sleeping problems, nightmares and reduced appetite than immigrants. More asylum seekers than refugees maintained that life would be better over time. Surprisingly, more refugees than asylum seekers indicated problems judging life ten years from now.

Involuntary psychiatric admissions are widespread among patients with an immigrant background, although the exact rules by law are different from country to country [27]. In Norway some 75% of immigrants are referred under compulsion, whereas 50% of ethnic Norwegians. In a three-year follow up of referrals to two psychiatric clinics in two different cities 32% of the immigrants were involuntarily admitted. The characteristics of these admissions were: significantly higher in men than in women, 73% versus 27%. The mean length of stay was shorter for the voluntarily admitted immigrants. Not at all surprising, immigrant patients with psychotic disorder were involuntarily admitted to a greater extent than non-psychotic patients, and even greater than in ethnic Norwegians. Many of the misunderstandings and attitudes interpreted as aggressive or violent behaviour in immigrant patients may decrease if the treatment of the patient both outside the hospital and at referrals gave him a feeling of getting through to staff with his message.

In another study the level of non-Western immigrants' use of acute psychiatric care compared with ethnic Norwegians was studied over an 8-year period [28]. One of the purposes of the study was to test the impression among clinicians in the wards that an increasing number of immigrants were referred for treatment in an acute setting. In table 3 below the total population in the catchment area is shown for each year, and also the proportion of non-Western immigrants calculated in two ways. There were relatively fewer women among the non-Western immigrants compared to the ethnic Norwegians, 6% versus 50%, respectively. The table shows that no increase in the proportion of non-Western immigrants was observed.

	2000	2001	2002	2003	2004	2005	2006	2007
A – Total population	94581	95080	96260	96716	98086	100824	103670	107848
B - Non-Western immigrants	19481	19593	19558	20048	20315	23020	21729	-
B / A %	20.6	20.6	20.3	20.7	20.7	22.8	21.0	
B / (A-B) %	25.9	30.9	25.5	26.1	26.1	29.6	26.5	

B/A shows the proportion of non-Western immigrants as a percentage of the total population
B/A-B shows the proportion of non-Western immigrants as a percentage of the ethnic Norwegian population in the catchment area

Table 3. Total catchment area population and non-Western immigrants as a percentage of the total population and total minus non-Western immigrant population

The number of referrals changed from year to year, as can be seen in table 4 below. 19 patients were referred in year 2000, whereas 40 in 2007, but the increase in proportion was not so impressive as can be seen from the two lowest rows in the table.

	2000	2001	2002	2003	2004	2005	2006	2007
A - Ethnic Norwegian	122	89	107	148	128	193	246	184
B - Non-Western immigrants	19	17	21	25	30	34	41	40
C - Other immigrants	3	8	3	2	6	2	11	14
B / A %	15.6	19.1	19.6	17.0	23.4	17.6	16.7	21.7
B / (A+C) %	15.2	17.5	19.1	16.7	22.4	17.4	16.0	20.2

Table 4. Number of referrals to acute psychiatric care in a sector of Oslo according to status as non-Western or other immigrant

The age of the immigrants was lower in all years, table 5. This is a consequence of the observation that people who emigrate usually are young, and if older people emigrate, then they come with a larger family group.

	2000	2001	2002	2003	2004	2005	2006	2007
Ethnic Norwegian	38.1	36.7	39.4	37.0	39.1	41.1	38.6	43.4
Non-Western immigrant	35.2	32.7	35.2	35.1	30.6	35.6	34.8	36.5

Table 5. Mean age of ethnic Norwegians and non-Western immigrants among patients referred to an acute psychiatric care facility in Oslo

Mean length of stay in the acute department was lower for ethnic Norwegians, indicating that at least no discrimination of immigrants occurred. They all seemingly got a length of stay commensurate with the illness they had at referral. As the fraction of psychotic illnesses among non-Western immigrants was higher, a longer stay may very well be good treatment. If the prevalence of mental disorders is the same or higher in immigrants than in the original population, this study indicates that they are under-represented among referred patients from the catchment area population. This seems to be the case especially for women.

Immigrants may have problems accessing psychotherapeutic treatment in an outpatient setting, as a prerequisite for psychotherapy would be sufficient language skills. It would be expected that immigrants to a greater extent get pharmaco-therapeutic treatment, but this question has not been studied in Norway.

5. Who should or could adapt within a new setting

What do we know about the ability of diverse groups of immigrants to integrate and assimilate a new culture? Is multiculturalism a positive solution or a cul-de-sac?

In a large group of Puerto Rican, Cuban, Mexican and other Latino immigrants to the US a registration of psychiatric disorders during the past year was done by Alegria et al. [29]. When adjusting for age, sex, nativity and age of arrival of immigrants, there were no significant differences between the four Latino groups. On the other hand, family conflict and burden were consistently related to the risk of mood disorders.

Successful adaptation into the US society is a multidimensional process. It includes maintenance of family harmony, integration in advantageous US neighbourhoods, and positive perceptions of social standing.

5.1 Ghettoization

Letting immigrants settle in urban disadvantaged areas, as is often allowed or specifically wished by the immigrants, may contribute to slower integration. Language skills and knowledge of health care systems and rules of everyday life are not learned. You may in many such areas meet immigrants who have spent several years there without being able to communicate in the language of their new home country. Such instances of ghettoization you find with people from many countries, not at all only among disadvantaged groups. Examples are Chinatowns, Italian or Greek district, Jewish or Muslim settlements, or

Moroccan or African dominated areas. Although the integration may be slow, such areas also contribute to a more diversified culture, which is used to a great extent by the native population.

Spreading the newly arrived immigrants to more remote areas, with very few immigrants at each place is done in Norway. The effect is controversial. The small immigrant groups may or may not be readily accepted at the new dwelling, and over time there has been a movement back to urban areas. It is not settled whether the adaptation of immigrants must be any different from the adaptation of young, not well-to-do natives during the first years.

5.2 Case

A Palestinian young man seeks asylum in a European country. His background is education at college level and he was the only family member getting an education above high school. His asylum application was rejected, but he appealed. He had to live in a special camp for asylum seekers as long as the decision was pending. His frustration ended in a referral to an acute psychiatric clinic for purported psychosis and suicidal ideation. Initially his mental status was difficult to evaluate and staff had diverse hunches. After some weeks observations and psychotherapeutic evaluations, including psychometric testing, no severe mental illness or post-traumatic stress reactions could be confirmed. His frustration at the unresolved situation, and the probable expulsion was understandable. Given an asylum, he would most probably find a job and assimilate as an immigrant.

5.3 Is there a healthy migrant effect?

Stafford et al. [30] have studied a purported healthy migrant effect in Canada. Immigrants to Canada report less depression compared to the non-immigrant population. The likelihood of depression decreased with increasing percentage of immigrants in the area for visible minority persons but not for white minority persons. A corollary to this finding would be not to press immigrants to settle in remote areas of the country.

6. Unreturnable asylum seekers

The burdens described above give special problems for asylum seekers who cannot be returned. Either because there is doubts about the identity of the asylum seeker or because returning these people to countries where they could be threatened with life sentences or a death penalty, is not accepted in the country of dwelling. The mental problems they have accrued are perpetuated, as shown for instance by Mueller et.al in European Journal of Public Health 2010; 21: 2. Taking care of unreturnable asylum seekers is an unsolved problem in Europe. Different solutions for other groups of the "sans papier" have been tried out.

6.1 Case

A mullah from Northern Iraq fled to Norway with his family because of threats of persecution, as he had been the leader of an opposition group to the then government in Iraq. If returned to Northern Iraq, where his group had its main action area, he would certainly be detained and probably sentences because of the violent actions of his group. Thus with the civilized rule of not returning people who would get a life or death sentence, he is staying. However, he is continuing his work of splinter group action over the Internet, editing a site the content of which would have been illegal in Iraq. And he is also threatening politicians in his country of residence. This is an example of stalemate immigrant policy.

7. Work as a means of inclusion in the new society

Work and educational experience and level among immigrants are not always appreciated. This has been studied in a large sample (N=2685) from Canada [31]. Four years after they arrived in Canada 52% of the immigrants were judged to be overqualified for their jobs based on their educational levels, with a lesser extent being overqualified based on experience, 44%, or their expectations, 43%. When the authors included job satisfaction and perception of employment situation in their calculations, over-qualification increased mental health problems. Asian Americans report similar results for mental, but not for physical health with a negative relation between increasing employment frustration and self-rated mental health [32]. The mainstay of American immigration policy has been giving or demanding work from the new citizens. This policy has probably increased the speed of adaptation and integration, and at the same time reduced the risk of mental illness. Immigrants from some countries have differing views on what they can do, and some have problems getting their former qualifications accepted, and develop a negative or paranoid attitude to the country of residence. Some cultures do not allow women to take on work, which would be in contrast to the expectations of the host country. On the other hand, when young girls are allowed to take an education, they perform better in schools and universities than their young brothers. Mental illness has a great impact on labour supply [33]. It is an established fact that mental illness negatively influences labour market performance, especially in cases with long-term psychotic and some neurotic diseases. In the study by Ojeda et al. with recent US data, she shows that mental illness is associated with lower rates of work among US-born males but not immigrant males and females. This is contrary to the belief of health and social care workers and researchers alike. Most people with mental illness work, but symptom severity reduces labour supply among natives especially. A more solid family and social network among natives may be the reason why labour supply with mental illness is reduced. Another adaptation is indicated in the next section.

The use of precarious employment in illegal immigrants, which abounds in countries like Spain, Italy and the US, is a greater threat to the workers [34]. Even when they initially do not have mental health problems, many develop this during the time with work where they are grossly exploited. The illegal immigrants to Spain were from Romania, Morocco, Ecuador and Colombia.

7.1 Cases

After the coup against president Allende in 1973, many politically active persons had to flee. A group came to Norway via the help of the Norwegian embassy in Santiago. One year later I saw, as a then high school teacher, three Chileans washing the school windows on long ladders. They had got this job at the public job centre. One was an architect, the other two astrophysicists. More qualified jobs were not attainable at the time.

Immigrants often start their work career with precarious jobs and meagre employment conditions. In a sample of more than 2000 workers a Spanish group observed that immigrant workers in Spain were present at work also when sick, i.e. sickness presenteeism compared to Spanish born workers [35]. Among the immigrant workers men, those with a stay < 2 years, with a university degree and salaries between 750 -1200 € per month had higher rates of sickness presenteeism. The authors conclude that immigrant workers should have the same standards of social security as Spanish born workers. This is not always easy to achieve. Polish construction workers in Norway often work as subcontractor employees with the firm based in Poland. Despite fierce protests from Norwegian trade unions, this way of giving immigrants lower pay is difficult to eradicate. The clandestine workers in Italy and Spain for instance fair even worse on the labour market.

The unemployment rate of immigrants is higher than for native born, as seen in the figure from the Economist. In Spain and Belgium the rate is much higher, whereas in the US it is fairly equal. The situation in the former East-European countries Hungary and Czech Republic is special. They have attracted few low skilled immigrants, and the small group of immigrants are specially invited high-skilled labour. The disadvantage of being immigrant is not very high, judged by the numbers in the figure, thus lending hope for many over time. From the Economist July 16th 2011, page 89

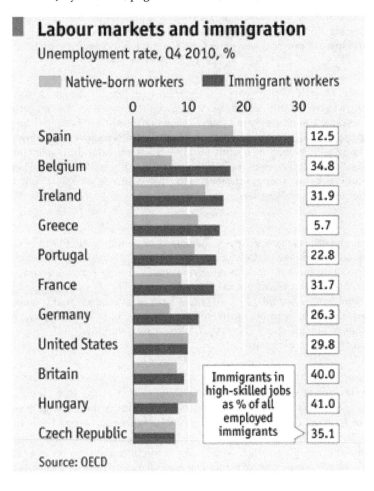

Fig. 1.

8. Adaptation to copious social welfare systems

Some countries in Northern Europe have copious social welfare systems as the result of social democratic achievements in Parliament and Unions over the last hundred years. The basis of these welfare systems has been for instance that sickness leave with up to full pay for up to a year is regarded as a right. It is cumbersome enough to be sick as you still would need your salary for your daily life. Everybody is a member of the public health care and social security system. You get what you need of treatment and contributions as a solidarity action from all. In some countries you would call this socialism. The confirmation of an existing illness is the joint responsibility of the patient and his medical doctor. The rules did not foresee that someone would present a non-existent illness to the doctor, and for the doctors some symptoms are not readily observable. Thus he has to rely on the patient telling the truth.

Some groups of immigrants accept such welfare payments without any of the urge to do your best and not exploit the system, as has been the main axis in the use of the welfare systems in host countries. Especially people coming from countries with an anomic culture, easily accept being financially supported for longer periods of time through public means. The solidarity aspect of public arrangements and entitlements may be forgotten.

8.1 Case
Somali man, age 37, arrived five years ago, married with three children. He has not learned any usable Norwegian, despite compulsory language courses over several hundred hours. Public agencies have subsequently not found any work or other activity for him giving more access to adaptation to the Norwegian society. On the contrary he is according to his family obligations doing well as long as he gets monthly transfers from the social welfare system. He and his family would get even more if he pro forma divorced his wife. Then she would get higher allowances as a single mother. Such behaviour is, however, not found in all Somali or other refugees to Norway.

8.2 Cases
The Norwegian health care system gives allowances to women giving birth every month for each child into to the teenage period. Single mothers also get an allowance for the extra costs of upbringing. There have recently been several cases among people of Roma decent and others presenting birth certificates and other documentation of non-existing children. The rules do not readily disclose this, so allowances have been paid for many years. Such cases are unwanted effects of a public social welfare system built on solidarity and truthful interaction with treatment and welfare staff. These cases amounted to fraud against public sources of more than 1 million euro.

8.3 Addendum
This chapter has not given a clear answer to the question in the title "the psychology of immigration, relief or burden?". Depending on the group of immigrants we look at, the answer may be both yes and no to both the immigration process being a relief and a burden.
- Some leave their home country to save the life of one self and family. Getting accepted in the new country gives relief. After some years, a few return because they miss the good side of their country of birth. The mental health of this group is fairly good, despite symptoms of PTSD in some.

- Some leave because there is no chance of a job or a decent life in the home country. The immediate relief depends on getting a more acceptable life in the host country. Illegal immigrants (sans papier) are an example of people who have to endure further hardship. The mental health of this group is unresolved and some develop more signs of disease than before emigrating.
- Some leave to join the family or to get married (of free will or forced by family). Older immigrants miss the routines and respect of life in birth country. Forced marriage is a route to undiscovered depression and somatoform disease. The old may be, also undiscovered, depressed.

Emigration is a significant step in the life of every person. Many factors must be in place to make good living in the new country. The fact that so few emigrated persons return permanently and that it is doubtful whether emigration in its own right increases the rate of mental illness, we may conclude that emigration is an important, but positive change in life. It is a challenge for the host country to get most out of their immigrant groups. US and Canadian experiences are the good examples, as those countries are built on emigration.

9. References

[1] Banfield, E.C., *The moral basis of a backward society.* 1958.
[2] Oedegaard, O., *The incidence of mental diseases as measured by sensus investigations versus admission statistics.* Psychiatr Q, 1952. 26(2): p. 212-8.
[3] Daniels, R., *Coming to America: a history of immigration and ethnicity in American life.* Book, 2002.
[4] Lagrange, H., *Le Déni des cultures.* Seuil, Paris, 2010: p. 350.
[5] Niyogi, S., *Bengali-American fiction in immigrant identity work.* Cultural Sociology, 2011. 5(2): p. 243-62.
[6] Antonovsky, A., *Unraveling the mystery of health. How people manage stress and stay well.* 1 ed1988, San Fransisco: Jossey-Bass Publishers. 218.
[7] Antonovsky, A., *The structure and properties of the sense of coherence scale.* Soc Sci Med, 1993. 36(6): p. 725-33.
[8] Gany., F.M., S.M. Shah, and J. Changrani, *New York city's immigrant minorities.* Cancer, 2006. 107(8 Suppl): p. 2071-81.
[9] Andersen, S. and J.E. Berg, *The use of a sense of coherence test to predict drop-out and mortality after residential treatment of substance abuse.* Addiction Research & Theory, 2001. 9(3): p. 239-51.
[10] Berg, J.E. and S. Andersen, *Mortality 5 years after detoxification and counselling as indicated by psychometric tests.* Substance Abuse, 2001. 23(1): p. 1-10.
[11] Wolter, H. and S. Stark, *Complementary system of health care in cooperation with migrant communities - requirements for successful integration in health care.* Gesundheitswesen, 2009. 71(6): p. 358-62.
[12] Gould, G., et al., *A multidisciplinary primary healthcare clinic for newly arrived humanitarian entrants in regional NSW: model of service delivery and summary of preliminary findings.* Aust N Z J Public Health, 2010. 34(3): p. 326-9.
[13] Goth, U.S. and J.E. Berg, *Migrant participation in Norwegian health care. A qualitative study using key infromants.* Eur J General Practice, 2010.
[14] Goth, U.S., J.E. Berg, and H. Akman, *The intercultural challenges of general practitioners in Norway with migrant patients.* Int J Migration, Health Social Care, 2010. 6(1): p. 26-32.

[15] Wong, S., G. Yoo, and A. Stewart, *The changing meaning of family support among older Chinese and Korean immigrants.* J Gerontol B Psychol Sci Soc Sci, 2006. 61(1): p. S4-9.

[16] Tan, J., L. Ward, and T. Ziaian, *Experiences of Chinese immigrants and Anglo-Australians ageing in Australia. A cross-cultural perspective on successful ageing.* J Health Psychology, 2010. 15(5): p. 697-706.

[17] Chen, W., *Internet-usage patterns of immigrants in the process of intercultural adaptation.* Cyberpsychol BEhav Soc Netw, 2010. 13(4): p. 387-99.

[18] Yeung, A., et al., *Integrating psychiatry and primary care improves acceptability to mental health services among Chinese Amreicans.* Gen Hosp Psychiatry, 2004. 26: p. 256-60.

[19] van Bergen, D., et al., *Suicidal ideation in thnic minority and majority adolescents in Utrecht, the Netherlands.* Crisis, 2008. 29(4): p. 202-8.

[20] Fernando, S., *Mental health, race and culture.* Book, 1991/2002.

[21] Selten, J. and A. Sijben, *Verontrustende opnamecijfers voor schizofrenie bij migranten uit Suriname, de Nederlands Antillen en Marokko.* Ned Tijdschr Geneeskd, 1994. 138(7): p. 345-50.

[22] Selten, J., et al., *Incidence of psychotic disorders in immigrant groups to The Netherlands.* Br J Psychiatry, 2001. 178: p. 367-72.

[23] Veen, N., et al., *Use of illicit substances in a psychosis incidence cohort: a comparison among different ethnic groups in the Netherlands.* Acta Psychiatr Scand, 2002. 105: p. 440-3.

[24] Berg, J.E. and E. Johnsen, *Innlegges innvandrere oftere enn etniske nordmenn i akuttpsykiatriske avdelinger? (Are non-Western immigrants referred to acute psychiatric care units more often than ethnic Norwegians?)* Tidskr Nor Lægeforen, 2004. 124(5): p. 634-6.

[25] Berg, J.E. and V.C. Iversen, *Use of psychometric tests in an acute psychiatric department according to ethnicity.* J Psychiatric Intensive Care, 2009. 5(2): p. 99-107.

[26] Iversen, V.C., J.E. Berg, and A.E. Vaaler, *Expectations of the future: Immigrant, asylum seeker, or refugee - does it matter?* J Psychiatric Intensive Care, 2010. 6(1): p. 23-30.

[27] Iversen, V.C., et al., *Clinical differences between immigrants voluntarily and involuntarily admitted to acute psychiatric units: a 3-year prospective study.* Journal of Psychiatric and Mental Health Nursing, 2011.

[28] Berg, J.E., *The level of non-Western immigrants' use of acute psychiatric care compared with ethnic Norwegians over an 8-year period.* Nordic J Psychiatry, 2009. 63(3): p. 217-22.

[29] Alegria, M., et al., *Understanding differences in past year psychiatric disorders for Latinos livng in the US.* Soc Sci & Med, 2007. 65: p. 214-30.

[30] Stafford, M., B.K. Newbold, and N.A. Ross, *Psychological distress among immigrants and visible minorities in Canada: a contextual analysis.* Int J Social Psychology, 2011. 57.

[31] Chen, C., P. smith, and C. Mustard, *The prevalence of over-qualification and its association with health status among occupationally active new immigrants to Canada.* Ethnicity & Health, 2010. 15(6): p. 601-19.

[32] de Castro, A., T. Rue, and D. Takeuchi, *Associations of employment frustration with self-rated physical and mental health among Asian American immigrants in the US labor force.* Public Health Nursing, 2010. 27(6): p. 492-503.

[33] Ojeda, V.D., et al., *Mental illness, nativity, gender and labor supply.* Health Economics, 2010. 19: p. 396-421.

[34] Porthé, V., et al., *La precariedad laboral en immigrantes en situación irregular en Espana y su relación con la salud.* Gac Sanit, 2009. 23(Suppl 1): p. 107-14.

[35] Agudelo-Suárez, A., et al., *Sickness presenteeism in Spanish-bron and immigrant workers in Spain.* BMC Public Health, 2010. 10: p. 791.

Epidemiology of Psychological Distress

Aline Drapeau[1,2,3], Alain Marchand[4,5] and Dominic Beaulieu-Prévost[6]
[1]Département de psychiatrie - Université de Montréal
[2]Centre de recherche Fernand-Seguin - Hôpital Louis. H. Lafontaine
[3]Département de médecine sociale et préventive - Université de Montréal
[4]École de relations industrielles - Université de Montréal
[5]Institut de recherche en santé publique - Université de Montréal
[6]Département de sexologie - Université du Québec à Montréal
Canada

1. Introduction

Psychological distress is widely used as an indicator of the mental health of the population in public health, in population surveys and in epidemiological studies and, as an outcome, in clinical trials and intervention studies. Yet the concept of psychological distress is still vague for some. Indeed, a closer look at the scientific literature shows that the expression "psychological distress" is often applied to the undifferentiated combinations of symptoms ranging from depression and general anxiety symptoms to personality traits, functional disabilities and behavioural problems. The aim of this chapter is to provide a critical review of the clinical features, assessment and prevalence of psychological distress and of the empirical evidence on the risk and protective factors associated with psychological distress in the general population and in two specific populations. Workers and immigrants deserve special attention since they are exposed to specific risk and protective factors that may modify the impact of more general factors. This chapter will underline several issues that are central to a better understanding of the epidemiology of psychological distress and that need to be addressed in future research.

2. Clinical features of psychological distress

Psychological distress is largely defined as a state of emotional suffering characterized by symptoms of depression (e.g., lost interest; sadness; hopelessness) and anxiety (e.g., restlessness; feeling tense) (Mirowsky and Ross 2002). These symptoms may be tied in with somatic symptoms (e.g., insomnia; headaches; lack of energy) that are likely to vary across cultures (Kleinman 1991, Kirmayer 1989). Additional criteria have been used in the definition of psychological distress but these criteria do not make consensus. In particular, tenants of the stress-distress model posit that the defining features of psychological distress are the exposure to a stressful event that threatens the physical or mental health, the inability to cope effectively with this stressor and the emotional turmoil that results from this ineffective coping (Horwitz 2007, Ridner 2004). They argue that psychological distress vanishes when the stressor disappears or when an individual comes to cope effectively with this stressor (Ridner 2004). There is plenty of evidence confirming the effect of stress on distress, however, including stress in the definition of distress fails to recognise the presence of distress in the absence of stress.

The status of psychological distress in the psychiatric nosology is ambiguous and has been debated at length in the scientific literature. On the one hand, psychological distress is viewed as an emotional disturbance that may impact on the social functioning and day-to-day living of individuals (Wheaton 2007). As such, it has been the object of numerous studies seeking to identify the risk and protective factors associated with it. On the other hand, distress is a diagnostic criterion for some psychiatric disorders (e.g., obsessive-compulsive disorders; post-traumatic stress disorder) and, together with impairment in daily living, a marker of the severity of symptoms in other disorders (e.g., major depression; generalized anxiety disorder) (Phillips 2009, Watson 2009). Thus, psychological distress would be a medical concern mostly when it is accompanied by other symptoms that, when added up, satisfy the diagnostic criteria for a psychiatric disorder. Otherwise, in line with the stress-distress model, it is viewed as a transient phenomenon consistent with a "normal" emotional reaction to a stressor. Horwitz (Horwitz 2007) illustrates this point by quoting a series of studies conducted among adolescents and showing the high fluctuation of depressive symptoms over intervals as short as one month. He argues that this fluctuation reflects the relatively brief sorrow that follows from failing a test, loosing a sporting match or breaking up with a boyfriend or girlfriend. The transient nature of psychological distress has been disputed by Wheaton and his colleagues (Wheaton 2007) who have investigated the stability of psychological distress among adults based on seven longitudinal studies lasting from 1 to 10 years. They found that psychological distress was moderately stable and argued that this finding runs counter to the assertion that distress is a transient phenomenon. However, they could not account for the role of personality in this relative stability of psychological distress over time. In effect, neuroticism has been shown to be associated with psychological distress and some argue that it may partly account for chronic distress (Jorm and Duncan-Jones 1990).

Psychological distress is usually described as a non-specific mental health problem (Dohrenwend and Dohrenwend 1982). Yet, according to Wheaton (Wheaton 2007), this lack of specificity should be qualified since psychological distress is clearly characterized by depression and anxiety symptoms. In effect, the scales used to assess psychological distress, depression disorders and general anxiety disorder have several items in common. Thus, although psychological distress and these psychiatric disorders are distinct phenomena, they are not entirely independent of each other (Payton 2009). The relationship between distress and depression - and to a lesser extent, anxiety - raises the issue of whether psychological distress lays in the pathway to depression if left untreated (Horwitz 2007). Unfortunately, the course of psychological distress is largely unknown.

Finally, defining psychological distress as a normal emotional reaction to a stressor raises the issue of delineating "normality" in different populations and different situations. Indeed, it is widely agreed that the individual and collective experience of disease is partly bounded by cultural norms and that although negative states of mind such as feeling sad, depressed or anxious tend to be universal, the expression of these states of mind may vary in intensity and in form across and within societies (Kirmayer 1989, Kleinman 1991, Westermeyer and Janca 1997). This transcultural variation is especially noteworthy in somatic symptoms. According to Kirmayer et al. (Kirmayer 1989), "somatic symptoms provide the most common expression of psychological distress worldwide" but the type of somatic symptoms associated with distress may differ across cultures. For example, among Chinese, emotions are related to specific organs and can cause physical damage to these organs: anger is associated with the liver, worry with the lungs and fear with the kidneys (Leung 1998). Haitians tend to view depression as a consequence of either a medical condition - usually anaemia or malnutrition - or worry. Thus, somatisation is related to mood disorder and it is expressed by feeling empty or heavy-headed, insomnia, fatigue or low energy, and poor appetite (Desrosiers and St Fleurose 2002). Similarly, in Arab culture, depression and somatisation are closely intertwined and depressive symptoms are expressed in physical terms, especially involving the chest and abdomen (Al-Krenawi and Graham 2000). Given the transcultural variation in the expression of distress, the transcultural validity of the scales used to assess psychological distress has been questioned. This point will be illustrated in the next section.

3. Assessment of psychological distress

Psychological distress is assessed with standardized scales that are either self-administered or administered by a research interviewer or a clinician. In principle, the development of a scale must be based on a comprehensive definition of the construct to be measured. As mentioned earlier, a major problem with the construct of psychological distress is its diversified meaning in the scientific literature. Indeed, several scales comprising a wide array of psychological, somatic and behavioral symptoms were developed without clear conceptual basis and are used to assess "psychological distress". In this chapter, the most widely accepted definition of psychological distress (i.e., "a state of emotional suffering characterized by symptoms of depression and anxiety") was adopted. In consequence, scales designed to measure an unspecified construct or a related construct such as depression or anxiety will not be discussed.

The development of a scale is a lengthy process. In short, it consists in four main steps. First, a set of items is selected from existing scales or formulated based on the definition of the construct under study and on the conceptual framework sustaining this construct in the targeted population. For instance, the assessment of the quality of life in adolescents and in seniors would require different conceptual frameworks because the main components of the quality of life in these two age groups differ considerably. Second, from the initial pool of items, a smaller set is identified based on the pattern of endorsement of these items in a representative sample of the targeted population. Third, this smaller set of items is submitted to several statistical analyses (e.g., factorial analysis; sensitivity and specificity analyses; receiver operating curve – ROC – analysis; test-retest analysis) to verify the validity and reliability of the scale. Fourth, a final version of the scale is constructed based on findings from the validation analyses. This process seems linear but, in effect, disappointing results at one step may require going back to preceding steps.

Two important issues must be stressed regarding the assessment of psychological distress. The first issue is the length of the time window used for the detection of distress symptoms. This time window ranges from the past 7 days to the past 30 days depending on the scale. The second issue is the cut-point used to discriminate individuals with a lower vs. higher level of distress. In most studies, psychological distress is analyzed as a continuous variable. However, the individual scores must be dichotomized to estimate the prevalence of distress and dichotomous scores are sometimes used as a solution to the notably asymmetrical distribution of the scores of psychological distress. Clearly, the length of the time window and the selection of the cut-point impact on the estimation of the prevalence of psychological distress and may also affect the identification of the less influential risk and protective factors. In principle, the length of the time window and the cut-point are set in the course of the development of the scale. Now and then, different time windows and cut-points are applied for a specific scale. In particular, the modification of a cut-point may be legitimate when it is demonstrated that the initial cut-point lacks validity for the population under study.

Several scales satisfy the definition of psychological distress adopted here. A full description of these scales and of their psychometric characteristics is out of the scope of this chapter. Therefore, only the most validated and popular instruments will be discussed to give an overview of the way psychological distress is generally assessed. Three families of scales were chosen for discussion: (a) the General Health Questionnaire; (b) the Kessler scales; and (c) the scales derived from the Hopkins Symptom Checklist. These scales share several items in common.

3.1 The General Health Questionnaire (GHQ)

The GHQ was designed to assess psychological distress in population surveys and epidemiological studies, and to screen for non-psychotic mental disorders in clinical settings (Goldberg and Williams 1991). It initially contained 60 items describing depression, anxiety and somatic symptoms and social impairment. The GHQ now exists in four additional versions that differ by the number of items (12, 20, 28 and 30). The GHQ-28 is frequently used in clinical studies, whereas the GHQ-12 is the most popular version in epidemiological studies and population surveys. The GHQ-12 includes the following items: able to concentrate; lost sleep over worry; playing a useful part in society; capable of making decisions; constantly under strain; couldn't overcome difficulties; enjoy normal activities; face up to problems; unhappy and depressed; losing confidence in yourself; thinking of yourself as worthless; feeling reasonably happy. The inclusion of social impairment symptoms, especially in the longer versions, seems in contradiction with the prevalent definition of psychological distress. However, due to its widespread use and recognition as an indicator of distress, the GHQ is often considered as the Gold standard for the measurement of psychological distress (Furukawa et al. 2003).

The items use a 4-point severity/frequency scale (0-3) to rate the extent to which respondents have experienced each symptom over the past two weeks; the expressions "recently" and "during the last few weeks" are occasionally used instead of the two weeks reference period. The items scores can be added to create a total score of distress. An alternative scoring system uses a dichotomous scale (0-0-1-1) instead of the 4-point scale. The GHQ scales have been validated with clinical (Segopolo et al. 2009) and non-clinical samples (Nerdrum, Rustøen, and Rønnestad 2006). Validated versions of the GHQ exist in more than 40 languages (McDowell 2006) and the cross-cultural validity of these scales was established in some countries (Furukawa and Goldberg 1999, Goldberg, Oldehinkel, and Ormel 1998). The GHQ-12 was shown to be measurement invariant (i.e., to measure the same construct) across gender (Shevlin and Adamson 2005) and between adults and adolescents (French and Tait 2004). However, there is some evidence that, as a screening instrument, the GHQ-12 tends to underestimate the prevalence of affective disorders in women and overestimates it in men (Cleary, Bush, and Kessler 1987). Martin et al. (Martin and Newell 2005) and Shevlin et al. (Shevlin and Adamson 2005) have questioned the uni-dimensionality of the GHQ following factorial analyses indicating that the GHQ-12 has at least two dimensions. This multidimensionality would cast doubt on the use of the total score of the GHQ-12 as a unidimensional index of psychological distress. However, a recent study based on confirmatory factor analysis suggests that the GHQ-12 is unidimensional and that the appearance of multidimensionality is due to a methodological artefact, i.e., a substantial degree of response bias for the negatively phrased items (Hankins 2008).

3.2 The Kessler scales
One of the most recent scale of psychological distress is the K10 (Kessler et al. 2002), a 10-item unidimensional scale specifically designed to assess psychological distress in population surveys. The K10 was designed with item response theory models to optimize its precision and sensitivity in the clinical range of distress, and to insure a consistent sensitivity across gender and age groups (Kessler et al. 2002). The scale evaluates how often respondents experienced anxio-depressive symptoms (e.g., nervousness, sadness, restlessness, hopelessness, worthlessness) over the last 30 days. Each item is scaled from 0 (none of the time) to 4 (all of the time) and the total score is used as an index of psychological distress. A 6-item version, called the K6, is also available. Since the K6 perform as well as the K10, Kessler et al. (Kessler et al. 2010) recommends the use of this shorter version.
Several studies showed no substantial bias for the K10 in relation to gender, education (Baillie 2005) or age (OConnor and Parslow 2010). The K6 also achieves an adequate level of measurement invariance across gender and age groups and over a 12-year period (Drapeau et al. 2010). The K6 was validated with teens (Green et al. 2010). The two Kessler scales were shown to outperform the GHQ-12 in detecting depressive and anxiety disorders in terms of overall ROC curve performance (95%CI of AUC being 0.89 to 0.91 for K10, 0.88 to 0.90 for the K6, and 0.78 to 0.82 for the GHQ) (Furukawa et al. 2003). In terms of dimensionality, most studies confirm the single-factor structure of the Kessler scales. Two studies provide some evidence for a two-factor structure for the K6 or a three- to four-factor structure for the K10 (Arnaud et al. 2010, Brooks, Beard, and Steel 2006). However, the very strong correlations between the factors in these studies still suggested considerable commonality between them. The inclusion of the K6 in the World Health Organization World Mental Health Survey Initiative has foster the translation and validation of this scale in 13 countries from the five continents (Furukawa et al. 2008, Kessler and Üstün 2008, Kessler et al. 2010). Additional validation studies have been conducted in Italy (Carra et al. 2011), Netherlands (Donker et al. 2010, Fassaert et al. 2009) and with Native Americans (Mitchell and Beals 2011). No substantial cultural bias has been identified so far.

3.3 The Symptom checklists
The Brief Symptom Inventory (BSI) (Derogatis and Melisaratos 1983, Derogatis 1993), the SCL-25 (Derogatis et al. 1974), the SCL-5 (Tambs and Moum 1993) and the more recent Brief Symptom Inventory-18 (Derogatis 2001) were all derived from the Hopkins Symptoms Checklist-58 items (HSCL-58) (Derogatis et al. 1974). The HSCL-58 contains a large array of symptoms but the BSI, the SCL-25 and the SCL-5 focus on anxio-depressive symptoms and somatic symptoms. The BSI contains 18 items that are rated on a 5-point scale (0 to 4). The scale focuses on the symptoms experienced during the last 7 days. The theoretical 3-factor structure of the BSI-18 is occasionally supported, but 1-factor and 4-factor structures have also been identified (Andreu et al. 2008, Prelow et al. 2005). The lack of stability of the factorial structure is problematic since it suggests problems of measurement invariance.

Effectively, studies of the BSI-18 conducted in the USA suggest that its factorial structure is different for Hispanic women vs. Afro-American or Caucasian women (Wiesner et al. 2010, Prelow et al. 2005). More specifically, the BSI-18 seems to have a 3-factor structure for Afro-American and Caucasian women and a 1-factor structure for Hispanic women. The official version of the BSI-18 exists only in English and few translations have been validated up to now.

The SCL-25 focuses on the symptoms experienced during the last 14 days and it is often used in studies conducted among immigrants (Hoffmann et al. 2006, Mollica et al. 1987, Rousseau and Drapeau 2004, Thapa and Hauff 2005). Many translations have been made and some have been validated (Strand et al.). The SCL-5 includes two anxiety items and three depression items. The correlation with the SCL-25 is quite high (r=0.92) and the performance of the SCL-5 to identify cases of serious mental disorder (in terms of sensitivity, specificity, predictive values and ROC curves) is almost as good as the that of the SCL-25 (Strand et al. 2003, Tambs and Moum 1993).

4. Prevalence of psychological distress

The prevalence of psychological distress is difficult to pinpoint due to the variety of the scales assessing distress, of the time windows used in the documentation of symptoms and of the cut-points applied to dichotomize the score of distress and identify individuals with pathological distress. It roughly ranges between 5% and 27% in the general population (Benzeval and Judge 2001, Chittleborough et al. 2011, Gispert et al. 2003, Kuriyama et al. 2009, Phongsavan et al. 2006) but it can reach higher levels in some segments of the population exposed to specific risk factors such as workers facing stressful work conditions and immigrants who must adapt to the host country while holding family responsibilities in the homeland. The International Labour Office stated that psychological distress affected between 15 and 20% of workers in Europe and North America (International Labour Office 2000) and one out of five workers may experience repeated episodes of psychological distress (Marchand, Demers, and Durand 2005a). The rate of the prevalence of psychological distress observed among immigrants ranges from 13% to 39% (Levecque, Lodewyckx, and Bracke 2009, Ritsner, Ponizovsky, and Ginath 1999, Sundquist et al. 2000).

Two characteristics of the prevalence of psychological distress are noteworthy: the widespread gender difference and the variation over the lifespan. The prevalence of psychological distress is higher in women than in men in most countries (Caron and Liu 2011, Jorm et al. 2005, Phongsavan et al. 2006) and in all age groups (Cairney and Krause 2005, Darcy and Siddique 1984, Myklestad, Roysamb, and Tambs 2011, Paul, Ayis, and Ebrahim 2006, Storksen et al. 2006, Walters, McDonough, and Strohschein 2002). Yet this gender difference is not universal. For instance, no gender difference was observed in Mexican Americans (Aranda et al. 2001), in African, Asian, Central American and South American immigrants in Norway (Thapa and Hauff 2005), in rural Australians (Kilkkinen et al. 2007) and in older Chinese (Chou 2007). The widespread gender difference points to three alternative hypotheses. The first hypothesis is that psychological distress may be partly attributable to gender-related personality traits or biological components, such as those found in depression and anxiety disorders (Parker and Hadzi-Pavlovic 2004). The second hypothesis is that, in most societies, women are more exposed or more vulnerable to the socio-cultural risk factors associated with psychological distress (Cleary and Mechanic 1983, Gove, Hughes, and Style 1983). Attempts to verify this hypothesis have produced mixed findings. Women seem more responsive to stress emanating from their social network (Kessler and McLeod 1984) or their parental role (Umberson et al. 1996) and they tend to be more exposed to marital stress (Aranda et al. 2001, McDonough and Walters 2001), domestic stress (Evans and Steptoe 2002) and parental stress (McDonough and Walters 2001, Umberson et al. 1996). However, women and men tend to experience an equal level of distress when faced with the similar stress (Ensminger and Celentano 1990, Walters, McDonough, and Strohschein 2002). Ensminger et al. (Ensminger and Celentano 1990) found intriguing pattern of gender differences in distress regarding parental status. This gender difference was observed in single parents but not in individuals heading two-parent households. Ensminger et al. (Ensminger and Celentano 1990) conclude that gender difference in psychological distress is most likely related to role configuration rather than to intrinsic gender differences. Finally, the third hypothesis is that, in most cultures, the expression of emotions differs across gender. Some items of the scales used to assess psychological are indeed more frequently endorsed by women than by men but this difference in items functioning does not appear to account completely for the gender difference in psychological distress (Drapeau et al. 2010, Leach, Christensen, and Mackinnon 2008).

In general, the prevalence of psychological distress tends to decrease over the lifespan starting from late adolescence (Caron and Liu 2011, Gispert et al. 2003, Phongsavan et al. 2006, Walters, McDonough, and Strohschein 2002). The decreasing trend is more or less apparent depending on the age range covered by the studies and it is usually attributed to differential exposure to risk factors and to survival bias. There is some indication that the prevalence of psychological distress might follow a U-shaped distribution although the location of the peaks of this distribution is unclear. Schieman (Schieman, Van Gundy, and Taylor 2001) found that the prevalence of psychological distress peaks at 18-29 years old and 80-89 years old whereas Pevalin (Pevalin 2000) noted a curve rising up to middle age, declining to about 60 and rising again in both gender. Focusing on seniors, Paul et al. (Paul, Ayis, and Ebrahim 2006) and Cairney and Krause (Cairney and Krause 2005) noted an increase of the prevalence of psychological distress after 65 years old. Jorm (Jorm 2000) reviewed eight studies dealing with the distribution of distress over the lifespan and concluded that the evidence was inconsistent. He attributes this inconsistency to possible age biases in the measurement of distress, to the effect of neuroticism which tends to decrease with age, and to confounding by cohort effect.

5. Epidemiology of psychological distress

Empirical evidence on the epidemiology of psychological distress mostly rests on cross-sectional data collected in large scale population surveys and in studies focusing on specific segments of the population defined by age, gender, ethnicity or social roles. Longitudinal data are scarce. In principle, longitudinal data are especially useful to clarify the time sequence between psychological distress and putative risk and protective factors, and the combined evolution of these factors and distress over time. However, their usefulness decreases as the time interval between waves of data collection increases.

The objectives of a number of studies published in the scientific literature are essentially descriptive. These studies provide data on the distribution of psychological distress across socio-demographic categories of people and allow for the identification of groups at higher risk of distress. Other studies aims to verify hypotheses derived from theoretical frameworks. These studies serve to better understand the mechanisms underlying the relationships between psychological distress and various factors. These theoretical frameworks typically stem from the stress-distress model and the role-identity model, which are complementary to a large extent. Stressors that occur outside of the context of specific roles (e.g., chronic health problems) are felt to impact on the psychological well-being only if they disrupt social roles. These point-of-views do not take into account the enduring stress related to disadvantaged life conditions such as poverty.

Pearlin (Pearlin 1989) posits that the stress process is embedded in three levels of social structure: social stratification (i.e., gender, age, socio-economic class, ethnicity), social institutions providing roles and statuses, and interpersonal relationships. Social structures determine the expression of distress, the exposure to specific stressors and the strategies used to cope with this stress. According to Pearlin, social roles entail five categories of strains: role overload (i.e., ineffective coping capacity vis-à-vis the demands inherent to a role); interpersonal conflicts within role sets (e.g., husband-wife); inter-role conflict (e.g., wife-mother-worker); role captivity (i.e., filling an unwanted role); and role restructuring within a role set (Pearlin 1989). According to Thoits, the saliency of specific social roles is central to the relationship between stress and distress in that stressful events or situations that threatens the role-identities most valued by an individual are more likely to impair his or her mental health (Thoits 1991). In her view, individuals who hold social roles and who perform adequately in those roles develop role-identities that contribute to their self-esteem by reinforcing their sense of who they are and of what is expected of them and by enhancing their sense of meaning and purpose in life. Thus the lack of social roles is a risk factor for psychological distress because it deprives individuals of a social identity. The role-identities theory has two main corollaries. First, the cultural value of specific social roles may vary across and within societies. Thoits (Thoits 1991) argues that, for instance in Western societies, the role of mother tends to be more salient than the role of father. Second, the accumulation of social roles should be protective since if one role fails to foster the self-esteem and the sense of meaning and purpose in individuals, the others can take over. Two hypotheses have been raised to explain why exposure to stress and coping strategies are likely to vary across the lifespan (Folkman et al. 1987). The developmental hypothesis contends that there are inherent changes in the ways people cope as they aged. The contextual hypothesis stipulates that age differences in coping are the result of changes in what people must cope with as they age.

A large number of risk and protective factors have been investigated in relation to psychological distress but the empirical evidence regarding the epidemiology of psychological distress ranges from convincing, to conflicting and questionable. The discrepancies between findings from different studies can sometimes be attributed to variation in the design of the studies (e.g., sample size; selection criteria; mode of data collection; assessment of psychological distress; type and measurements of other variables; statistical analysis). However, they may also reflect true epidemiological differences between groups or countries. Indeed, most studies have been carried out in Western countries and findings from these studies may not be readily generalized to countries with a different socio-cultural ideology or lower standards of living. The discrepancies between studies may also be attributable to selection and information biases. Selection biases may occur when non participation in a study and attrition are not random with regard to a factor related to the rationale underlying the study, for instance when highly distressed individuals are more likely to refuse to take part in a study or to drop out of a longitudinal study. Information biases may arise when some categories of respondents fail to report their distress symptoms, maybe to comply with what they feel is socially desirable, and when the scale used to assess psychological distress lacks validity for the groups under study.

In this section, data on the epidemiology of psychological distress is presented in three parts. The first part reviews the empirical evidence pertaining to the general population, stressing - whenever possible - gender and age differences. The effect of some factors (e.g., poverty; social isolation; childhood trauma) is so powerful that it is felt over the lifespan. Other factors tend to have a more short-term effect or their effect varies considerably across life-stages. The second and third parts summarize findings pertaining respectively to workers and to immigrants.

5.1 In the general population

To summarize the empirical evidence on the epidemiology of psychological distress in the general population, risk and protective factor are split in three categories: (1) socio-demographic factors; (2) stress-related factors; and (4) personal resources. The *socio-demographic* factors regroups the characteristics of individuals that are inborn (e.g., gender; age; ethnicity) or that reflect the role of individuals in the social structure. These factors are the most common indicators of the populations at risk of psychological distress that could be targeted for prevention or intervention programs. The *stress* category covers the events and life conditions that exert a stress on the psychological well-being of individuals. The *social resources* category encompasses the resources that are available to individuals to prevent the occurrence of psychological distress. These three types of factors may be complementary. For instance, poverty is viewed as a stressful life condition whereas income is viewed as a personal resource.

Some factors are not considered in this summary of the epidemiology of distress either because the evidence is lacking or because they are usually interpreted in terms of social and economic factors that can be assessed more directly. Health behaviour such as smoking and alcohol intake are associated with increased odds and mean level of distress (Chittleborough et al. 2011, Kuriyama et al. 2009, , Myklestad, 2011 #718; Phongsavan et al. 2006) but the interpretation of this association is awkward. Smoking and alcohol may be a form of self-medication to dilute the burden of distress but they may also generate some distress. Few studies have explored the role of residential environment, which is usually described by opposing urban and rural areas. Findings are inconclusive and the rural-urban distinction is generally used as a proxy for economic disadvantage and for barriers to access to resources (Caron and Liu 2011, Myer et al. 2008).

5.1.1 Socio-demographic factors

A part from gender and age, which were discuss in the section on prevalence, ethnicity and social roles, especially the roles of worker and spouse are the main socio-demographic factors associated with variations in psychological distress. Ethnicity is viewed as a proxy for the cultural background of individuals. As a cultural marker, it is meant to account – albeit imperfectly - for the cultural norms, values and beliefs that influence the behaviour and attitude of people belonging to a specific ethnic group or country. Ethnicity may also signal membership in a minority that is stigmatized. The impacts of this ethnic stigmatisation include a loss of self-esteem and a lower access to the social resources that contribute to the health and psychological well-being of individuals, such as adequate housing, income and employment. Discrimination has been shown to be a risk factor for psychological distress in several studies (Gonzalez-Castro and Ubillos 2011, Yip, Gee, and Takeuchi 2008). Findings from the study carried by Thapa and Hauff (Thapa and Hauff 2005) suggest that women and men may react differently to specific manifestations of discrimination: the mean level of distress was higher in men who were denied a job whereas it was higher in women who were denied housing. Thus it is not ethnicity per se that constitutes a risk factor but instead the socio-economic implications of membership in an ethnic minority.

The empirical evidence regarding ethnicity is conflicting. These conflicting findings may result from the way ethnicity and psychological distress are measured and analysed. For instance, two studies carried out in Australia have produced opposite results although both studies used the K10 to assess psychological distress among adults and applied a similar cut-point (i.e., ≥ 22). However, the measurement of ethnicity was different. Chittleborough et al. (Chittleborough et al. 2011) found that the odds of distress was higher in immigrants than in born Australians with the exception of immigrants from the United Kingdom (UK) whereas Phongsavan et al. (Phongsavan et al. 2006) found no significant difference between English speakers and non English speakers. Odds ratios were not altered by the addition of other variables in the studies. In all likelihood, English speakers would roughly equate with born Australians and immigrants from the UK whereas non English speakers would coincide with other immigrants. The measurement of membership into an ethnic minority through country of birth, self-reported ethnicity and language spoken at home may fail to capture the rationale underlying the concept of ethnic minority. Alternatively, members of some ethnic minorities may be more resilient than what is usually assumed. The transcultural validity of standardized scales has been questioned repeatedly but, as discussed previously, the most popular scales used to assess psychological distress (e.g., GHQ and K6 or K10) have shown their construct validity across various ethnic groups.

Bratter and Eschbach (Bratter and Eschbach 2005) have used data from the National Health Interview Survey conducted in the United States of America (USA) to investigate the association between ethnicity and psychological distress. The large sample size (n = 162 032) recruited over the five cross-sectional annual waves (from 1997 to 2001) of the survey allowed them to stratify respondents in 10 self-reported "race/ethnic" groups. Only two ethnic minorities (Native Americans and Puerto Ricans) reported a higher mean level of psychological distress than "Whites". In the other minorities, the mean level was either lower than (Asian and Mexican) or similar to (African Americans, Cubans and other Hispanics) that of the mainstream population. The lack of statistically significant difference between Black and White Americans has been confirmed in other studies (Nemeroff, Midlarsky, and Meyer 2010). According to Bratter and Eschbach (Bratter and Eschbach 2005), these findings question the conceptual distinction between ethnic minorities and majorities in mental health studies and the assumption that membership in an ethnic minority is a risk marker for mental illness. They argue that although disadvantaged ethnic groups may be more exposed to the risk factors associated with psychological distress, they are not necessarily more vulnerable. In effect, individuals may belong to the ethnic majority and still be stigmatised because of their ethnic background (e.g., Black majority in South Africa; Myer et al. 2008).

Overall, the role of worker (Gispert et al. 2003, Phongsavan et al. 2006, Schieman, Van Gundy, and Taylor 2001, Walters, McDonough, and Strohschein 2002) act as a protective factor against psychological distress. According to Warr and Jackson (Warr and Jackson

1987), the role of worker fosters the psychological well-being not only because it is a valued social role but also because working provides financial resources and opportunities for control, skill use, socialisation and externally generated goals. Unemployed are viewed as a group at risk of psychological distress because they do not have access to these benefits although some work-related advantages (e.g., skill utilisation; socialisation) may be obtained outside the work environment. McKee-Ryan et al. (McKee-Ryan et al. 2005) carried out a meta-analysis to test the hypothesized influence of unemployment on psychological well-being. Psychological distress was one of the measures of mental illness used in the 52 selected studies. This meta-analysis confirmed that, in general, unemployment is a risk factor for mental illness though the detrimental effect of unemployment varies across categories of unemployed. Indeed, the motive for unemployment must be taken into account. Jorm et al., (Jorm et al. 2005) and Lincoln et al. (Lincoln et al. 2011) have found no overall significant difference in distress between unemployed and employed but a higher mean level of distress in individuals out of the labour market compared to employed individuals. Findings from the study conducted by Marchand et al. (Marchand, Drapeau, and Beaulieu-Prévost 2011) show that individuals unemployed because of family responsibilities report a mean level of distress similar to workers and lower than those without a job due to permanent or temporary disabilities and job seekers. In general, living with a spouse is also associated with a lower level of psychological distress (Caron and Liu 2011, Jorm et al. 2005) except perhaps in seniors (Cairney and Krause 2005, Paul, Ayis, and Ebrahim 2006, Préville et al. 2002). However, although individuals who are divorced, separated or widowed tend to report a higher mean level of distress than those who are married, the mean level of distress is similar in never married and married (Walters, McDonough, and Strohschein 2002). At first glance, the lack of difference in married vs. singles may seem in contradiction with the finding that people living alone tend to report a higher mean level of psychological distress than those living with others (Paul, Ayis, and Ebrahim 2006, Phongsavan et al. 2006); but singles may live with friends and family. Finally, the influence of the role of parent on psychological distress is more controversial partly because the assessment of the parental role is intricate. For example, the number of children seems to act as a protective factor for the mental health of men but not of women (Jorm et al. 2005) whereas the age of the youngest child does not appear to affect psychological distress (Walters, McDonough, and Strohschein 2002).

5.1.2 Stress- related factors

In general, the empirical evidence supports the hypotheses derived from the stress-distress model: exposure to stressful events or life conditions tends to vary across social groups and the impact of the exposure to specific stressors on mental health is more or less severe depending on the resources available to cope with this stress among people belonging to these groups. Some studies focus on specific stresses consistent with the role-identify theory (e.g., life transition such as job loss, marital breakdown; family and work-related conflict) whereas others cover a wide range of stressors. In addition, most studies have targeted a specific age group such as adolescent, young adults, working age adults and seniors since, in agreement with the stress-distress model, exposure to different types of stress is likely to vary across the lifespan.

Murphy and Athanasou (Murphy and Athanasou 1999) conducted a meta-analysis on the effect of gaining or losing employment on mental health. Sixteen studies were identified and the outcome measure of 11 of these studies was psychological distress. In all but two studies, job loss was associated with an increase in psychological distress. A number of alternative explanations may account for the increase in distress following job loss. The hypothesis that more distressed individuals were more likely to lose their job, was discarded by studies that control for the level of distress before the loss of employment. The hypothesis that those with a stressing or unsatisfying job would be less likely to experience an increase in distress following the loss of their job could not be verified in the studies selected by Murphy and Athanasou (Murphy and Athanasou 1999). The socio-economic context at the time of the job loss, the cultural meaning of the role of worker and the financial compensation following job loss were not investigated.

Jorm and his colleagues found several age and gender differences in the factors associated with psychological distress among Australian workers (Jorm et al. 2005). For instance exposure to stress tended to vary across the three age groups under study (20-24; 40-44; 60-64). More precisely, the probability of a recent end of a relationship, a recent problem with someone, and a recent job threat declined with increasing age. Childhood adversity, personal or family injury or illness, problem with someone, problem at work and conflicting relationship with friends or family were risk factors for psychological distress for both women and men. However, gender differences occurred in three types of stress: job insecurity was a risk factor for men but not for women whereas death in the family and end of a relationship were risk factors for women but not for men. These findings support the assumption that the role of worker is still more prominent for men than for women whereas family-related roles are more crucial for women than for men.

For seniors, chronic stress, recent life events and childhood trauma emerge as major risk factors for psychological distress (Cairney and Krause 2005). For adolescents, stress related to academic performance increases the odds of psychological distress (Darcy and Siddique 1984, Myklestad, Roysamb, and Tambs 2011, Ystgaard, Tambs, and Dalgard 1999) but there is some evidence that this type of stress may be more detrimental for girls than for boys. Thus the impression of failing in the role of students affects the psychological well-being of adolescents. Being bullied at school (Myklestad, Roysamb, and Tambs 2011) and family conflict (Wilkinson-Lee et al. 2011, Ystgaard, Tambs, and Dalgard 1999) increase the mean level of distress in both girls and boys although when detailed stressful situations are taken into account family conflicts seem to affect girls more than boys (Ystgaard, Tambs, and Dalgard 1999). Parental divorce seems to have a stronger effect in adolescent girls; time lapse since divorce does not appear to modify the association with distress (Storksen et al. 2006). Størksen et al. attributed the effect of divorce on distress to the enduring family conflicts following a divorce since divorce per se is quite common in Norway. In their opinion, parental divorce must be seen as a stressful situation instead of as a stressful event. Rickwood and d'Espaignet (Rickwood and d'Espaignet 1996) investigated the evolution of the prevalence of psychological distress from the age of 16 to 25 and found that for both women and men it reaches a peak at the final year at school and drops afterwards. Graduation from high school marks the end of adolescence and the beginning of adulthood for most youths living in industrialized countries (Gaudet 2007). From a psychosocial point of view, the transition from adolescence to early adulthood stands as a major life transition since, over a short period of time, high school graduates experience abrupt changes in their lifestyle and social identity and face new sources of stress, social network and social support that may foster or strain their psychological well-being (Creed, Muller, and Patton 2003, Needham 2007, Schulenberg, Sameroff, and Cicchetti 2004).

Poverty is associated with poor mental and physical health because it prevents people from purchasing adequate food, clothing and services, it affects self-esteem and the sense of control over one's life, it can be a cause of social exclusion and it can increase the likelihood of stressful events. Kessler (Kessler, Price, and Wortman 1985) defines two mechanisms explaining the relationship between socio-economic status and distress. Social selection posits that emotionally vulnerable individuals tend to drift to the lower socioeconomic strata of the society (i.e., distress causes SES drift) whereas social causation implies that economical hardship leads to distress by influencing the stresses to which one is exposed or the resources available to cope with stressful experiences (i.e., SES causes distress). He argues that: lower-class people might be highly exposed to the types of stressful experiences which can cause distress; and that they might be more likely to become distressed when exposed to these stresses. Lower income and socio-economic status have repeatedly been shown to be a risk factor for distress (Caron and Liu 2011, Myer et al. 2008, Phongsavan et al. 2006). Individuals with a low income tend to have a lower education, to be more frequently unemployed and to belong to ethnic minorities but the risk factors associated with psychological distress tend to be the same for low and higher income groups (Caron and Liu 2011). Thus people with a low income would not be more vulnerable to general risk factors but they would be more exposed to them. Benzeval and Judge (Benzeval and Judge 2001) have investigated the relationship between poverty and health over time in adults based on the British Household Panel Survey, a longitudinal population survey conducted every year between 1991 and 1997. They found that the odds of distress was higher in individuals whose current income was in the bottom 40% of the population income distribution whereas the five-year average income and the number of years below the average income or in the bottom fifth of the population distribution were not a risk factor for psychological distress. Thus there seems to be some sort of a ceiling effect to the detrimental effect of poverty. For adolescents, perceived poverty (Hamilton, Noh, and Adlaf 2009) may be more distressing than true financial difficulties as reported by parents (Myklestad, Roysamb, and Tambs 2011) although the latter may take more importance as adolescents move towards adulthood (Myklestad, Roysamb, and Tambs 2011). Sakurai et al. (Sakurai et al. 2010) have investigated three components of socio-economic status (SES) (i.e., subjective social status; education; income) in Japanese aged 20 to 74 years old. They found that low income increased the odds for distress for both women and men, that education did not affect the odds of distress for either gender and that women who felt that their social status was low were at higher risk of distress than those who felt that it was higher. In their opinion, the weaker (and not statistically significant) association of distress with education and income may reflect the fact that these indicators of socio-economic status are not as relevant to Japanese. Sakurai et al. (Sakurai et al. 2010) contend that the relationship between low income and distress in men but not in women reflects the Confucian gender role ideology were men are the sole bread-earners for their families. Perceived failure in this role may decrease men's self-esteem, causing greater distress.

In adults, chronic health problems and limitations in daily activities whether in self or in a close family member play an important role in the epidemiology of psychological distress (Gispert et al. 2003, Mandemakers and Monden 2010, Zabora et al. 2001). This association could be attributed to the diminished quality of life, the disruption of social roles, and the side effects of medication (Chittleborough et al. 2011). The detrimental impact of some chronic health problems may vary across the life span (Myklestad, Roysamb, and Tambs 2011), across gender (Gispert et al. 2003) and ethnic groups (Bratter and Eschbach 2005).

5.1.3 Personal resources

Personal resources may be split in two categories: inner resources and external resources. Inner resources encompass those resources that have a strong component of personality such as self-esteem and sense of control over one's life. These resources are relatively stable over the life span although they may be shattered temporarily or permanently in case of a traumatic event. High levels of self-esteem and sense of control over one's life are associated with lower mean level of psychological distress in adults (Gadalla 2009, Jorm et al. 2005, Walters, McDonough, and Strohschein 2002) and seniors (Cairney and Krause 2005). The sense of control over one's life tends buffer the effect of poor health and daily stress on distress but not the effect of poverty (Gadalla 2009). External resources include social network, social support, income and education.

In general, social support appears to be more essential to the psychological well-being of individuals than social network (Cairney and Krause 2005, Caron and Liu 2011, Gadalla 2009, Préville et al. 2002). In addition, there is some evidence that the type and source of support may act differently in women and men and across the lifespan. The study conducted by Kuriyama et al. (Kuriyama et al. 2009) in Japanese aged 40 and over illustrates the complexity of the relationship between the type of support and psychological distress. In this study, the odds of psychological distress were higher in women and men who lacked someone to provide advice when in trouble, and in women who had no one to consult about their health, to drive them to hospital and to take care of them. For adolescents, support from a group of friends is generally associated with a lower level of distress (Myklestad, Roysamb, and Tambs 2011, Ystgaard, Tambs, and Dalgard 1999). However, when friends at school and outside of school are distinguished, support from friends at school act as a protective factor for boys but not for girls and support from friends outside of school has no influence on psychological distress (Myklestad, Roysamb, and Tambs 2011). Operario et al. (Operario et al. 2006), found that high distress was associated with girls who reported low parental warmth and who turned to their peers for support during family conflict; boys were not affected by parental warmth or peers support. The type of social support and social network that are associated with distress in the adult population do not seem to have the same protective effect in seniors (Paul, Ayis, and Ebrahim 2006). Number of contact have no effect on psychological distress among seniors (Cairney and Krause 2005) whereas perceived social support, are associated with a decrease distress.

The protective effect of higher income and education against psychological distress has been confirmed in most studies for women and for men, for all age groups and across countries (Caron and Liu 2011, Chittleborough et al. 2011, Huang et al. 2009, Jorm et al. 2005, Nemeroff, Midlarsky, and Meyer 2010, Walters, McDonough, and Strohschein 2002). There is some evidence that education might interact in the relationships between psychological distress and income or disability. For example, the effect of education may be more protective for individuals with an average or higher income (Caron and Liu 2011). Education is assumed to buffer the effect of disability because more educated people may be better equipped (have better cognitive skills) to deal with the consequences of disability, such as disruption of social roles, increased difficulties in daily living, loss of income. However, although. Mandemakers and Monden have shown that disability impacts more on the psychological distress of young adults with a low education than of better educated ones whatever the level of disability, they found that the better economic resources and cognitive abilities did not account for the interaction effect of education (Mandemakers and Monden 2010).

5.2 In workers

There is growing and convincing evidence that occupations and work organisation conditions affect the psychological well-being of workers. The investigation of work-related psychological distress rests on three main theoretical models. The Job Demand-Control Model (Karasek 1979) posits that work demands (i.e., workload; time constraints, pace of work; conflicting, emotional and physical demands) exert considerable stress on workers and that the level of decision latitude at work (i.e., high levels of skill utilization and decision authority) moderates the effect of this stress on the mental health of workers. The Demand-Control-Support Model (Karasek and Theorell 1990) expands on the Job Demand-Control Model by emphasizing the impact of social support in the workplace on the interaction between decision latitude and work demands. The Effort-Reward Imbalance Model (Siegrist 1996) underscores the importance of an equilibrium between demands and rewards (i.e., wage; social recognition; security; motivation; career perspective) in the experience of work-related stress and the onset and development of psychological distress. According to this model, an imbalance between demands and rewards is especially detrimental to the mental health of workers overcommitted to their job. Most empirical studies support the hypothesized influence of high work demands, low decision latitude, poor social support at work, and minimal rewards on the psychological distress observed in workers (Marchand, Demers, and Durand 2005b). However, the interaction between these factors have not been corroborated (Bonde 2008, Marchand and Durand 2011). The Job Demand-Control Model, Demand-Control-Support Model and Effort-Reward Imbalance Model have mostly been investigated in relationship with the type of occupations and work organisation condition.

5.2.1 Occupations

A number of longitudinal and cross-sectional studies worldwide have identified variations in psychological distress across occupations. Findings from these studies are difficult to compare because of differences in the classification of occupations. Data from a French study, the GAZEL cohort, showed that the mean level of psychological distress tends to be higher in semi-professionals (e.g., administrator; associate engineers), supervisors, office workers, blue-collar workers and craftsmen (Niedhammer et al. 1998). In the Netherlands, data from the Maastricht cohort study revealed that "occupation" explained 2.7% of the variance in psychological distress among workers (Bultmann et al. 2001). In this study, the prevalence of distress was higher for 10 out of the 131 occupations and the occupations at higher risk were mainly blue and white collar workers. Similarly, in Canadian studies conducted by Marchand and his colleagues, "occupation" accounted for 1% to 3% of the variance in psychological distress (Marchand, Demers, and Durand 2005b, 2005a, 2006). The Whitehall Study, which followed a large sample of London civil servants found that employees in higher grades or management positions were at lower risk of psychological distress than those lower in the hierarchy (Stansfeld et al. 2003). Similar results were obtained for the GAZEL cohort (Paterniti et al. 2002).

5.2.2 Work organisation conditions

Work organisation conditions seem more important than occupations per se to explain variations in psychological distress. Work organisation conditions can be defined around four organisational dimensions related to task design, demands, social relations and gratifications (Marchand, Demers, and Durand 2005a).

The nature and content of tasks vary across occupations and across organizations. Task can be more or less repetitive and make more or less use of an individual's skills and qualifications. The work organisation can also allow more or less control (i.e., autonomy, decision authority) to individuals in the performance of work-related tasks. Monotonous and repetitive jobs are associated with a higher risk of psychological distress (Johansson 1989, Shiron, Westman, and Melamed 1999) whereas skills utilization and control over the task completion are associated with lower risk of distress (Albertsen, Nielsen, and Borg 2001, Bourbonnais et al. 2005, Karasek and Theorell 1990). Altogether, the larger one's decision latitude is (i.e., high skill use and high decision authority), the lower the risk of distress in workers. However, findings from some studies suggest that too much skills utilization and decision authority can lead to more psychological distress (Marchand, Demers, and Durand 2005b, 2006). Organisational demands and personal involvement in the job yield to psychological and cognitive loads that can affect one's mental health. The stress generated by these demands is not necessarily negative since it may, within a certain limit, increase one's mastering and social identification at work. Nevertheless, beyond this limit, physical, psychological and contractual demands can foster psychological distress.

Physical demands take the form of several occupational health and safety risks manifest in the work environment (e.g., high levels of noise, dust, heat, cold, toxic vapours, neurotoxic substances) and the workplace can give rise to some risks of injuries and death. In addition, workers can be confronted to a high level of physical efforts (e.g., transporting heavy loads, uncomfortable work postures). Overall, physical demands are a risk factor for psychological distress (de Jonge, Mulder, and Nijhuis 1999, Marchand, Demers, and Durand 2005b). Similarly, psychological demands can generate elevated stress and increase the odds of psychological distress (Albertsen, Nielsen, and Borg 2001, Bourbonnais et al. 2005, Marchand, Demers, and Durand 2005b, Paterniti et al. 2002). Psychological demands are typified by task rhythm, workload, time constraints, and conflicting and emotional demands (e.g., client aggression, exposure to the suffering of others). Contractual demands are defined by unusual work schedules and number of working hours. Workers dealing with work schedules that are alternating, irregular or on night shift, experience a difficult situation. Shift work, being on call, and unpredictable work schedules require workers to adapt to variations in the circadian rhythm, which can promote sleep problems and diverse nervous reactions that can increase the feeling of distress. These types of work schedules can also lead to negative effects on family life and social isolation, which will further endanger the mental health of workers. All in all, work schedule and work hours increase the risk of psychological distress (Hayasaka et al. 2007, Hilton et al. 2008, Marchand, Demers, and Durand 2005b, Matthews, Power, and Stansfeld 2001, Sekine et al. 2006, Spurgeon, Harrington, and Cooper 1997).

Conflicting relationships at work, either with co-workers or supervisors, can create a stressful experience that may impact on the mental health of workers. In this vein, the social support received at work has been the subject of considerable attention and refers to social interactions providing instrumental and emotional support from colleagues and superiors. The social support at work fulfils the need of individuals to be acknowledged and endorsed in the execution of their task; it is a source of pleasure and compensation for the efforts invested at work. Studies using global scales of social support at work generally report lower levels of psychological distress when the social support is higher (Albertsen, Nielsen, and Borg 2001, Bourbonnais et al. 1998, Marchand, Demers, and Durand 2005a, 2006, McDonough 2000, Pomaki, Maes, and Ter Doest 2004). Social relations also encompass the style of supervision. Some research suggests that the clarity and the consistency of instructions given by the supervisor is an important element in the reduction of psychological distress of white collars workers (Stansfeld et al. 1999). Abusive supervision (i.e., authoritarian and aggressive styles) brings about an elevated level of psychological distress in exposed workers (Tepper 2000). Finally problems with violence or harassment at work on the part of colleagues or supervisors are worthy of investigation, since several studies highlight the major impact of these problems on psychological distress (Marchand, Demers, and Durand 2005b, McDermut, Haaga, and Kirk 2000, Mueller, De Coster, and Estes 2001, Piotrkowski 1998, Richman et al. 1999).

Finally, gratifications available in the workplace bring to the individuals an important source of recognition, motivation, valorisation, and of identification to their work. Thus a low level of gratifications can engender dissatisfaction and stress, which might affect mental health. These gratifications involve not only remuneration, but also career perspectives, job security and self-esteem at work. Some studies report a lower level of psychological distress in workers satisfied with the rewards obtained within their workplace (de Jonge et al. 2000, Demerouti et al. 2000, Tepper 2000). Conversely, several studies support the hypothesis that job insecurity and possibly the mode and the level of remuneration could in themselves be conductive to psychological distress (Bourbonnais et al. 1998, Ibrahim, Smith, and Muntaner 2009, Ikeda et al. 2009, Marchand, Demers, and Durand 2005a, 2006, McDonough 2000, Rugulies et al. 2006).

5.3 In immigrants

Resettling in an alien society entails a number of stressful experiences such as gaining employment, maintaining family cohesion within and across countries, recreating a social network and, sometimes, learning a new language. The level of stress generated by these experiences varies across categories of immigrants and is exacerbated by the cultural distance between the homeland and the host country and the lack of transferable skills (e.g., language, education, work experience). Immigrants may also have a hard time resettling if the host society is unable, because of a difficult socio-economic situation, or reluctant, because of inter-ethnic prejudices, to welcome strangers. Compared to other categories of immigrants, refugees may be disadvantaged because their exposure to political violence in their homeland or in refugees' camps may have weakened their physical and mental health. According to Silove (Silove 1999), exposure to political violence may harm a number of adaptive resources such as the feeling of safety, the capacity to form and nurture interpersonal bonds, the sense of identity and role functioning, the faith in justice, and the belief that life is meaningful and coherent. At first glance, immigrants and refugees would appear at higher risk of psychological distress than natives. However, this risk may be offset by the healthy migrant effect (Stafford, Newbold, and Ross 2011). In effect, immigrants form a selective group of individuals characterized by their determination to start a new - and hopefully better - life abroad and most countries select immigrants based on their health status and transferable skills. Similarly, healthier and better-educated refugees may be more likely to have survived the political violence in their home country and to have been selected for migration in refugees camp (Mollica et al. 2001).

Several factors affecting psychological distress in the general population also operate on the psychological distress of immigrants and refugees. In general, immigrant women report a higher mean level of distress than immigrant men (Gonzalez-Castro and Ubillos 2011, Lerner, Kertes, and Zilber 2005, Levecque, Lodewyckx, and Bracke 2009) although this difference may not be statistically significant in older immigrants (Chou 2007, Ritsner, Ponizovsky, and Ginath 1999). Similarly, financial hardship (Gonzalez-Castro and Ubillos 2011, Lerner, Kertes, and Zilber 2005, Sundquist et al. 2000), poor self-reported health (Chou 2007, Lerner, Kertes, and Zilber 2005) and recent stressful events (Lerner, Kertes, and Zilber 2005, Thapa and Hauff 2005) act as risk factors whereas family cohesion (Lerner, Kertes, and Zilber 2005, Yip, Gee, and Takeuchi 2008) and the sense of control over one's life (Lerner, Kertes, and Zilber 2005, Sundquist et al. 2000) play a protective role.

The influence of other long-established risk and protective factors is more uncertain. Most studies have found no statistically significant effect of age (Levecque, Lodewyckx, and Bracke 2009, Thapa and Hauff 2005, Yip, Gee, and Takeuchi 2008) on the psychological distress of immigrants whereas the evidence is mixed for unemployment (Lerner, Kertes, and Zilber 2005, Levecque, Lodewyckx, and Bracke 2009, Thapa and Hauff 2005), education (Chou 2007, Levecque, Lodewyckx, and Bracke 2009, Sundquist et al. 2000) and marital status (Chou 2007, Lerner, Kertes, and Zilber 2005, Thapa and Hauff 2005).

Deciphering the relationships between psychological distress and factors typical of immigrants is a difficult task because of the complex interplay of the context of migration, the ethno-cultural background of immigrants and the socio-cultural characteristics of the host country. Bronstein and Montgomery conducted a systematic review of the literature related to the epidemiology of psychological distress in refugee children based on 22 studies (Bronstein and Montgomery 2011). They concluded that the mean level of psychological distress was high in these children and that it tended to vary by age, gender, country of origin, pre-migratory traumatic experience and post-migratory support. A similar exercise has not been conducted among adult refugees but some of the conclusions reached by Bronstein and Montgomery also apply to adults. For instance, Chou et al. (Chou 2007) recorded a higher mean level of distress in refugees to Australia than in individuals who had migrated to be reunited with their family or who were selected for immigration based on their professional skills whereas Thapa and Hauff (Thapa and Hauff 2005) observed no statistically significant difference between refugees and immigrants in Norway, and Rousseau and Drapeau (Rousseau and Drapeau 2004) found that the association between psychological distress and the context of migration to Quebec varied depending on the home country of immigrants. The effect of past exposure to political violence on the psychological distress of refugees in the host country is also ambiguous. Sundquist et al. (Sundquist et al. 2000) detected no significant effect in refugees from four different countries, Thapa and Hauff (Thapa and Hauff 2005) found a significant effect for women but not for men and Rousseau and Drapeau (Rousseau and Drapeau 2004) noted that the effect depended on the type of exposure to political violence and on the country of origin of refugees. Thus, at the population level, refugees are not systematically at higher risk of psychological distress than other immigrants.

Three main indicators have been used to assess the level of acculturation of immigrants: self-defined ethnic identity, mastery of the mainstream language and relationships with natives from the host country. Defining oneself as a member of the host country while preserving close ties with the culture of origin tends to act as a protective factor against psychological distress (Birman and Taylor-Ritzler 2007), perhaps more so for women than for men (Lerner, Kertes, and Zilber 2005). Sundquist et al. (Sundquist et al. 2000) found that a poor mastery of the mainstream language was a risk factor for men but not for women. Finally, Gonzalez-Castro et al. (Gonzalez-Castro and Ubillos 2011) and Thapa and Hauff (Thapa and Hauff 2005) have found no significant effect of social support provided by members of the mainstream population on psychological distress.

6. Conclusion

In the past few decades, empirical evidence has accumulated regarding the epidemiology of psychological distress. Still, the use of scales comprising a wide array of undifferentiated symptoms has impeded our understanding of the risk and protective factors that impact on psychological distress. Nevertheless, when restricting the review of the scientific literature on studies based on scales that assess psychological distress defined as *a state of emotional suffering characterized by symptoms of depression and anxiety* sometimes accompanied by somatic symptoms, several characteristic features emerge. First, in the general population, stressful events and life conditions and the lack of valued social roles come up as significant risk factors for psychological distress whereas inner resources (e.g., self-esteem) and external resources (e.g., income) are important protective factors. Second, among workers, high work demands, low decision latitude, poor social support at work, and minimal rewards increase the risk of psychological distress. Work-related factors do not explain all the variations in psychological distress observed in workers but the integration of the various elements that make up the social environment of workers (i.e., work, family, social networks, local community-neighbourhood) has proved difficult both theoretically and empirically. Finally, the prevalence of psychological distress is especially high among immigrants and refugees. Although several factors affecting the psychological well-being of the general population also impact on the level of psychological distress of immigrants and refugees, specific factors related to the context of migration and the resettlement process seem to take their toll on the mental health of these individuals. In all likelihood, factors associated with psychological distress also affect other dimensions of mental health and mental illness and there is a need to identify the similarities and differences between the epidemiology of psychological distress and other mental health problems.

The empirical evidence points to a number of issues that must be addressed to better understand, and eventually to prevent, psychological distress. Knowledge about the course of psychological distress is especially lacking and it prevents the distinction between transient and pathological distress. The gender and age differences in psychological distress remain largely unexplained although it has been the focus of several studies. Exposure to specific risk factors seems to vary across gender and across age group but the effect of this differential exposure on psychological distress is unclear. The complex interplay of socio-demographic factors, stress-related factors and individual resources also need to be further investigated. The relative contributions of occupation and work organization conditions and factors acting outside of the work environment have been largely unexplored. For instance, conceptual frameworks concerning work-related factors leave no room for the way gender and migration status could moderate the relationship between these factors and psychological distress. Still, the main brake to a better understanding of the epidemiology of psychological distress is the almost complete lack of systematic reviews of the empirical evidence concerning the numerous risk and protective factors associated with distress.

7. Acknowledgement

The authors express their gratitude to the institutions, especially the Fonds de la recherche en santé mentale du Québec and the Canadian Institutes for Health Research, that have financed their researches in mental health and, more specifically in psychological distress, and to the numerous respondents, research associates and students who have taken part in their studies.

8. References

Al-Krenawi, A., and J.R. Graham. 2000. "Culturally sensitive social work practice with Arab clients in mental health settings." *Health and Social Work* no. 25:9-22.

Albertsen, K., M.L. Nielsen, and V. Borg. 2001. "The Danish psychosocial work environment and symptoms of stress: the main, mediating and moderating role of sense of coherence." *Work and Stress* no. 15:241-253.

Andreu, Y., M. J. Galdon, E. Dura, M. Ferrando, S. Murgui, A. Garcia, and E. Ibanez. 2008. "Psychometric properties of the Brief Symptoms Inventory-18 (Bsi-18) in a Spanish sample of outpatients with psychiatric disorders." *Psicothema* no. 20 (4):844-850.

Aranda, M.P., I. Castaneda, P.-J. Lee, and E. Sobel. 2001. "Stress, social support, and coping as predictors of depressive symptoms: Gender differences among Mexican Americans." *Social Work Research* no. 25:37-48.

Arnaud, B., L. Malet, F. Teissedre, M. Izaute, F. Moustafa, J. Geneste, J. Schmidt, P. M. Llorca, and G. Brousse. 2010. "Validity study of Kessler's psychological distress scales conducted among patients admitted to French emergency department for alcohol consumption-related disorders." *Alcoholism: Clinical and Experimental Research* no. 34 (7):1235-1245. doi: ACER1201 [pii] 10.1111/j.1530-0277.2010.01201.x.

Baillie, A.J. 2005. "Predictive gender and education bias in Kessler's psychological distress scale (K10) " *Social Psychiatry and Psychiatric Epidemiology* no. 40:743-748.

Benzeval, M., and K. Judge. 2001. "Income and health: the time dimension." *Social Science and Medicine* no. 52:1371-1390.

Birman, D., and T. Taylor-Ritzler. 2007. "Acculturation and psychological distress among adolescent immigrants from the former Soviet Union: exploring the mediating effect of family relationships." *Cultural Diversity and Ethnic Minority Psychology* no. 13 (4):337-346. doi: 2007-15428-008 [pii] 10.1037/1099-9809.13.4.337.

Bonde, J.P.E. 2008. "Psychosocial factors at work and risk of depression: a systematic review of the epidemiological evidence." *Occupational and Environmental Medicine* no. 65:438-445.

Bourbonnais, R., C. Brisson, R. Malenfant, and M. Vezina. 2005. "Health care restructuring, work environment, and health of nurses." *American Journal of Industrial Medicine* no. 47:54-64.

Bourbonnais, R., M. Comeau, M. Vezina, and G. Dion. 1998. "Job strain, psychological distress, and burnout in nurses." *American Journal of Industrial Medicine* no. 34:20-28.

Bratter, J.L, and K Eschbach. 2005. "Race/Ethnic Differences in Nonspecific Psychological Distress : Evidence from the National Health Interview Survey." *Social Science Quarterly* no. 86 (3):620-644.

Bronstein, I., and P. Montgomery. 2011. "Psychological distress in refugee children: A systematic review." *Clinical Child and Family Psychological Review* no. 14:44-56.

Brooks, R. T., J. Beard, and Z. Steel. 2006. "Factor structure and interpretation of the K10." *Psychological Assessment* no. 18 (1):62-70. doi: 2006-03905-007 [pii] 10.1037/1040-3590.18.1.62.

Bultmann, U., I. Kant, P.A. van den Brandt, and S.V. Kasl. 2001. "Differences in fatigue and psychological distress across occupations: results from the Maastricht Cohort Study of fatigue at work." *Journal of Occupational and Environmental Medicine* no. 43:976-983.

Cairney, J., and N. Krause. 2005. "The social distribution of psychological distress and depression in older adults." *Journal of Aging and Health* no. 17 (6):807-835. doi: 17/6/807 [pii] 10.1177/0898264305280985.

Caron, J., and A. Liu. 2011. "Factors associated with psychological distress in the Canadian population: a comparison of low-income and non low-income sub-groups." *Community Mental Health Journal* no. 47 (3):318-330. doi: 10.1007/s10597-010-9306-4.

Carra, G., P. Sciarini, G. Segagni-Lusignani, M. Clerici, C. Montomoli, and R. C. Kessler. 2011. "Do they actually work across borders? Evaluation of two measures of psychological distress as screening instruments in a non Anglo-Saxon country." *European Psychiatry* no. 26 (2):122-127. doi: S0924-9338(10)00116-1 [pii] 10.1016/j.eurpsy.2010.04.008.

Chittleborough, C. R., H. Winefield, T. K. Gill, C. Koster, and A. W. Taylor. 2011. "Age differences in associations between psychological distress and chronic conditions." *International Journal of Public Health* no. 56 (1):71-80. doi: 10.1007/s00038-010-0197-5.

Chou, K. L. 2007. "Psychological distress in migrants in Australia over 50 years old: a longitudinal investigation." *Journal of Affective Disorders* no. 98 (1-2):99-108. doi: S0165-0327(06)00296-5 [pii] 10.1016/j.jad.2006.07.002.

Cleary, P.D., B.T. Bush, and L.G. Kessler. 1987. "Evaluating the use of mental health screening scales in primary care settings using Receiver Operating Characteristic Curves." *Medical Care* no. 25:S90-S98.

Cleary, P.D., and D. Mechanic. 1983. "Sex differences in psychological distress among married people." *Journal of Health and Social Behavior* no. 24:111-121.

Creed, P.A., J Muller, and W. Patton. 2003. "Leaving high school: The influence and consequences for psychological well-being and career-related confidence." *Journal of Adolescence* no. 26:295-311.

Darcy, C., and C.M. Siddique. 1984. "Psychological distress among Canadian adolescents." *Psychological Medicine* no. 14:615-628.

de Jonge, J., H. Bosma, R. Peter, and J. Siegrist. 2000. "Job strain, effort-reward imbalance and employee well-being: a large-scale cross-sectional study." *Social Science and Medicine* no. 50:1317-1327.

de Jonge, J., M. Mulder, and F. Nijhuis. 1999. "The incorporation of different demand concept in the job demand-control model: effects on health care professionals." *Social Science and Medicine* no. 48:1149-1160.

Demerouti, E., A.B. Bakker, F. Nachreiner, and W.B. Schaufeli. 2000. "A model of burnout and life satisfaction amongst nurses." *Journal of Advanced Nursing* no. 32:454-464.

Derogatis, L. R. 1993. *BSI Brief Symptom Inventory. Administration, Scoring, and Procedures Manual (4th Ed.)*. Minneapolis, MN: National Computer Systems.

— — —. 2001. Brief Symptom Inventory (BSI)-18 : Administration, scoring and procedures manual. Minneapolis, MN: NCS Pearson.

Derogatis, L. R., R. S. Lipman, K. Rickels, E. H. Uhlenhuth, and L. Covi. 1974. "The Hopkins Symptom Checklist (HSCL): a self-report symptom inventory." *Behavioral Science* no. 19 (1):1-15.

Derogatis, L. R., and N. Melisaratos. 1983. "The Brief Symptom Inventory: an introductory report." *Psychological Medicine* no. 13 (3):595-605.

Desrosiers, A., and S. St Fleurose. 2002. "Treating Haitian patients." *American Journal of Psychotherapy* no. 56:508-521.

Dohrenwend, B.P., and B.S Dohrenwend. 1982. "Perspectives on the past and future of psychiatric epidemiology." *American Journal of Public Health* no. 72:1271-1279.

Donker, T., H. Comijs, P. Cuijpers, B. Terluin, W. Nolen, F. Zitman, and B. Penninx. 2010. "The validity of the Dutch K10 and extended K10 screening scales for depressive and anxiety disorders." *Psychiatry Research* no. 176:45-50.

Drapeau, A., D. Beaulieu-Prévost, A. Marchand, R. Boyer, M. Préville, and S. Kairouz. 2010. "A life-course and time perspective on the construct validity of psychological distress in women and men. Measurement invariance of the K6 across gender." *BMC Medical Research Methodology* no. 10 (68):doi:10.1186/1471-2288-10-68.

Ensminger, M.E., and D.D. Celentano. 1990. "Gender differences in the effect of unemployment on psychological distress." *Social Science and Medicine* no. 30:469-477.

Evans, O., and A. Steptoe. 2002. "The contribution of gender-role orientation, work factors and home stressors to psychological well-being and sickness absence in male- and female-dominated occupational groups." *Social Science and Medicine* no. 54:481-492.

Fassaert, T., M.A.S. de Wit, W.C. Tuinebreijer, H. Wouters, A.P. Verhoeff, A.T.F. Beekman, and J. Dekker. 2009. "Psychometric properties of an interviewer-administered version of the Kessler psychological distres scale (K10) among Dutch, Moroccan and Turkish respondents." *International Journal of Methods in Psychiatric Research* no. 18:159-168.

Folkman, S., R.S. Lazarus, S. Pimley, and J. Novacek. 1987. "Age differences in stress and coping processes." *Psychology and Aging* no. 2:171-184.

French, D. J., and R. J. Tait. 2004. "Measurement invariance in the General Health Questionnaire-12 in young Australian adolescents." *European Child and Adolescent Psychiatry* no. 13 (1):1-7. doi: 10.1007/s00787-004-0345-7.

Furukawa, T. A., N. Kawakami, M. Saitoh, Y. Ono, Y. Nakane, Y. Nakamura, H. Tachimori, N. Iwata, H. Uda, H. Nakane, H. Watanabe, Y. Naganuma, Y. Hata, M. Kobayashi, Y. Miyake, T. Takeshima, and T. Kikkawa. 2008. "The performance of the Japanese version of the K6 and K10 in the World Mental Health Survey in Japan." *International Journal of Methods in Psychiatric Research* no. 17 (3):152-158. doi: 10.1002/mpr.257.

Furukawa, T., and D. P. Goldberg. 1999. "Cultural invariance of likelihood ratios for the General Health Questionnaire." *Lancet* no. 353 (9152):561-2. doi: S0140-6736(98)05470-1 [pii] 10.1016/S0140-6736(98)05470-1.

Furukawa, T.A., R.C. Kessler, T. Slade, and G. Andrews. 2003. "The performance of the K6 and K10 screening scales for psychological distress in the Australian National Survey of Mental Health and Well-Being." *Psychological Medicine* no. 33:357-362.

Gadalla, T.M. 2009. "Determinants, correlates and mediators of psychological distress. A longitudinal study." *Social Science & Medicine* no. 68:2199-2205.

Gaudet, S. 2007. Emerging adulthood: A new stage in the life course. In *Policy Research Initiative*, edited by Government of Canada. Ottawa (Canada).

Gispert, R., L. Rajmil, A. Schiaffino, and M. Herdman. 2003. "Sociodemographic and health-related correlates of psychiatric distress in a general population." *Social Psychiatry and Psychiatric Epidemiology* no. 38:677-683.

Goldberg, D. P., T. Oldehinkel, and J. Ormel. 1998. "Why GHQ threshold varies from one place to another." *Psychological Medicine* no. 28 (4):915-921.

Goldberg, D.P., and P. Williams. 1991. *A User's Guide to the General Health Questionnaire.* Great Britain: NFER-NELSON Publishing Company.

Gonzalez-Castro, J. L., and S. Ubillos. 2011. "Determinants of psychological distress among migrants from Ecuador and Romania in a Spanish city." *International Journal of Social Psychiatry* no. 57 (1):30-44. doi: 57/1/30 [pii] 10.1177/0020764010347336.

Gove, W.R., M. Hughes, and C.B. Style. 1983. "Does marriage have positive effects on the psychological well-being of the individual?" *Journal of Health and Social Behavior* no. 24:122-131.

Green, J. G., M. J. Gruber, N. A. Sampson, A. M. Zaslavsky, and R. C. Kessler. 2010. "Improving the K6 short scale to predict serious emotional disturbance in adolescents in the USA." *International Journal Methods in Psychiatric Research* no. 19 Suppl 1:23-35. doi: 10.1002/mpr.314.

Hamilton, H. A., S. Noh, and E. M. Adlaf. 2009. "Adolescent risk behaviours and psychological distress across immigrant generations." *Canadian Journal of Public Health* no. 100 (3):221-225.

Hankins, M. 2008. "The factor structure of the twelve item General Health Questionnaire (GHQ-12): the result of negative phrasing?" *Clinical Practice and Epidemiology in Mental Health* no. 4:10. doi: 1745-0179-4-10 [pii] 10.1186/1745-0179-4-10.

Hayasaka, Y., K. Nakamura, M. Yamamoto, and S. Sasaki. 2007. "Work environment and mental health status assessed by the General Health Questionnaire in female Japanese doctors." *Industrial Health* no. 45:781-786.

Hilton, M.F., H.A. Whiteford, J.S. Sheridan, C.M. Cleary, D.C. Chant, P.S. Wang, and R.C. Kessler. 2008. "The prevalence of psychological distress in employees and associated occupational risk factors." *Journal of Occupational and Environmental Medicine* no. 50:746-757.

Hoffmann, C., B. H. McFarland, J. D. Kinzie, L. Bresler, D. Rakhlin, S. Wolf, and A. E. Kovas. 2006. "Psychological distress among recent Russian immigrants in the United States." *Journal of Social Psychiatry* no. 52 (1):29-40.

Horwitz, A.V. 2007. "Distinguishing distress from disorder as psychological outcomes of stressful social arrangments." *Health* no. 11:273-289.

Huang, J. P., W. Xia, C. H. Sun, H. Y. Zhang, and L. J. Wu. 2009. "Psychological distress and its correlates in Chinese adolescents." *Australian and New Zealand Journal of Psychiatry* no. 43 (7):674-680. doi: 912416347 [pii] 10.1080/00048670902970817.

Ibrahim, S., P. Smith, and C. Muntaner. 2009. "A multi-group cross-lagged analyses of work stressors and health using Canadian national sample." *Social Science and Medicine* no. 68:49-59.

Ikeda, T., A. Nakata, M. Takahashi, M. Hojou, T. Haratani, N. Nishikido, and K. Kamibeppu. 2009. "Correlates of depressive symptoms among workers in small and medium-scale manufacturing enterprises in Japan." *Journal of Occupational Health* no. 51.

International Labour Office. 2000. Mental Health in the Workplace. Geneva.

Johansson, G. 1989. "Job demands, and stress reactions in repetitive and uneventful monotony at work." *International Journal of Health Services* no. 192:365-377.

Jorm, A.F. 2000. "Does old age reduce the risk of anxiety and depression? A review of epidemiological studies across the adult life span." *Psychological Medicine* no. 30:11-22.

Jorm, A.F., and P. Duncan-Jones. 1990. "Neurotic symptoms and subjective well-being in a community sample: different sides of the same coin." *Psychological Medicine* no. 20:647-654.

Jorm, A.F., T.D. Windsor, K.B.G. Dear, K.J. Anstey, H. Christensen, and B. Rodgers. 2005. "Age group differences in psychological distress: the role of psychosocial risk factors that vary with age." *Psychlogical Medicine* no. 35:1253-1263.

Karasek, R.A. 1979. "Job demands, job decision latitude, and mental strain: Implication for job redesign." *Administrative Science Quarterly* no. 24:285-309.

Karasek, R.A., and T. Theorell. 1990. *Healthy work: stress, productivity, and the reconstruction of the working life.* New York: Basic Books.

Kessler, R. C, and T. B Üstün. 2008. *The WHO World Mental Health Surveys : global perspectives on the epidemiology of mental disorders.* New York: Cambridge University Press.

Kessler, R. C., J. G. Green, M. J. Gruber, N. A. Sampson, E. Bromet, M. Cuitan, T. A. Furukawa, O. Gureje, H. Hinkov, C. Y. Hu, C. Lara, S. Lee, Z. Mneimneh, L. Myer, M. Oakley-Browne, J. Posada-Villa, R. Sagar, M. C. Viana, and A. M. Zaslavsky. 2010. "Screening for serious mental illness in the general population with the K6 screening scale: results from the WHO World Mental Health (WMH) survey initiative." *International Journal Methods Psychiatric Research* no. 19 Suppl 1:4-22. doi: 10.1002/mpr.310.

Kessler, R.C., R.H. Price, and C.B. Wortman. 1985. "Social factors in psychopathology: Stress, social support, and coping processes." *Annual Review in Psychology* no. 36:531-572.

Kessler, Ronald C., Gavin Andrews, L.J. Colpe, E. Hiripi, Daniel Mroczek, S.-L. T. Normand, Elle E. Walters, and A.M. Zaslavsky. 2002. "Short screening scales to monitor population prevalences and trends in non-specific psychological distress." *Psychological Medicine* no. 32:959-976.

Kessler, Ronald C., and J.D. McLeod. 1984. "Sex differences in vulnerability to undesirable life events." *American Sociological Review* no. 49:620-631.

Kilkkinen, A., A. Kao-Philpot, A. O'Neil, B. Philpot, P. Reddy, S. Bunker, and J. Dunbar. 2007. "Prevalence of psychological distress, anxiety and depression in rural communities in Australia." *Australian Journal of Rural Health* no. 15:114-119.

Kirmayer, L.J. 1989. "Cultural variations in the response to psychiatric disorders and psychological distress." *Social Science and Medicine* no. 29:327-339.

Kleinman, A. 1991. *Rethinking Psychiatry. From Cultural Category to Personal Experience.* New York: The Free Press.

Kuriyama, S., N. Nakaya, K. Ohmori-Matsuda, T. Shimazu, N. Kikuchi, M. Kakizaki, T. Sone, F. Sato, M. Nagai, Y. Sugawara, M. Akhter, M. Higashiguchi, N. Fukuchi, H. Takahashi, A. Hozawa, and I. Tsuji. 2009. "Factors associated with psychological distress in a community-dwelling Japanese population: the Ohsaki Cohort 2006 Study." *Journal of Epidemiology* no. 19 (6):294-302. doi: JST.JSTAGE/jea/JE20080076 [pii].

Leach, L.S., H. Christensen, and A.J. Mackinnon. 2008. "Gender differences in the endorsement of symptoms for depression and anxiety. Are gender-biased items responsible?" *Journal of Nervous and Mental Disease* no. 196:128-135.

Lerner, Y., J. Kertes, and N. Zilber. 2005. "Immigrants from the former Soviet Union, 5 years post-immigration to Israel: adaptation and risk factors for psychological distress."

Psychological Medicine no. 35 (12):1805-1814. doi: S0033291705005726 [pii] 10.1017/S0033291705005726.

Leung, J.P. 1998. "Emotions and mental health in Chinese people." *Journal of Child and Families Studies* no. 7:115-128.

Levecque, K., I. Lodewyckx, and P. Bracke. 2009. "Psychological distress, depression and generalised anxiety in Turkish and Moroccan immigrants in Belgium: a general population study." *Social Psychiatry and Psychiatric Epidemiology* no. 44 (3):188-197. doi: 10.1007/s00127-008-0431-0.

Lincoln, K. D., R. J. Taylor, D. C. Watkins, and L. M. Chatters. 2011. "Correlates of Psychological Distress and Major Depressive Disorder Among African American Men." *Research on Social Work Practice* no. 21 (3):278-288. doi: 10.1177/1049731510386122.

Mandemakers, J. J., and C. W. Monden. 2010. "Does education buffer the impact of disability on psychological distress?" *Social Science and Medicine* no. 71 (2):288-297. doi: S0277-9536(10)00306-0 [pii] 10.1016/j.socscimed.2010.04.004.

Marchand, A., A. Demers, and P. Durand. 2005a. "Do occupation and work conditions really matter? A longitudinal analysis of psychological distress experiences among Canadian workers." *Sociology of Health and Illness* no. 27:602-627.

— — —. 2005b. "Does work really cause distress? The contribution of occupational structure and work organization to the experience of psychological distress." *Social Science and Medicine* no. 60:1-14.

— — —. 2006. "Social structures, agent personality and workers' mental health: A longitudinal analysis of the specific role of occupation and of workplace constraints-ressources on psychological distress in the Canadian workforce." *Human Relations* no. 59:875-901.

Marchand, A., A. Drapeau, and D. Beaulieu-Prévost. 2011. "Psychological distress in Canada: The role of employment and reasons for non-employment." *International Journal of Social Psychiatry* no. doi:10.1177/0020764011418404.

Marchand, A., and P. Durand. 2011. "Psychological distress, depression, and burnout: similar contribution of the job demand-control and job demand-control-support models?" *Journal of Occupational and Environmental Medicine* no. 53:185-189.

Martin, C. R., and R. J. Newell. 2005. "The factor structure of the 12-item General Health Questionnaire in individuals with facial disfigurement." *Journal of Psychosomatic Research* no. 59 (4):193-199. doi: S0022-3999(05)00386-7 [pii] 10.1016/j.jpsychores.2005.02.020.

Matthews, S., C. Power, and S.A. Stansfeld. 2001. "Psychological distress and work and home roles: a focus on socio-economic differences in distress." *Psychological Medicine* no. 31:725-736.

McDermut, J.F., D.A.F. Haaga, and L. Kirk. 2000. "An evaluation of stress symptoms associated with academic harassment." *Journal of Traumatic Stress* no. 13:397-411.

McDonough, P. 2000. "Job insecurity and health." *International Journal of Health Services* no. 30:453-476.

McDonough, P., and V. Walters. 2001. "Gender and health: reassessing patterns and explanations." *Social Science and Medicine* no. 52:547-559.

McDowell, I. 2006. *Measuring Health. A Guide to Rating Scales and Questionnaires* Third Edition ed. New York: Oxford University Press.

McKee-Ryan, F.M., Z. Song, C.R. Wanberg, and A.J. Kinicki. 2005. "Psychological and physical well-being during unemployment. A meta-analytic study." *Journal of Applied Psychology* no. 90:53-76.

Mirowsky, J., and C.E. Ross. 2002. "Selecting outcomes for the sociology of mental health: Issues of measurement and dimensionality." *Journal of Health and Social Behavior* no. 43:152-170.

Mitchell, C. M., and J. Beals. 2011. "The utility of the Kessler Screening Scale for psychological distress (K6) in two American Indian communities." *Psychological Assessment*:1-11. doi: 2011-08824-001 [pii] 10.1037/a0023288.

Mollica, R.F., N. Sarajic, M. Chernoff, J. Lavelle, I.S. Vukovic, and M.P. Massagli. 2001. "Longitudinal study of psychiatric symptoms, disability, mortality, and emigration among Bosnian refugees." *Journal fo the American Medical Association (JAMA)* no. 290:635-642.

Mollica, R.F., G. Wyshak, D. de Marneffe, F. Khuon, and J. Lavelle. 1987. "Indochinese versions of the Hopkins Symptom Checklist-25: A screening instrument for the psychiatric care of refugees. ." *American Journal of Psychiatry* no. 44:497-500.

Mueller, C.W., S. De Coster, and S.B. Estes. 2001. "Sexual harassment in the workplace. Unanticipated consequences of modern social control in organizations." *Work and Occupations* no. 28:411-446.

Murphy, G.C., and J.A. Athanasou. 1999. "The effect of unemployment on mental health." *Journal of Occupational and Organizational Psychology* no. 72:83-99.

Myer, L, DJ Stein, A Grimsrud, and al. 2008. "Social determinants of psychological distress in a nationally-representative sample of South African adults." *Social Science and Medicine* no. 66:1828-1840.

Myklestad, I., E. Roysamb, and K. Tambs. 2011. "Risk and protective factors for psychological distress among adolescents: a family study in the Nord-Trondelag Health Study." *Social Psychiatry and Psychiatric Epidemiology*. doi: 10.1007/s00127-011-0380-x.

Needham, B.L. 2007. "Gender differences in trajectories of depressive symptomatology and substance use during the transition from adolescence to young adulthood." *Social Science and Medecine* no. 65 (6):1166-1179.

Nemeroff, R., E. Midlarsky, and J. F. Meyer. 2010. "Relationships among social support, perceived control, and psychological distress in late life." *International Journal of Aging and Human Development* no. 71 (1):69-82.

Nerdrum, P, T Rustøen, and M. H Rønnestad. 2006. "Student Psychological Distress : A psychometric study of 1750 Norwegian 1st year undergraduate students." *Scandinavian Journal of Educational Research* no. 50:95-109.

Niedhammer, I., M. Goldberg, A. Leclerc, I. Bugel, and S. David. 1998. "Psychosocial factors at work and subsequent depressive symptoms in the Gazel cohort." *Scandinavian Journal of Work, Environment and Health* no. 24:197-205.

OConnor, D. W., and R. A. Parslow. 2010. "Mental health scales and psychiatric diagnoses: responses to GHQ-12, K-10 and CIDI across the lifespan." *Journal of Affective Disorders* no. 121 (3):263-267. doi: S0165-0327(09)00310-3 [pii] 10.1016/j.jad.2009.06.038.

Operario, D., J. Tschann, E. Flores, and M. Bridges. 2006. "Brief report: Associations of parental warmth, peer support, and gender with adolescent emotional distress." *Journal of Adolescence* no. 29:299-305.

Parker, G., and D. Hadzi-Pavlovic. 2004. "Is the female preponderance in major depression secondary to a gender difference in specific anxiety disorders?" *Psychological Medicine* no. 34:461-470.

Paterniti, S., I. Niedhammer, T. Lang, and S.M. Consoli. 2002. "Psychosocial factors at work, personality traits and depressive symptoms: Longitudinal results from the GAZEL Study." *British Journal of Psychiatry* no. 181:111-117.

Paul, C., S. Ayis, and S. Ebrahim. 2006. "Psychological distress, loneliness and disability in old age." *Psychology, Health and Medicine* no. 11 (2):221-232. doi: NKP4H48802610027 [pii] 10.1080/13548500500262945.

Payton, A.R. 2009. "Mental health, mental illness, and psychological distress: same continuum or distinct phenomena?" *Journal of health and Social Behavior* no. 50 (June):213-227.

Pearlin, L.I. 1989. "The sociological study of stress." *Journal of Health and Social Behavior* no. 30:241-256.

Pevalin, D.J. 2000. "Multiple applications of the GHQ-12 in a general population sample: an investigation of long-term retest effects." *Social Psychiatry and Psychiatric Epidemiology* no. 35:508-512.

Phillips, M.R. 2009. "Is distress a symptom of mental disorders, a marker of impairment, both or neither?" *World Psychiatry* no. 8:91-92.

Phongsavan, P., T. Chey, A. Bauman, R. Brooks, and D. Silove. 2006. "Social capital, socio-economic status and psychological distress among Australian adults." *Social Science and Medicine* no. 63 (10):2546-2561. doi: S0277-9536(06)00331-5 [pii] 10.1016/j.socscimed.2006.06.021.

Piotrkowski, C.S. 1998. "Gender harassment, job satisfaction, and distress among employed white and minority women." *Journal of Occupationnal Health Psychology* no. 3:33-43.

Pomaki, G., S. Maes, and L. Ter Doest. 2004. "Work conditions and employees' self-set goals: goal processes enhance prediction of psychological distress and well-being." *Personality and Social Psychology Bulletin* no. 30:685-694.

Prelow, H. M, S. R Weaver, R. R Swenson, and M. A Bowman. 2005. "A preliminary investigation of the validity and reliability of the Brief-Symptom Inventory-18 in economically disadvantaged Latina American mothers." *Journal of Community Psychology* no. 33:139-155.

Préville, M, R Hébert, G Bravo, and R Boyer. 2002. " Predisposing and facilitating factors of severe psychological distress among frail elderly." *Canadian Journal on Aging* no. 21 (1):195-204.

Richman, J.A., K.M. Rospenda, S.J. Nawyn, J.A. Flaherty, M. Fendrich, M.L. Drum, and T.P. Johnson. 1999. "Sexual harassment and generalized workplace abuse among university employees: Prevalence and mental health correlated." *American Journal of Public Health* no. 89:358-363.

Rickwood, D., and E.T. d'Espaignet. 1996. "Psychological distress among older adolescents and young adults in Australia." *Australian and New Zealand Journal of Public Health* no. 20:83-86.

Ridner, S.H. 2004. "Psychological distress: concept analysis." *Journal of Advanced Nursing* no. 45:536-545.

Ritsner, M, A Ponizovsky, and Y Ginath. 1999. "The effect of age on gender differences in the psychological distress ratings of immigrants." *Stress medicine* no. 15:17-25.

Rousseau, C., and A. Drapeau. 2004. "Premigration exposure to political violence among independent immigrants and its association with emotional distress." *Journal of Nervous and Mental Disease* no. 192 (12):852-856. doi: 00005053-200412000-00008 [pii].

Rugulies, R., U. Bultmann, B. Aust, and H. Burr. 2006. "Psychosocial work environment and incidence of severe depressive symptoms: prospective findings from a 5-year follow-up of the Danish Work Environment Cohort Study." *American Journal of Epidemiology* no. 163:877-887.

Sakurai, K., N. Kawakami, K. Yamaoka, H. Ishikawa, and H. Hashimoto. 2010. "The impact of subjective and objective social status on psychological distress among men and women in Japan." *Social Science and Medicine* no. 70 (11):1832-1829. doi: S0277-9536(10)00090-0 [pii] 10.1016/j.socscimed.2010.01.019.

Schieman, S., K. Van Gundy, and J. Taylor. 2001. "Status, role, and resource explanations for age patterns in psychological distress." *Journal of Health and Social Behavior* no. 42 (1):80-96.

Schulenberg, J.E., A.J. Sameroff, and D. Cicchetti. 2004. "The transition to adulthood as a critical juncture in the course of psychopathology and mental health." *Development and Psychopathology* no. 16:799-806.

Segopolo, M. T., M. M. Selemogwe, I. E. Plattner, N. Ketlogetswe, and A. Feinstein. 2009. "A screening instrument for psychological distress in Botswana: validation of the Setswana version of the 28-item General Health Questionnaire." *International Journal of Social Psychiatry* no. 55 (2):149-156. doi: 55/2/149 [pii] 10.1177/0020764008093448.

Sekine, M., T. Chandola, P. Martikainen, M. Marmot, and S. Kagamimori. 2006. "Socioeconomic inequalities in physical and mental functioning of Japanese civil servants: explanations from work and family characteristics." *Social Science and Medicine* no. 63:430-445.

Shevlin, M., and G. Adamson. 2005. "Alternative factor models and factorial invariance of the GHQ-12: a large sample analysis using confirmatory factor analysis." *Psychological Assessment* no. 17 (2):231-236. doi: 2005-07704-011 [pii] 10.1037/1040-3590.17.2.231.

Shiron, A., M. Westman, and S. Melamed. 1999. "The effects of pay systems on blue-collar employees' emotional distress: The mediating effects of objective and subjective work monotony." *Human Relations* no. 52:1077-1097.

Siegrist, J. 1996. "Adverse health effects of high-effort/low-reward conditions." *Journal of Occupationnal Health Psychology* no. 1:27-41.

Silove, D. 1999. "The psychosocial effects of torture, mass human rights violations, and refugee trauma: Toward an integrated conceptual framework." *Journal of Nervous & Mental Disease* no. 187:200-207.

Spurgeon, A., M.J. Harrington, and C.L. Cooper. 1997. "Health and safety problems associated with long working hours: a review of the current position." *Occupationnal and Environmental Medicine* no. 54:367-375.

Stafford, M., B.K. Newbold, and N.A. Ross. 2011. "Psychological distress among immigrants and visible minorities in Canada: a contextual analysis." *International Journal of Social Psychiatry* no. doi: 10.1177/0020764010365407

Stansfeld, S.A., R. Fuhrer, M.J. Shipley, and M.G. Marmot. 1999. "Work characteristics predict psychiatric disorder: prospective results from the Whitehall II study." *Occupationnal and Environmental Medicine* no. 56:302-307.

Stansfeld, S.A., J. Head, R. Fuhrer, J. Wardle, and V. Cattell. 2003. "Social inequalities in depressive symptoms and physical functioning in the Whitehall II study: exploring a common cause explanation." *Journal of Epidemiology and Community Health* no. 57:361-367.

Storksen, I., E. Roysamb, T.L. Holmen, and K. Tambs. 2006. "Adolescent adjustment and well-being: Effects of parental divorce and distress." *Scandinavian Journal of Psychology* no. 47:75-84.

Strand, B.H., O.S. Dalgard, K. Tambs, and M. Rognerud. 2003. "Measuring the mental health status of the Norwegian population: A comparison of the instruments SCL-25, SCL-10, SCL-5 and MHI-5 (SF-36." *Nordic Journal of Psychiatry* no. 57:113-118.

Sundquist, J, L Burfield-Bayard, LM Johansson, and al. 2000. "Impact of ethnicity, violence and acculturation on displaced migrants: psychological distress and psychosomatic complaints among refugees in Sweden." *Journal of Nervous and Mental Disease* no. 188:357-365.

Tambs, K., and T. Moum. 1993. "How well can a few questionnaire items indicate anxiety and depression?" *Acta Psychiatrica Scandinavia* no. 87 (5):364-367.

Tepper, B.J. 2000. "Consequences of abusive supervision." *Academy of Management Journal* no. 43:178-190.

Thapa, S. B., and E. Hauff. 2005. "Gender differences in factors associated with psychological distress among immigrants from low- and middle-income countries--findings from the Oslo Health Study." *Social Psychiatry and Psychiatric Epidemiology* no. 40 (1):78-84. doi: 10.1007/s00127-005-0855-8.

Thoits, P.A. 1991. "On merging identity theory and stress research." *Social Psychology Quarterly* no. 54:101-112.

Umberson, D., M.D. Chen, J.S. House, K. Hokins, and E. Slaten. 1996. "The effect of social relationships on psychological well-being: Are men and women really so different?" *American Sociological Review* no. 61:837-857.

Walters, V., P. McDonough, and L. Strohschein. 2002. "The influence of work, household structure, and social, personal and material resources on gender differences in health: an analysis of the 1994 Canadian National Population Health Survey." *Social Science and Medicine* no. 54:677-692.

Warr, P., and P. Jackson. 1987. "Adapting to the unemployed role: A longitudinal investigation." *Social Science and Medicine* no. 25:1219-1224.

Watson, D. 2009. "Differentiating the mood and anxiety disorders: A quadripartite model." *Annual Review of Clinical Psychology* no. 5:221-247.

Westermeyer, J., and A. Janca. 1997. "Language, culture and psychopathology: Conceptual and methodological issues." *Transcultural Psychiatry* no. 34:291-311.

Wheaton, B. 2007. "The twain meets: distress, disorder and the continuing conundrum of categories (comment on Horwitz)." *Health* no. 11:303-319.

Wiesner, M., V. Chen, M. Windle, M. N. Elliott, J. A. Grunbaum, D. E. Kanouse, and M. A. Schuster. 2010. "Factor structure and psychometric properties of the Brief Symptom Inventory-18 in women: a MACS approach to testing for invariance across racial/ethnic groups." *Psychological Assessment* no. 22 (4):912-922. doi: 2010-24850-007 [pii] 10.1037/a0020704.

Wilkinson-Lee, A. M., Q. Zhang, V. L. Nuno, and M. S. Wilhelm. 2011. "Adolescent emotional distress: the role of family obligations and school connectedness." *Journal of Youth and Adolescence* no. 40 (2):221-230. doi: 10.1007/s10964-009-9494-9.

Yip, T., G. C. Gee, and D. T. Takeuchi. 2008. "Racial discrimination and psychological distress: the impact of ethnic identity and age among immigrant and United States-born Asian adults." *Developmental Psychology* no. 44 (3):787-800. doi: 2008-05171-013 [pii] 10.1037/0012-1649.44.3.787.

Ystgaard, M., K. Tambs, and O. S. Dalgard. 1999. "Life stress, social support and psychological distress in late adolescence: a longitudinal study." *Social Psychiatry and Psychiatric Epidemiology* no. 34 (1):12-19.

Zabora, J., K. Brintzenhofeszoc, B. Curbow, C. Hooker, and S. Piantadosi. 2001. "The prevalence of psychological distress by cancer site." *Psycho-Oncology* no. 10:19-28.

5

Culture, Psychiatry and Cultural Competence

Arabinda Narayan Chowdhury
Northamptonshire Healthcare NHS Foundation Trust,
Stuart Road Resource Centre, Corby, Northants NN17 1RJ
UK

1. Introduction

Why the study of culture and its clinical application is important in mental health training and service? Mental health and illness is a set of subjective experience and a social process and thus involves a practice of culture-congruent care. Series of anthropological, sociological and cross-cultural research has clearly demonstrated a very strong ground in favour of this contention.

An individual's cultural background colours every facets of illness, from linguistic or emotional expression (Helman, 2007; Lewis-Fernandez, 1996) to the content of somatic complaints (Goldber & Bridges, 1988) and delusional (Yip, 2003) or hallucinatory experiences (Kim, 2006; Cowen, 2011). Cause, course and outcome of major psychiatric disorders are influenced by cultural factors (Kleinman, 1988; Kirmayer, 2001; Littlewood & Lipsedge, 1997). Wide variations in the prevalence of many psychiatric disorders across geographic regions and ethnocultural groups have been documented (Maercker, 2001). In mental health, dysfunctional behaviour is a key issue in diagnosis, viz. distinction from normal to disordered behaviour. The social and cultural context here is important because identification of abnormal dysfunctional behaviour is basically a social judgement (Kirmayer & Young, 1999). Different cultural and ethnic groups have different perception and practices about health as per their ecocultural adaptation (Weisner, 2002). Social and cultural factors are major determinants of the use of health care services and alternative sources of help. Recent changing global demography demands the recognition and response to cultural diversity in psychiatric practice (intercultural clinical work). Culturally based attitudes and assumptions direct the perspectives that both patient and clinicians constantly encounter in therapeutic communications (Moffic, 1983).

Ethnicity, ethno-cultural identity, social class, cultural dimension of gender, cultural explanation and meaning of sufferings or illness, cultural codes of expression of distress, cultural value system and support network, cultural belief about religion and spirituality, cultural specificity in coping mechanism and ways of inter-cultural assimilation are the few broad issues in cultural psychiatry that helps to understand the clinical manifestation of psychopathology. Lack of awareness of important cultural differences can undermine the development of a therapeutic alliance and the negotiations and delivery of effective treatment. Following is a brief discussion on three important issues, viz. relationship between culture and mental health, cultural competence and cross-cultural communication and lastly the outline of cultural formulation in clinical assessment.

2. Cultural psychiatry

"Psychiatry may outline a science of the psyche and its disturbances but it also reflects a cultural interpretation about personal experience, responsibility, social behaviour, and the requirements for social order. The cultural character of the psychiatric enterprise itself, just as much as the characteristics of its disorders, constitute the subject matter of cultural psychiatry" (Fabrega, 2001).

2.1 Cultural psychiatry: Definition and concept

It is a special field of psychiatry concerned with the cultural aspects of human behaviour, mental health, psychopathology and treatment (APA, 1969). Alarcon (2009) puts it as: "Cultural psychiatry deals with the description, definition, assessment, and management of all psychiatric conditions, inasmuch as they reflect and are subjected to the patterning influence of cultural factors. It uses concepts and instruments from the social and biological sciences, to advance a full understanding of psychopathological events and their management by patients, families, professionals and the community at large." Within the framework of bio-psych-socio-cultural paradigm in psychiatry, cultural psychiatry is mainly focused on socio-cultural aspects of human behaviour. Tseng (2001) proposes three levels of approach: **Clinical level:** that aims to promote culturally competent mental health care for patients of diverse ethnic and cultural backgrounds, viz., culturally relevant assessment and culturally appropriate care. **Research level:** is the exploration of how ethnic or cultural factors influence behaviour and psychopathology as well as the process of healing (ethnopharmacology) and at **Theoretical level:** aims to expand our knowledge of human behaviour and mental problems transculturally to facilitate the development of more universally applicable and cross-culturally valid theories of psychopathlogy.

Recent advances in medical sociology, psychiatric anthropology and cross-cultural psychology make the domain of cultural psychiatry more broad and challenging (Kelly, 2010; Al-Issa, 1995). Following are the few issues of clinical importance from the trans-cultural point of view: Personality-culture interaction, psychosocial conflicts and problems related to rapid social change, attitudes and beliefs towards behavioural deviance in changing societies, multicultural communication styles, assessment of stress and cultural variation of coping and resilience, cultural change and psychic adaptation in the era of globalization and migration, technological advancement in communication and media, ecological changes and its impact on mental health, cultural principles in psychiatric diagnosis, clinical guidelines in cross-cultural mental health assessments, applications of therapeutic techniques to various ethnic groups, ethnopsychopharmacology and alternative (ethnobotany) or folk care, cultural determinants of public health policy, and the cultural implications of the new managed care approaches in the service delivery.

2.2 What is culture?

Culture is defined as a set of behavioural norms, meanings, and values or reference points utilized by members of a particular society to construct their unique view of the world, and ascertain their identity. It includes a number of variables such as language, traditions, values, rituals, customs, etiquette, taboos or laws, religious beliefs, moral standards and practices, gender and sexual orientation, and socio-economic status (GAP, 2002). All these issues are reflected in cultural products like common sayings, legends and folk lore, drama, plays, art, philosophical thoughts and religious faith (Tseng & Strelzer, 2006). So, Culture is **learned** through active teaching, and passive acting, **shared** among its group members, **patterned** as having definite sets of beliefs and practices that guide different areas of individual and social life, **adaptive,** through change across variable environments and **symbolic** with many arbitrary signs that represent something special to the group. Culture is learned by the process of *enculturation* and is *transmitted* from generation to generation through family units and social environments. Culture operates at two levels: at the macroscopic level it represents the social and institutional pattern of a society at large and at the microscopic level it influences the individual thinking and behaviour, both consciously and unconsciously.

2.3 Various experiences with the cultural system

A **cultural system** may be defined as the interaction of different elements of culture with the individual or groups. It is a dynamic process and different from social system. Sometimes both systems together are referred as socio-cultural system.

Enculturation, an anthropological term, is the process by which a person learns the requirements of his/her own culture, and acquires values and behaviours that are appropriate or necessary in that culture (Grusec & Hastings, 2007). The process of enculturation is related to socialization. Enculturation is operative through child-rearing patterns, language development, and institutionalized education and through different abiding social systems. It is a learning process through introjections and absorption of value systems from parents, family members, neighbors, friends, school, social evens, traditional literature and media.

Acculturation: is a process in which members of one cultural group adopting the cultural traits or social patterns of another group. Acculturation is an important process of cultural change in immigrated population (Berry, 1997) and influences their mental health (Bhui et al., 2005).

Acculturative Stress: It refers to the psychological, somatic, and social difficulties that may accompany acculturation processes. This was first described by Redfield et al. (1936) as, "psychic conflict" that may arise from conflicting cultural norms. Acculturative adaptation to a new culture is a complex and dynamic process whereby individuals continuously negotiate among accepting, adapting to, or denying the characteristics of a majority culture, as well as retaining, changing, or rejecting certain components of their own culture. This involves serious changes in multiple areas of functioning (e.g., values, behaviours, beliefs, attitudes, etiquette, moral judgement etc.), and for individuals, families, and groups engaged in this process, these adjustments are often experienced as stressful. The nature of familiarity and length of exposure to the new culture are important risk variables for the acculturative stress.

Assimilation: is the process whereby a minority group gradually adapts to the customs and values of the prevailing culture. It is a two-way process – firstly, an individual or a group of diverse ethnic and racial minority or immigrant individuals comes to adopt the beliefs, values, attitudes, and the behaviours of the majority or dominant culture and secondly, at the same time, they relinquishes the value system of their cultural tradition and becomes a member of the dominant society. Assimilation is a slow and a gradual process. The term has political and social implications also. *Assimilation Index* tells us how a migrant has assimilated (with the host culture) so that he/she is no longer seemed to be an immigrant. Vigdor (2008), from Manhattan Institute for Policy Research , uses Assimilation Index value that can distinguish immigrants from U.S. natives, calculated on the basis of economic (employment, occupations, education, homeownership); cultural (ability to speak English, marriage to natives, number of children) and civic (naturalization, military service) information.

Cultural identity: is the identity of a group or culture or of an individual as far as one is influenced by one's belonging to a group or culture. The usual cultural identifiers are place, gender, history, nationality, ethnicity, language, religious faith, and aesthetics. Recognition of cultural identity is important for a culture-fare mental health care (Groen, 2009; Kent & Bhui, 2003).

Deculturation or Cultural Uprooting: Deculturation results when members of nondominant cultures become alienated (either by accident or by force) from the dominant culture and from their own minority society (Berry & Sam, 1980). As the deculturation is the loss of one's traditional culture without integration into a new culture so it is like a tree that has lost its roots- so called uprooting and there is a culture loss without replacement. The consequence of deculturation may results in increased stress and psychopathology (Cheetham et al., 1983) and cultural bereavement (Bhugra & Becker, 2005).

Cultural diffusion: is the spreading of ideas or products from one culture to another. This concept was first introduced by Krober (1940). There are three categories of cultural diffusion: *Direct diffusion* is when two cultures are very close to each other, resulting in intermarriage, trade, and even warfare. *Forced diffusion* occurs when one culture subjugates (conquers or enslaves) another culture and forces its own customs on the conquered people. Colonisation is the unique example. The term *Ethnocentrism* or *Cultural imperialism* is often applied to forced diffusion. *Indirect diffusion* is when cultural ideas are spread through a middleman or even another culture (e.g. spread of fast food MacDonald culture in Middle East). Recently, by technological advancements, media, TV, movies, culture may be transmitted to people far away without any direct contact.

Diaspora: is the movement, migration, or scattering of people away from an established or ancestral homeland .The term *Diaspora* carries a sense of displacement and a sense of hidden hope or desire to return to homeland. Safran (1991) described six criteria of Diasporas from migrant communities: the group maintains a myth or collective memory of their homeland; they regard their ancestral homeland as their true home, to which they will eventually return; being committed to the restoration or maintenance of that homeland; and they relate their identity with the culture of their homeland.

Cultural Paranoia: The concept was introduced by Grier & Cobbs (1968) in their book 'Black Rage', where they said that Black clients may not disclose personal information to White therapists for fear that they may be vulnerable to racial discrimination and this condition was regarded not a form of psychopathology but a healthy and adaptive response by African Americans towards the white Americans. This concept was further elaborated by Ridley (1984) but challenged by others (Homer & Ashby, 1986, Bronstein, 1986). Culture deeply influence our cognitive reference, perceptual experiences and belief system and thus have strong influence on persecutory ideas, shared delusions (Sen & Chowdhury, 2006) and even treatment seeking and hospitalization (Whaley, 2004).

Cultural Mistrust: It "involves the inclination among blacks to mistrust whites, with mistrust most evident in the areas of education and training, business and work, interpersonal and social relations, politics and law" (Terrell & Terrell, 1981). It may pose a great obstacle to health service delivery (Cort, 2004).

Culture shock: is the difficulty people have adjusting to a new culture that differs markedly from their own, usually occurs during visiting a new place or during a short-term sojourn (international students). Thorough phases of initial excitement and then negotiation and adjustment, people usually master the new environment. There are many symptoms and signs of culture shock, including general unease with new situations, irrational fears, difficulty with sleeping, feeling sick, anxiety and depression, preoccupation with health, and homesickness (Oberg, 1960). *Cultural confusion* results from a growing lack of consensus about what is proper or appropriate in a given circumstances. It is the initial phase of culture shock when people become confused, tired and disoriented in a new foreign environment.

Cultural Accommodation: It is the process by which individuals may take on values and beliefs of the host culture and accommodate them in the public sphere, while maintaining the parent culture in the private sphere.

Cultural Negotiation: It is an adjustment process that takes place at individual, interpersonal, and systemic levels. It occurs when individuals (e.g., adjusting immigrants in a new society or bicultural individuals having two cultural backgrounds) navigate diverse settings (e.g., school, home, work, community) and shift their identities and values depending on the norms of each environment. This allows individuals to fulfil differing expectations, obligations, and roles and to maintain relationships inside and outside their own cultural communities. Cultural negotiation helps to balance differing value systems, familial and community expectations, peer relationships, and identities.

Cultural Equivalence: Cultural equivalence is the term used in research methodology that is used to minimize the cultural bias and measurement error in the development and/or adaptation of assessment tools (Vandevijver & Tanzer, 2004). Five dimensions (conceptual, content, linguistic, technical, and normative equivalencies) are important and to be used to minimize measurement error in cross cultural applications.

2.4 Some useful concepts in cultural psychiatry

Race: Old concept of geographical race is now abandoned. Race is a socially and culturally constructed category not a biological validity. It is now believed that inequalities between racial groups are not consequences of biological inheritance but rather products of historical and contemporary social, economic, educational and political circumstances (AAA, 1999).

Ethnicity: It refers to social group of people whose members identify with each other from other groups by a common historical path, behaviour-norms and their own mark of group identities. The group members share a common language, religion, and a sense of a historical continuity of traditions and root culture. Ethnic variations of disease prevalence and ethnic health inequalities are important issues in mental health.

Minority: A racial, religious, political, national, or other group (relatively small) thought to be different from the larger group in a society. The status of a minority may be acquired by: (a) Native people after they have been invaded, taken over or destroyed by militarily, technologically or economically superior outsiders- the whole range of colonization is the example, e.g., .Native Americans in North America, native aborigines in Australia and Canada. (b) Racial background and historical path of migration to a host country - African-Americans in USA/ East Indians in Europe/ Tibetans in India. (c) Ethnic origin- like Hutterite in USA or Dalits in India and (d) Religious affiliation- Muslims in India/Hindus in Bangladesh.

Society: Composed of a large social grouping that shares the same geographical or virtual territory, subject to the same political authority and dominant cultural expectations and organized by an administrative structure and regulated by certain rules or systems. Several cultures or subcultures may exist within a single society.

Subculture: A cultural group within a larger culture, often having beliefs or interests at variance with those of the larger culture. The smaller subcultures usually have the same racial background as the majority group, but they choose to have distinctly different sets of beliefs, value systems and life style. E.g. Amish in USA. In mental health the term often used with different connotations likes drug subculture, criminal subculture, urban subculture or youth subculture etc.

Social Class: refers to the social stratification in a society. Sociologists use *Socio-Economic-Status (SES)* that includes variables like education, occupation and income. In mental health, social class is considered primarily the product of the perceptions and beliefs held by people in different subgroups in a society like upper class, middle working class and lower class, which are associated with certain lifestyles, values and ethics. An extreme example is the caste system in India. These classes seldom changes radically but SES is changeable across the social ladder.

Primary Cultural Characteristics: things that a person cannot easily change, but if they do, a stigma may occur for themselves, their families or society. It includes nationality, race, colour, gender, age and religious affiliation.

Secondary Cultural Characteristics: includes educational status, SES, occupation, political beliefs, urban vs. rural residence, enclave identity, sexual orientation, gender issues, marital status, parental status, length of time away from the country of origin, migration status.

Worldview: the way individuals or groups look at the universe to form basic assumptions and values about their lives and world around them. It is the fundamental cognitive orientation of an individual or a society involving philosophy, cosmology, relationship with nature, existential meaning, moral and ethical reasoning, social relationships, magico-religious beliefs, values, emotions and ethics (Palmer, 1996).

Cultural Relativism: The concept of cultural relativism was first postulated by the German-American anthropologist Franz Boas (1858- 1942) in 1887 and later the term was coined by Alain LeRoy Locke (1885-1954), an American philosopher in 1924. Cultural relativism maintains the view that all cultures are equal in value and therefore should not be judged on the basis of another cultural perspective. It supports the belief that mental health should be understood through the context of normative behaviour within a specific culture. Proponents argue that issues like abortion, euthanasia, female circumcision and physical punishment in child rearing should be accepted as cultural practice without judgement from the outside world. Opponents argue that cultural relativism may undermine condemnation of human right violations, and family violence cannot be justified or excused on a cultural basis. There is some ongoing debate between universalistic and relativistic opinions about how cultures influence the manifestation of mental illness. According to the universalistic view the core psychiatric disorders are universal and what may vary across cultures are the symptomatic manifestation of the disorder or the threshold of labelling pathological versus normal behaviour.

Cultural diversity: encompasses the cultural differences that exist between people, such as language, dress and traditions, and the way societies organize themselves, their conception of morality and religion, and the way they interact with the environment. The Universal

Declaration on Cultural Diversity was adopted by UNESCO (2001) and declared cultural diversity as "common heritage of humanity", where the main focuses are: (a) the diversity of people's backgrounds and circumstances is appreciated and valued, (b) similar life opportunities are available to all, and (c) strong and positive relationships exist and continue to be developed in the workplace, in schools and in the wider community and society. Careful and ethical consideration of cultural diversity is a key issue in mental health because it aims to integrate cultural awareness, and cultural sensitivity into clinical practice and training, which have impacts on the quality of mental health service provision to individuals from minority ethnic communities (Bhui & Bhugra, 2002a). In this era of globalization and interconnected world we are living in a multicultural society and thus the core principle of mental health today is the unity within diversity (Brody, 2001).

2.5 Some key issues in cultural psychiatry

Following are the few important socio-anthropological issues, that mental health professionals should have in his/her mind during the cultural history taking in cross-cultural context.

Cultural variations of Family Systems: Family system functions as a unit, and every family member plays a unique role in the system. So change in any one member of the system will influence, by a ripple effect, the whole family system. Issues like kinship system, family structure, primary axis, interpersonal-dynamics, one-parent family, and family violence are important psychologically. Family organization (extended/nuclear) and relational roles (patriarchal or matriarchal systems) vary across cultural or subcultural groups.

Child development and enculturation process: upbringing process, cultural rituals and ethics in child rearing, gender-based customs, schooling, childhood trauma or abuse- all have significant impact on personality development.

Marriage system: gender role, its cultural meaning and responsibilities, socio-cultural implication of bride wealth or dowry system.

Culture and Personality development: socio-cultural environment, acquisition of values, beliefs and expectations, development of emotionality in the socialization process.

Social Customs: habitual ways of behaving carried out by tradition and enforced by social sanctions- customs relating to exposure of body parts, food choices, sexuality, substance abuse/ drinking, social interaction and restrictions etc.

Rituals: is a set of actions, performed mainly for their symbolic value, e.g., traditional practice of certain sets of or prescribed ceremonies like rituals with birth, puberty, wedding and death. In some cultures there are varieties of health rituals exists.

Etiquette: refers to the code of expected social behavior according to conventional norm within a society or a group, same as 'manners' in social interactions. To know the etiquette of a target culture is beneficial in cross-cultural communication.

Taboos: a social prohibition or restriction on certain things or behaviour, breaking of which is socially unacceptable because of the belief that it might result in ill effect. In every culture there are some superstitious beliefs and set rules of avoidance of some behaviours or objects.

Culture and Gender: Gender refers to the ways in which cultures differentiate and define roles based on biological sex and reproductive functions. Men and women do have some fundamentally different experiences of their bodies, of their social worlds and of their life course. There are also important gender differences in styles of emotional expression, symptom experience, social expectations and help seeking. Gender equality and freedom differs from culture to culture. In mental health, gender difference influence rates of common mental disorders, there are gender specific risk factors and gender bias occurs in the treatment of mental illness (WHO, 2011; Emslie et al., 2002).

Attitudes and views about ageing: in some culture aged persons are more respected and listen to, have role in decision making, aged persons are more vulnerable to neglect and exploitation, have less access to health care.

Beliefs about health-illness-healing: beliefs in bad deed or *karma*/ancestral or God's punishment/ evil eye or sorcery / witchcraft/ possession/ supernatural force may influence illness experience and help seeking. In some cultures there may be strong resistance to blood transfusion or blood tests. Culture strongly influences illness beliefs and thus enhances 'psychic infectivity' in some psychiatric epidemics (Chowdhury, 1992a). Ethnomedicine or the study of cross-cultural health system (Banerjee & Jalota, 1988) is one of the central topics in cultural psychiatry.

Views about Birth, Death and Mourning: influence emotional reactions, grief and bereavement. Numerous cultural rituals involve the phenomenon of death. Some of these rituals may preclude the conduct of an autopsy.

Value system: Values are powerful drivers of how we think and behave. Values are a significant element of culture, where they form a part of the shared rule- set of a group. If someone transgresses other's value it may lead to betrayal responses (distress, loss of trust and seeking justice). Health professionals should be cautious of the values in practice. There are many categories of value like personal, social, political, economic and religious.

Idioms of Distress: Culture heavily influences how people understand and respond to distressing events. Distress is not expressed in the same way in all cultures or communities. In some culture distress is expressed by 'somatisation': people complain of physical symptoms which are mainly caused by emotional or mental worry, anxiety, or stress. The term 'idioms of distress' has been used to describe specific illnesses that occur in some societies and are recognized only by members of those societies as expressions of distress. A good example is the term 'nerve' which is used in many societies to designate both physical pain and emotional discomfort and is clinically presented with bodily pain, fatigue, insomnia or feelings of sadness, tension, and weepiness (Scheper-Hughes, 1992).

Disease and Illness: Disease, a biological construct, represents all the manifestations of ill health in response to some pathological process and is translated into nosological descriptions of signs/symptoms under medical framework. Illness, a socio-cultural construct, having a symbolic nature, and primarily represented by the subjective, emotional, behavioural, interpretative and communicative responses of the affected individual (Eisenberg, 1977). Cultural explanation and ethnomedical worldview influence the perception of illness and health, healing (Boyd, 2000) and sick role and illness behaviour (Chowdhury & Dobson, 2002).

Explanatory Model of Illness (EMI): Patient's illness beliefs influence their symptom formation and degree of disability (Fig.1). Klienman (1992) suggested that by exploring the *explanatory model* of illness we can better understand our patients and families: "Explanatory Models are the notions about an Episode of sickness and its treatment that is employed by all those engaged in the clinical process." He provided a very simple 'What, Why, How and Who' questions to elicit patient's explanation about illness (Box 1). Weiss (1997) further developed this into different clinical sets of Explanatory Model Interview Catalogue for different cultural and clinical groups across different countries. Explanatory model is a very useful clinical tool not only in mental health assessment (Bhui & Bhugra, 2002b; McCabe & Priebe, 2004) but also in other areas of medicine (Ross et al., 2002; Hallenbeck, 2003).

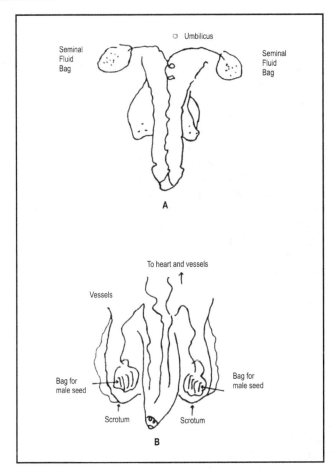

Fig. 1. *Body-heat* **explanatory model of Indian Koro patients** (Chowdhury, 2008). Increased body heat was implicated for the sudden 'pulling-in' of the penis. A. Drawing by a 22 year boy with Dhat syndrome - showing the *penile pull* was active from both the seminal fluid bag in the abdomen. B. Drawing by a 34 year male school teacher with Scrotal Filaria – showing that the *pulling force* was operative from the heart

2.6 Culture and psychopathology

How does Culture relate to Psychopathology? Tseng (2003) provides a very practical clinical construct about how culture influence psychopathology. He provided seven types of effects as follows:

2.6.1 Pathogenic Effects: refers to situations where culture is a direct causative factor in forming or generating psychopathology, e.g. *stress* can be created by culturally formed anxiety, culturally demanded performance or culturally prescribed roles and duties. So culture is considered to be a causative factor, because culture-specific beliefs and ideas contribute directly to the formation of particular stress inducing certain type of psychopathology. Culture-Bound Syndromes are the example.

Culture Bound Syndromes (CBS)

Culture-bound or culture-specific syndromes cover an extensive range of disorders occurring in particular cultural communities or ethnic groups. The behavioural manifestations or subjective experiences particular to these disorders may or may not correspond to diagnostic categories in DSM-IV-TR or ICD-10. They are usually considered to be illnesses and generally have local names. They also include culturally accepted idioms or explanatory mechanisms of illness that differ from Western idioms. There is some conceptual confusion with the term 'Culture-bound'. In the widest sense everything is culture-bound. Here the word 'bound' implicates that the symptoms describe is confined to one specific culture, but in reality they may be found in multiple cultures (may be by different name). So Levine and Gaw (1995) suggested more precise term for CBS as "folk diagnostic categories". Some researchers, in a wider sense, debated the Eurocentric role of culture-boundness even with cultural psychiatry in the global context (Jadav, 2004).

Awareness of culture-bound syndromes is important to help psychiatrists and physicians to make culturally appropriate diagnoses (Chowdhury et al., 2003). The concept is also interesting to medical and psychiatric anthropologists because the culture-bound syndromes provide examples of how culturally salient symptoms can be elaborated into illness experiences. CBS was included in the fourth version of Diagnostic and Statistical Manual (APA, 1994) and provided symptomatic descriptions of 25 culture-bound syndromes in the Glossary of Culture-Bound Syndromes in appendix I (Table 1). Simons and Hughes (1985) provided a comprehensive list and description of CBS as reported globally. Though CBS is mainly implicated to non-Western cultures but in recent years, there is increased recognition by cultural psychiatrists of syndromes in western culture (Littlewood, 2002) that are heavily culture-related like anorexia nervosa (Swaptz, 1985); obesity (Ritenbaugh, 1982), drug-induced dissociative states, multiple personality or personality disorders (Alarcon et al., 1998) and premenstrual tension syndrome (Johnson, 1987).

Guarnaccia and Rogler (1999) provided a set of four key questions for clinical analysis of CBS in the context of culture and psychopathology. These are:

1. *Nature of the phenomenon?* The character of CBS in the context of a given culture and what are the defining features of the phenomenon?
2. *Location in the social context:* who are affected? What is the social structural location and who are at risk or any situational trigger?
3. *Relationship to Psychiatric Disorder:* Empirical relation of CBS with designated psychiatric disorder? Any comorbid psychiatric disorder? The CBSs often coexist with other psychiatric disorder, as many psychiatric disorders do with each other. Delineation of comorbidity factor will in help in clinical decision making.
   Example: Epidemiological study in Puerto Rico (Guarnaccia et al., 1993) showed high rate of psychiatric disorder among those reporting ataque de nervios (63% vs. 28% of the sample) - 3.5 times more likely to meet criteria for an anxiety disorder and 2.75 times more likely to meet the criteria for an affective disorder than those who had not reported an attack de nervios.
4. *Different comorbidities:* Difference in the symptomatic, emotional and contextual aspects of cultural syndromes, may show different subtypes of the designated psychiatric disorder.
   Example: Koro or genital retraction syndrome has offered a unique opportunity to study comorbidity in CBS, as over the years Koro has been reported from diverse culture and ethnicity (Chowdhury, 1996; 1998). For example: Koro with high sex guilt and

depressive reaction (Chowdhury, 1992b, Chowdhury & Rajbhandari, 1995) or with heightened sexual anxiety and anxiety disorder (Chowdhury, 1990) or with hypersuggestability and hysterical reaction (Chowdhury, 1994a) and even sometimes with medical comorbidities (Chowdhury, 1989; Puranik & Dunn, 1995).

Name (Geographical/cultural location)	Presentation
Amok (Malaysia, Indonesia, Philippines, Brunei, Singapore)	Dissociative episode- violent and homicidal behaviour, usually preceded by brooding over real or imagined insults.
Ataque de nervios (Nervous attack) (Latin-America)	Brief, intense release of emotion believed to be caused by family conflict or anger.
Bilis (Rage)	Outburst of anger.
Boufée deliriante (West Africa and Haiti)	Outburst of agitated, aggressive behaviour, marked confusion, psychomotor excitement, often with visual and auditory hallucinations or paranoid ideation.
Brain fag or brain fog (West Africa)	Usually among high school or university students. Symptoms: difficulties in concentrating, remembering, and thinking.
Dhat syndrome (Indian subcontinent)	Sexual/ general weakness due to loss of semen through urine or faeces.
Falling out/blacking out (Southern USA, Caribbean)	Episodes of sudden collapse and fainting, often with hysterical blindness.
Ghost sickness American Indian (Novajo)	A syndrome, associated with dead or dying, attributed to ghosts (chindi) or witchcraft. Symptoms are general weakness, loss of appetite, feeling of suffocation, recurring nightmares and a pervasive feeling of terror.
Hwa-byung (Anger sickness) (Korea)	Epigastric pain, usually female, shortness of breath, flushing, indigestion, palpitations, vomiting, cold hands, dysphoria from an imagined abdominal mass, thought to be caused by suppressed or unresolved anger, disappointment or grudges.
Koro (China, Malaysia, India, SEA)	Acute fear- genitalia will retract into the body (also breast into the chest in female), causing death.
Latah (Malaysia, Indonesia)	Hypersensitivity to sudden fright, often with echopraxia, echolalia, command obedience, and dissociative or trancelike behaviour.
Locura (Latinos in USA/ Latin America)	Chronic psychosis with incoherence, agitation, auditory and visual hallucinations, inability to follow rules of social interaction, and possible violence- attributed to an inherited vulnerability or life adversities.
Mal-de-ojo (Evil eye) (Mediterranean, Hispanic)	A common idiom of disease, attributed to any misfortune, and social disruption.
Nervios (Latinos in USA/ Latin	Refers to a general state of vulnerability to stressful life experiences and difficult life circumstances. A wide range of symptoms: emotional distress, somatic disturbance,

Name (Geographical/cultural location)	Presentation
America)	and inability to function. Common symptoms: headaches, brain aches, irritability, stomach disturbances, sleep difficulties, nervousness, easy tearfulness, inability to concentrate, trembling, tingling sensations, and mareos (dizziness with occasional vertigo-like exacerbation).
Pibloktoq (Arctic hysteria) (Arctic circle, Inuhuit Eskimos)	Symptoms: hysterical (screaming, uncontrolled wild behaviour), depression, coprophagia, echolalia, insensivity to extreme cold. Common in winter and among women.
Gi-gong (Psychotic reaction) (China)	An acute, time-limited episode characterized by dissociative, paranoid, or other psychotic or nonpsychotic symptoms that occur after participating in the Chinese folk health-enhancing practice of *qi-gong*.
Rootwork (African American, Caribbean, White population in Southern USA)	Cultural interpretations that explain illness as the result of hexing, witchcraft, voodoo, or the influence of an evil person.
Sangue dormido (Portuguese in Cape Verde)	Literally "sleeping blood" with symptoms of pain, numbness, tremor, paralysis, convulsions, stroke, blindness, heart attack, infection, and miscarriage.
Shenjang shuairuo (Neurasthenia) (India, China)	Mental and physical fatigue, poor concentration and memory, headache, dizziness, changes in sleep, appetite, sexual function.
Shen kui (China)	Anxiety, panic and sexual complaints with no physical findings, attributed to loss of semen or 'vital essence'.
Shin-byung (Korea)	A syndrome characterized by anxiety and somatic complaints like general weakness, dizziness, fear, loss of appetite, insomnia, and gastrointestinal problems, followed by dissociation and possession by ancestral spirits.
Spell (African American, White population in Southern USA)	A trance state in which individuals "communicate" with deceased relatives or with spirits.
Susto (Latinos in USA, Mexico, Central America, South America)	Attributed to an illness precipitated after a frightening event that causes the soul to leave the body, leading to symptoms of unhappiness and sickness.
Taijin Kyofusho (Social phobia) (Japan)	Guilt about embarrassing others- an intense fear that one's body, body parts, or bodily functions are displeasing, embarrassing, or offensive to other people.
Zar (Ethiopia, Somalia, Egypt, Sudan, Iran, and Middle East)	Experience of spirit possession- presented with dissociative episodes with laughing, shouting, hitting the head against a wall, singing, or weeping.

Table 1. DSM IV (2000) list of some common CBSs (Trujillo, 2008; Hall, 2008)

2.6.2 Pathoselective Effects: cultural choice to stress reaction that shapes the nature of psychopathology, e.g., Running amok in Malaysia, familial suicide in some cultures.

2.6.3 Pathoplastic Effects: the ways in which culture contributes to modeling or plastering of the manifestation of psychopathology- this acts in two ways: *Shaping the content of the symptoms*: content of delusions, hallucinations, obsessions or phobias is subject to psychosocial context in which the pathology is reported. *Modeling the clinical picture as a whole* - Taijin-kuofu-sho in Japan and Brain fag syndrome in Nigeria. Culture plays a pathoplastic role in some psychiatric epidemics also (Chowdhury et al., 1993).

2.6.4 Pathoelaborating Effects: Certain behaviours (either normal or pathological) may become exaggerated to the extreme by *cultural reinforcement*: Latah in Malaysia is being utilized by people for social amusement; *hara-kiri* – formal way of suicide by a soldier in Japan to avoid capture or humiliation by enemy is an honourable way of ending one's life. Verbal insult for non-payment of loan may be a justified reason for attempting self-harm in some Asian communities. Cultural notion of body-image/ shape, diet and body weight regulation to an extreme degree are good example of this category in recent health-conscious and commercially driven urban culture.

2.6.5 Pathofacilitative Effects: Many psychiatric disorders are intimately tied to psychological and sociocultural variables in their development, e.g., suicidal behaviour (Chowdhury, 2002), alcoholism (Chowdhury et al., 2006), and substance abuse, e.g., initial social tolerance towards involvement of unemployed youths in drug trafficking activities resulted in high incidence of heroin dependence and HIV infection in Monipore, India (Chowdhury, 1994b).

2.6.6 Pathodiscriminating Effects: Sociocultural labeling of behaviour as normal or abnormal- several mental conditions or behaviours, e.g., personality disorder, sexual deviation and substance abuse are accepted or rejected as per the social discrimination according to cultural factors.

2.6.7 Pathoreactive Effects: Culture influences how people label a disorder and how they emotionally react to it. Prognosis of schizophrenia is better in less developed, rural, farming societies than industrialized nations. The social environment, attitudes of family and community determine how well the person will rehabilitate into social and family life, thus affecting the prognosis. Excessive and often overrepresentation of risk from mental patients in the media and the public reaction thereof (stigmatizing mental patients) in the Western world is a good example of this category (BBC, 1999; Edney, 2004).

3. Cultural competency in health care

All our clinical interactions take place in the context of culture. Culture always matters in health care, if the culture is ignored or overlooked, individuals and families are at risk of not getting the required support, or worse yet, receiving service that is more harmful than helpful.

3.1 Culture gives context and meaning of symptom or distress
Culture is a filter through which people process their understanding, experiences and impact of life events. Culture influences people's values, actions, and expectations of

themselves and of others and thus influence their behaviour. Culture provides the world-view about health, healing, and wellness beliefs- both to clients and professionals. Culture influences the help-seeking behaviours of patients, their attitudes and expectation toward health care providers and thus influence treatment acceptance and compliance (Chowdhury, 1991).

Everyone has a culture. It is the core issue in identity, behavior and world views. Everyone lives in multiple cultural orbits: ethnic, religious, class, gender, race, language, and social network (Olsen et al., 2006). Cultures are not static. It changes and evolves over time as individuals change over time. It involves continuous change in response to varied circumstances, challenges and opportunities. Culture is not determinative. Different people take on and respond to the same cultural expectations in different ways. Assumptions therefore cannot be made about individuals based on a specific aspect of their cultural experience and identity.

3.2 What does it mean to be culturally competent?

Cultural competency (CC) is "a set of academic and personal skills that allow us to increase our understanding and appreciation of cultural differences between groups" (Cross et al., 1989). Becoming culturally competent is a developmental process. It includes the ability to understand the language, culture, and behaviors of other individuals and groups, and to make appropriate clinical recommendations. The goal of CC is to create a health care system and workforce that are capable of delivering the highest quality care to every patient regardless of race, gender, ethnicity, culture, or language proficiency (Betancourt et al., 2005).

3.3 Why is cultural competency important for health professionals?

CC is the ability to interact successfully with patients from various ethnic and/or cultural groups. The increasing cultural diversity of recent era demands the delivery of culturally competent services. Every health professions should be aware of these three issues: (a) **Lack of awareness:** about cultural differences can make it difficult for both providers and patients to achieve the best, most appropriate care in a culture-conducive way. (b) **Diversity:** Despite all our similarities, fundamental differences among people arise from nationality, ethnicity, and culture, as well as from family background, individual experiences and current cultural disposition. The differences and similarities among diversity should be recognized, celebrated, and respected. Understanding of cultural diversity improves mental health service within a framework of legitimate practice (James & Prilleltensky, 2002). (c) **Expectations:** Cultural, ethnic, linguistic, and economic differences influence how individuals or groups access and use health, education, and social services (Lauu, 2000). These differences affect health beliefs, practices, and behaviour on the part of both patient and provider, and also influence the expectations that patient and provider have of each other.

Often in the therapeutic setting there is lack of awareness of these differences, mentioned above, and their impacts, which may be devastating and may lead to:

1. **Miscommunication:** Patient-provider relationships are affected when understanding of each other's expectations is missing. The provider may not understand why the patient does not follow instructions: e.g., why the patient takes a smaller dose of sleeping medicine than prescribed (because of a belief that Western medicine is "too strong and may damage heart"); or why the family, rather than the patient, makes important

decisions about the patient's health care (because in the patient's culture, major decisions are made by the family as a group).

2. **Rejection:** Likewise, the patient may reject the provider (and the entire system) even before any one-on-one interaction occurs because of non-verbal cues that do not fit expectations. For example, "The doctor is not wearing a white coat - maybe he's not really a doctor; or, "The doctor smiles too much. Doesn't she take me seriously?"

3. **Cultural Distance:** A gap between the culture of two different groups, such as that between the culture of institutions/clinician and the service user or their families. Mental health service delivery faces this challenge especially to reach the ethnic minority clients (Littlewood & Lipsedge, 1988; Saha, 2006).

3.4 Rationale for cultural competency

Many studies and official reports showed disparity in health care due to *cultural incompetence*. The Report of Surgeon General on Mental Health (1999), USA, highlighted several disparities between racial and ethnic minorities and whites where Minorities (a) have less availability of, and access to, mental health services, (b) are less likely to receive needed mental health services, (c) often receive a lower quality of mental health care and (d) are underrepresented in mental health research. Some studies have clearly delineated that patient's race and gender affect physician's medical decision making (Cooper-Patrick et al., 1999; Weisse et al., 2001).

Meyer (1996) describes four major reasons why we need CC in healthcare. These are: (1) Difference in clinical presentation among different ethnic and racial groups, (2) Language and communication difficulties, (3) Ethical issues and decision making- western medicine versus traditional/folk medicine or practice and (4) Trust/respect – cultural variation of levels of trust towards authority. So CC virtually offers a wide range of service development in a culture-fair way (Anderson et al, 2003) and is providing definite advantage in service delivery in a multicultural society as follows:

1. CC = Quality of Care and service outcome,
2. CC = Disparity Reduction (Eliminating disparities in the health status of people of diverse racial, ethnic, and cultural backgrounds),
3. CC = Risk Management (more understanding of the client's behaviour to mitigate risk),
4. CC = Linguistic Competence - One necessary aspect of cultural competence is linguistic competence,
5. CC = Responding to demographic changes in the society,
6. CC = Help to reduce the likelihood of liability or malpractice claims,
7. CC = A Fundamental Social (often legal) Responsibility- reflects the basic value-base of the public mental health approach, which should be responsive to individual needs and preferences,
8. CC=Meets the obligation to respect UNO's Cultural Diversity and Racial Discrimination protocol.

3.5 Types of CC: There are two types- Individual and Organizational

3.5.1 Component of Organizational CC: The organization should have (1) clearly articulated vision regarding the importance of diversity and inclusion to the business of the organization, (2) should do Climate survey to assess the degree to which individuals and members of the groups perceive they are valued, rewarded and have opportunities for growth and should provide (3) ongoing education, mentoring and evaluation throughout the organization for employees and managers to understand the expectations and skills necessary for developing a culturally competent   organization. A culturally competent organization ensures that a commitment to CC can be seen throughout all levels of the hierarchy.

3.5.2 Components of Individual CC

CC exists on a continuum from incompetence to proficiency.

At individual level CC comprises five components (Papadopoulos et al., 2004):

1. **Cultural desire:** genuine motivation to engage in the process of cultural competence and commitment to self-evaluation and criticism to develop cross-cultural knowledge.

2. **Cultural Awareness** of one's own cultural worldview (values, beliefs and practice) to reduce the risk of cultural bias and conflict in therapeutic assessment and decision making.

3. **Attitude** towards cultural differences, i.e., appreciating and accepting differences. Two ways of enabling attitudes are by: *Sensitivity training*: Reflect on culture, racism, sexism, etc. / Case studies and *Awareness training*: Population level statistics or ethnic disease prevalence data can alert the presence of minority groups and their needs in the area served.

4. **Knowledge of different cultural practices and worldviews.** It is the most important part for the development of cultural competencies. The key focus here is the acquiring of *Inter-cultural knowledge*, i.e., deliberately seeking out various world views and explanatory models of disease. Knowledge promotes understanding between cultures, failure of which may lead to intentional or unintentional discrimination (Purnell, 2005). Following are the few areas of knowledge which are essential for the mental health professionals (Saldana, 2001): (A) *Knowledge about specific facts related to culture of the client:* (a) Clients' culture: history, traditions, values, family systems, artistic expressions; (b) roles of language, speech patterns, communication styles, help-seeking behaviors, and (c) impact of racism and poverty on behaviour, attitudes, values, and disabilities. (B) *Knowledge about the culture of service and institution:* (a) the impact of the social service policies on clients of colour; (b) available resources (i.e., agencies, persons, informal helping networks, research) available for ethnic minority clients and communities; (c) how power relationships within communities or institutions impact different cultural groups, and (d) how professional values may either conflict with or accommodate the needs of clients from different cultural background.

5. **Cross-cultural Skill:** Focused on the ability and desire to combine awareness and knowledge to interpret and incorporate culture-specific understandings into primary, secondary and tertiary healthcare settings. Four ways to achieve it are:

   a. *Cultural skill development:* Learning how to culturally assess a patient, explaining an issue from another's perspective; reducing resistance and defensiveness; and acknowledging interactive mistakes that may hinder the desire to communicate.

   b. *Cultural encounters:* Meeting and working with people of a different culture will help dispel stereotypes and may contradict academic knowledge. Culturally competent skill should help to be humble enough to fight stereotypes and remain open to the individuality of each patient.

   c. *Cultural empowerment:* Professional ability to openly discuss racial and ethnic differences and issues and to respond appropriately to culturally based cues, ability to utilize the concepts of empowerment on behalf of culturally different clients and communities and proactive to recognize and combat racism, racial stereotypes, and myths among individuals and institutions.

d. *Cross-Cultural communication:* One of the most important learning processes in the development of cultural competency.

3.6 Cross-cultural communication

Cross-cultural or Inter-cultural communication is the interaction with persons of different cultural, ethnic, racial, gender, religious, age and class backgrounds. It is a process of exchanging, negotiating, and mediating one's cultural differences through language, non-verbal gestures, and space relationships. Cultural background, health beliefs and treatment expectations affect health care encounters with every patient (Kai, 2005). Different cultures have different 'set rules' that influence the behaviour, pattern of speech, value judgement, concept of time and interpersonal space and emotional attitudes towards distress and dysfunctions. Intercultural communication involves understanding others and making you understood by others. Culturally competent communication reduces racial and ethnic disparity in health care (Taylor & Lurie, 2004).

Communication is an important component of patient care (Skelton et al., 2001). With globalization and increased influx of multicultural population groups, cross-cultural communication is becoming an integral part of medical education and care (Stumpf & Bass, 1992). It is currently getting increased attention from medical schools and accreditation organizations (Loudon et al, 1999). There is also increased interest in researching patient-doctor communication and recognizing the need to teach and measure this specific clinical skill (Teutsch, 2003).

Cross-cultural communication is an ongoing learning process and involves many barriers, blocks and new initiatives and skill (Mull, 1993). Health professionals should be aware of three limitations that may interferes with effective cross-cultural understanding (Ting-Toomey, 1999): *Cognitive constraints* - These are the existing frames of reference or world views that provide a backdrop where all new information is compared, contextualize and inserted. *Behaviour constraints* - Each culture has its own set rules about proper behavior which affect verbal and nonverbal communication. The *Emotional constraints* are the ways of emotional regulation which varies from culture to culture. So for every health professionals, these three personal agenda need constant updating, viz., cognitive competence, affective competence and role competence.

3.6.1 Cultural differences in communication

Recognition of cultural differences in communication is important in therapeutic negotiations. Following are the few examples (DuPraw & Axner, 1997):

1. *Different Communication Styles:* The way people communicate varies widely between, and even within, cultures. Three aspects of communication style are important: language use, non-verbal communication and degree of assertiveness in communication (reflect positivity and confidence). Language use differs from culture to culture. Across cultures, some words and phrases are used in different ways. Even in English, the word 'Yes' has many connotation depending on the way it is said.

    Nonverbal communication, or body language, is a vital form of communication. When we interact with others, we continuously give and receive countless wordless signals (Argyle, 1988). The *Static* non-verbal communications include: Distance, Orientation (face to face/ side-by-side) Posture (of formality/relaxed/tensed) and Physical Contact (shaking hands/ touching/ holding/ embracing/ pushing). The *Dynamic* nonverbal communications are: Facial Expressions (smile, frown, raised eyebrow/ yawn/ sneer), Gesture (hand movement), Eye Contact, Kinesis (movements – forward/backward, vertical or side-to-side), Touch (Tactile Communication), Personal Space (Proxemics): the space you place between yourself and others, Environment (arrange objects into your environment), Silence (its meaning underneath) and Time. All these issues are highly culture-dependent.

2. *Different Approaches to Completing/Handling Tasks:* The success of any medical assessment and treatment negotiation virtually depends on the willingness of the client to complete the task. There are different ways that people handle tasks in terms of time frame, following of instructions, value judgement of the therapeutic decision offered and feedback as and when necessary. This may reflect in treatment negotiation, adherence or compliance to the management plan in a psychiatric clinical setting. Cultural framework in relation to time management, sense of reciprocal responsibility and trust influence how one takes the task at hand.

3. *Different Decision Making Styles:* The roles individuals play in decision-making vary widely from culture to culture. This is an important issue in accepting the treatment decision. In some culture a strong value is placed on holding decision-making responsibilities oneself and in some cultures decision needs affirmation from the family members (Asian Culture) or from the clan head before starting treatment (Some African culture).

4. *Different Attitude toward Disclosure:* Disclosure is a very sensitive as well as crucial issue in medical assessment. Frank reporting of sensitive personal issues varies from culture to culture. Potential problem may arise in areas like history taking on Drug/HIV or sexual history or history of abuse or domestic violence.

3.6.2 Factors that impede cross-cultural communications

Lack of Understanding: One of the major barriers to effective cross-cultural communication is the lack of understanding of client's culture.

Personal Values: Health professional's personal values may constitute a significant barrier, which may be due to class-bound values or culture-bound values (Sue & Sue, 1977).

Judgmental Attitudes: Tendency to evaluate other's values, beliefs and behaviours in a negative way.

Prejudice: Tendency of 'pre-judging' someone's characteristics simply because they have been categorised as belonging to a particular group. It is usually associated with negative attitudes to that group and often has ethnic or racial overtones.

Discrimination: Differential treatment of an individual due to minority status; actual and perceived; e.g., "here we have no facility to serve people like that."

Generalization: reducing numerous characteristics of an individual or group to a general form that is oversimplification, e.g., "All Caribbeans are highly superstitious".

Stereotyping: an oversimplified conception, opinion or belief about some aspect of an individual or a group. To categorize and make assumptions about others based on identified characteristics (such as gender, race, ethnicity, age, religion, nationality, or socioeconomic status) is a serious mistake. e.g., "she's like that because she's Indian – all Indians are shy and nonverbal."

Ethnocentrism: The tendency to evaluate other groups according to the values and standards of one's own ethnic group, especially with the conviction that one's own ethnic group is superior to the other groups (as if "my way is the best in the world"). Ethnocentrism leads to make false assumption about cultural differences and helps to make premature judgement. It is an obstacle to intercultural communication (Dong et al., 2008). Clinical practice in Western psychiatry is very often criticised as an ethnocentric discipline (Ata & Morrison, 2005; Fernando, 1991).

Cultural imperialism: is the practice of extending the policies and practices of one group (usually the dominant one) to other or minority groups.

Cultural Imposition: is the intrusive application of the majority group's cultural view upon individuals and families - belief that everyone should conform to the majority; e.g., "we know the right thing for you, if you don't like it you may go elsewhere."

Cultural Blindness: Differences are ignored and one proceeds as though differences did not exist; e.g., "there's no need to worry about a person's culture – you do your job and that is enough".

Racism: Race has social meaning, assigns status, limits or increase opportunities and influence interaction between patient and clinicians. Racism has been described as prejudice combined with power (Abrums, 2004). United Nations (1965) 'International Convention on the Elimination of All Forms of Racial Discrimination' defines racism as: "Any distinction, exclusion, restriction or preference based on race, colour, descent, or national or ethnic origin which has the purpose or effect of nullifying or impairing the recognition, enjoyment or exercise, on equal footing, of human rights & fundamental freedoms in the political, economic, social, cultural or any other fields of public life". Racism may be overt or covert. "Institutionalised racism consists of the collective failure of an organisation to provide an appropriate and professional service to people because of their colour, culture or ethnic origin. It can be seen or detected in processes, attitudes and behaviour which amount to discrimination through unwitting prejudice, ignorance, thoughtlessness, and racist stereotyping which disadvantage minority ethnic people" (Lancet, 1999). Stokely Carmichael, a Trinidadian-American black activist, coined this term in 1960. Racism in health care is a very sensitive and challenging issue in UK, USA and other European countries (Bhopal, 2007), especially in work place, medical (Dennis, 2001; Mistry & Latoo, 2009), and psychiatric service delivery (McKenzie & Bhui, 2007. *Racial fatigue* is the state of potential emotional and psychological sequel of feeling isolated in a work or health environment because of racial discrimination, especially when the issues were consistently ignored and not discussed (*racial silence*) (Nunez-Smith et al., 2007).

Stigma: Stigma is a severe form of social disapproval or personal discontent with a person on the ground of their unique characteristics, which is judged as a sign of disgrace and something that sets a person apart from others. Goffman (1990) defined stigma as "the process by which the reaction of others spoils normal identity". Goffman described three forms of stigma: the experience of a mental illness, physical deformity and association with a particular race, religion or belief. Stigma derives from deeply ingrained individual and social attitudes and always leads to discrimination. Negative attitudes and stigma directly affects the clinical practice in psychiatry (Byrne, 1999). Stigmatization of individuals with mental illnesses is widespread (Chowdhury et al., 2001; Jadav et al., 2007) and serves as a major barrier to proper mental health care and the better quality of life (Mann & Himelein, 2004; Charles et al., 2007). Reduction of stigma against persons with mental illness is a serious preventive work (Arboleda & Sartorius, 2008; Crisp et al., 2000) at all levels of mental health work- from clinic, hospitals, institution to community (Penn & Couture, 2002). World Psychiatric Association started an international programme to fight stigma and discrimination against schizophrenia in 1996 and Royal College of Psychiatrist, London, completed an anti-stigma campaign (*Changing Minds*) with a five year (1998-2003) strategy.

3.6.3 Factors that facilitate cross-cultural communications

Cross cultural communication is the process of dealing with people from other cultures in a way that minimises misunderstandings and maximises the potential benefit out of therapeutic relationships. Payne (2004) provides some useful basic tips for effective cross-cultural communications. These are few important in a health service context: (a) *Slow Down* and speak clearly, normal pace, normal volume, no colloquialisms, or double negatives (i.e. 'not bad') ; (b) *Separate Questions*- short sentences one by one; (c) *Avoid Negative Questions; (d) Take Turns*- talk and listen; (e) *Write it Down*- for clarity if necessary; (f) *Check Meanings* - whether you are properly understood; (g) *Avoid Slang; (h) Be Supportive* – make the client comfortable, confident and trust you; (i) *Maintain Etiquette*- learn some cross-cultural issues before dealing a people from the target culture and (j) *Listen actively:* Listening is one of the most important skills in any communication, especially in the field of medicine (Robertson, 2005). The success of any therapeutic consultation depends on how well the patient and doctor communicate with each other (Gask & Usherwood, 2002). Following are the few rules to become an active listener: pay attention, avoid distractions, show that you are listening, engage yourself, provide feedback, defer judgment and respond appropriately. Some useful interview guides are shown in Box 1.

4. Clinical application of culture: Cultural assessment

4.1 Emic-etic perspective

Proper insight and understanding about culture's impact on mental health and treatment is crucially important to prevent disparities in assessment and treatment (Hwang et al, 2008). How we perceive the other culture is dependent on our view or looking lenses. There are two ways of looking at any given cultural system: Emic and Etic - terms coined by Kenneth Lee Pike, an American linguist and anthropologist in 1954 (Pike, 1967). These are linguistic terms- phonetic (sound of universal language) and phonemic (sound of specific language) respectively. *Etic* is used to address things that are considered universal, whereas *emic* is culture-specific. From clinical research point- an *emic* account is a description of behaviour or a belief that account comes from a person within the culture (insider). The *etic* approach implies that research is conducted by an outside observer. *Etic* approach may be more objective but may lose culturally relevant meaning in its interpretation. Emic-etic controversy in the research of culture and mental health is a long debate and challenge in psychiatry (Marano, 1982; Littlewood, 1998; Warner, 1999).

In their very influential publication on 'Culture and Psychiatry' Tseng and Streltzer (2004) very nicely summed up three basic areas of cultural interaction with the therapeutic system. These are:

1. *The culture of the Patient:* patient's understanding of illness, perceived cause, symptom experience and meaning and treatment expectations – all of which are being influenced by culture.
2. *The culture of the Physician:* pattern of attention, interaction and communication with the patient. Physician's culture explicitly or implicitly guides his/her attitude toward the patient, understating of the problem, support and treatment and care provision of the patient

3. *The culture of Medical Practice:* These are the framework of rules, regulations, customs and attitudes of the medical system and institutions in which the service to the client is provided. Tseng and Streltzer (2004) described it as " invisible cultural system" and in every society there are set rules for each medical disciplines and institutions, for its members and principles of care. All these culture-dependent medical customs influence doctor-patient relation and interaction (Tseng, 2003) and treatment expectations.

A. Explanatory Model of Distress: 8 questions of Kleinman et al., (1978)

1. What do you think has caused your problem?
2. Why do you think it started when it did?
3. What do you think your sickness does to you?
4. How severe is your sickness? Will it have a short or long course?
5. What kind of treatment do you think you should receive?
6. What are the most important results you hope to receive from this treatment?
7. What are the chief problems your sickness has caused for you?
8. What do you fear most about your sickness?

B. LEARN model (Berlin & Fowkes, 1983) for physicians-in-training
- Listen with sympathy and understanding to the patient's perception of the problem
- Explain your perceptions of the problem and your strategy for treatment.
- Acknowledge and discuss the differences and similarities between these perceptions.
- Recommend treatment while remembering the patient's cultural parameters.
- Negotiate agreement. It is important to understand the patient's explanatory model so that medical treatment fits in their cultural framework.

C. FICA model (Josephson & Peteet, 2004): screening for worldview and spirituality
- Faith and religious/spiritual beliefs
- Involvement in the practices associated with a faith or beliefs
- Community of support related to a faith or beliefs
- Address how these beliefs, practices, and community are to be integrated in health and mental health care

---

Box 1. Models of Effective Cross-Cultural Communication and Negotiation

4.2 Culture in mental health care

Group of Advancement of Psychiatry (GAP, 2002) clearly stressed the importance of culture in mental health and strongly advised that careful assessment of the cultural context of psychiatric problems must form a central part of any clinical evaluation. They categorized four areas of cultural importance in clinical psychiatry.

1. *Diagnostic and Nosological factor:* cultural competency training and cultural formulation in clinical assessment that enhances treatment and care planning.
2. *Therapeutic and protective role:* culturally determined attitudes and behaviour can operate as a cushion that prevents the occurrence of psychopathology and/or the spread of its harmful consequences. Role of extended families and social networks neutralize the impact of stigma, and traditional healing, role of religious beliefs and practices may enhance health recovery.

3. *Ethnopsychopharmacology:* Series of recent research has shown that there is a significant difference among ethnic groups in their response and vulnerability to side-effects of medications because of the genotypic variations, which influence the pharmacokinetics and pharmacodynamics of drug metabolism (Matthews, 1995). The role of cytochrome P450 enzymes in hepatic metabolism has been extensively studied (Lin et al., 1993). Asian patients often respond to substantially lower doses of psychotropics. Specific mutations of certain cytochrome P450 enzymes lead to poor or slow metabolism. Several ethnic variations in drug response has been documented, e.g., to neuroleptics (extrapyramidal side effects- Jann et al., 1989), Asian-Caucasians difference in tricyclic antidepressants serum level (Rudorfer et al., 1984); racial differences in red blood cell sodium and lithium levels (Hardman et al., 1998) and clozapine-induced agranulocytosis has been more commonly observed in Ashkenazi Jews, especially in those with a cluster of HLA types (Lieberman et al., 1990). Multiple psychosocial factors like gender, diet, consumption of cigarettes, caffeine, alcohol, herbs, psychoactive substances, sleep-activity-rest patterns and environmental-geographical effects influence ethnocultural differences in psychotropic drug metabolism and response (Jacobsen, 1994; Ng et al., 2008). Recent advances in genetic neuroscience; especially the psychosocial genomics (Box 2) unfolded a new horizon of understanding of culture/social-gene interactions: "how the subjective experiences of human consciousness, our perception of free will, and social dynamics can modulate gene expression, and vice versa" (Rossi, 2002a).

4. *Management and structuring clinical services:* Culture is an important element in the structure of management approaches and provision of services to the community. Three issues form the basis of this approach, viz., Cultural sensitivity, i.e. the awareness of culturally based needs in a given population, Cultural relevance, i.e. the implementation of measures that help to provide culturally sensitive services and Cultural competence, both of the organisation and its workforce to deliver the care in a culturally appropriate way.

5. The cultural formulation

Culture has a very important role in precipitating, perpetuating and preventive factors in relation to any illness (Bhugra & Osborne, 2006). The cultural assessment is thus helping providers understand where and how patients derive their ideas about disease and illness. Assessments help to determine beliefs, values and practices that might have an effect on patient care and health behaviors (Weiss, 2001). In fact, cultural assessment improves patient safety in healthcare organization (Nieva & Sorra, 2003). So Cultural Consultation service (Kirmayer et al., 2003) and Cross-cultural psychiatric assessment (Bhugra & Bhui, 1997) is now becoming a cornerstone of clinical assessment in multicultural health services and psychiatric training. Cultural formulation not only make the diagnostic process and treatment more culturally sensitive (Borra, 2008), but also becoming a part of therapeutic justice in the midst of growing cultural pluralism in recent societies (Lewis-Fernandez & Diaz, 2002).

5.1 DSM IV –Tr cultural formulation

APA published DSMIV in 1994 which included an 'Outline for Cultural Formulation' to provide a concise method of incorporating cultural issues into the therapeutic (diagnosis

Psycho-Social Genomics is the study of how psychological and social processes modulate gene expression and brain plasticity (Rossi, 2002a). Virtually it is an interdisciplinary field involving studies of stress, psychosomatics, psychoimmunology, psycho-neuro-endocrinology and psychobiology of creativity, optimal performance, dreaming, art, ritual, culture, and spiritual life. The main focus of psychosocial genomics is to explore how the levels of gene expression, neurogenesis, and healing are interrelated as a complex, adaptive system with the levels of human experiencing, behaviour, and consciousness (Rossi, 2002b). In other words, psychosocial forces and factors can shape neurobiology.

The contributions from psychosocial genomics have shown that socio-environmental experiences influence neurobiological structure and functions of brain across the life cycle (Garland & Howard, 2009). This is called '**Dynamic Gene Expression'**: the interplay between behavioural state-related gene expression (nature) and activity-dependent gene expression (nurture) bring about healing through neurogenesis and learning (Hofmann, 2003). Investigations of neuroplasticity demonstrate that the adult brain can continue to form novel neural connections and grow new neurons in response to learning or training even into old age. The discovery that gene expression is not static, but rather is influenced in an ongoing way by interactions with the environment – has led to the interest in the influence of psychosocial treatments on illnesses that are thought to have strongly biological underpinnings (Rossi, 2004).

Box 2. Psychosocial Genomics

and care) process (Lu, 2006). The DSM-IV-TR (APA, 2000) Outline for Cultural Formulation provides a systematic method of considering and incorporating sociocultural issues into the clinical formulation. Depending on the focus and extent of the evaluation, it may not be possible to do a complete cultural formulation during the first interview. However, when cultural issues emerge, they may be explored further during subsequent meetings with the patient. In addition, the information contained within the cultural formulation may be integrated with the other aspects of the clinical formulation. Though there are some criticism of DSM IV and culture (Littlewood, 1992; Rogler, 1993) and cultural formulation (Mezzich et al., 2009; Thakker & Ward, 1998), yet DSM IV-TR outline for cultural formulation is the only relatively standard protocol till available for assessment of culturally diverse individuals (Lim, 2002). Kirmayer and colleagues from the Transcultural Psychiatry Group at McGill University, Montreal, Canada provided a very useful expanded version of DSM IV outline for clinical use (Kirmayer et al., 2008).

5.2 Content of cultural formulation (DSM-IV-TR):

Following is a brief description of the five components of Cultural Formulation framework of DSM IV TR (Focus, 2006):

1. *Cultural identity of the individual:* Usual focus is on ethnicity, age, gender, acculturation/ biculturality, language (mother tongue and present use), socioeconomic status, sexual orientation, religious and spiritual beliefs, disabilities, political orientation, health literacy, migration, involvement with culture of origin and host culture.
2. *Cultural explanation of the individual's illness:* Usual focus is on patient's explanatory models or idioms of distress, perceived cause and cultural meaning of distress/symptoms, past help-seeking and present treatment expectations and preferences.

	Cultural Factors	Salient findings
1.	Ethnic and Cultural Identity	
	Original culture/ host culture Mother tongue/ present language Immigration/Migration history- first /second generation Level of tie with original culture Level of assimilation with host culture	
2.	Cultural background	
	Family role – extended/nuclear family Religious and/ or spiritual beliefs and practices Social support and network Experience of any discrimination and or prejudice due to race, religion, cultural identity, gender, sexuality, or disability? Experience of any trauma , its cultural explanation	
3.	Present problem	
	Symptoms – culture specific meanings Perceived cause Illness meaning and idioms of distress Cultural explanation of cause and cure Past help-seeking (culture-based)	
4	Treatment expectations	
	Perception of any cross-cultural barrier Cultural distance or animosity? Treatment expectations Involvement of family/ community/ traditional healer in the treatment process Therapeutic modality desired: Pharmaco-therapy/Psychotherapy/ Traditional/ Religious/Legal/Community	
5.	Cultural Formulation	

	Diagnosis: Medical (discuss and clarify the meanings of
	       diagnostic label)
	       Cultural (discuss with the client/ family)	

	Rate: level of illness severity	
	Rate: level of functioning	
	Rate: level and nature of stressors	
	Rate: level of social support	
	Any cultural issue related to symptoms of therapeutic importance (cause/ culture congruent mood, guilt, delusion or hallucination)	
	Clinician's cultural identity	
	Interpreter used	

Table 2. Short Cultural Formulation Note

3. *Cultural factors related to psychosocial environment and levels of functioning:* involves information on available social supports, levels of function or disability, the roles of family/kin systems and religion and spirituality in providing emotional, instrumental, and informational support.

4. *Cultural elements of the relationship between the individual and the clinician:* This include the ethnocultural identity and social status of physician, language, knowledge about the client's culture, transference and countertranferance issues, cross-cultural skill and ability and eagerness of the physician to understand client's problem form his/her cultural context.

5. *Overall cultural assessments:* how the cultural assessment will apply to diagnosis, treatment planning and care.

Cultural formulation should be as exhaustive as possible and the health professional should maintain a detailed note with ample narratives. It needs a special session to work out. Following is a brief interview note (Table 2) which may be helpful in a busy clinic to keep relevant cultural note with the clinical record of the client.

Currently experimentations and clinical trials are ongoing with the Cultural Formulation protocol in different academic institutions including DSM V and ICD 11 working groups and it is hoped that shortly we will get a more comprehensive, easy-to-use clinical protocol that would be useful for assessment and treatment planning. Initiatives from different cultures and countries are necessary to gain more cross-cultural knowledge and to mitigate Eurocentric bias.

6. Conclusion

In recent decades the horizon of psychiatry, rather mental health and wellbeing has broadened to an unprecedented extent because of many challenging and fascinating inputs from medical geography (Holley, 1998; Mayer, 1996) and ecology (Carey, 1970; Gadit, 2009), medical sociology (Rogers & Pilgrim, 2010; Cook & Wright, 1995), medical anthropology (Kleinman, 1988; Fabrega, 1992; Gaines, 1992), psychology and neurosciences. There is a significant change in the medical ethics of therapeutic system and procedures with more focus on human rights, race relation and equality and diversity, and immigration health within a national standards and legal framework. Globalization and technological improvement facilitated population movement and created a multicultural cliental in every sphere of civil life, be it work place, industry, corporate or health service. So culture is now becoming a primary issue in all communication and policy frameworks. Medical teaching and training primarily focus core medical subjects, inputs from sociology, anthropology or other social sciences are virtually negligible. This is a global scenario. In recent years some universities and national health agencies highlighted the need for cross-cultural training and cultural competence in health care. This is a good sign. Some international health organizations like WHO, World Psychiatric Association, American Psychiatric Association, Royal College of Psychiatrist, European Psychiatric Association, Society for the Study of Psychiatry and Culture and others are also advocating this need very proactively. A dozen of very scholarly journals dedicated to culture and mental health, to name a few, Culture, Medicine and Psychiatry, Transcultural Psychiatry, World Cultural Psychiatry Bulletin, International journal of Culture and Mental Health, Mental Health, Religion and Culture, Anthropology and Health Journal, Anthropology and Medicine, Ethnicity and Health, Journal of Immigrant and Minority Health, International Journal of Social Psychiatry etc. are also taking the cultural issues in the forefront of medicine and mental healthcare, and thus enriching our perception, attitude and thrust for cross-cultural knowledge in a very positive way. In recent decades quite a large number of books on culture and health (mental health) has been published and helped us to develop our therapeutic ambience in a more culture-conducive way. Cultural diversity, competency and cultural formulation has become a part of health care delivery system (Anderson et al., 2003) and medical education (Marzan & McEvoy, 2010) and psychiatry training programme (Lu & Primm, 2006) in some of the universities and health care organizations. It is now well evidenced-base that cultural competency in health care in general and mental health care in particular is a ethical, legal and clinical requirement (Johnson & Cert, 2004) which in turn prompted more health service research and culture-ethnicity-health studies in academia (Skultans & Cox, 2000; Lopez & Guarnaccia, 2000). But unfortunately this momentum in culture and mental health initiatives is observed mainly in the developed countries, significant progress in the developing part of the globe is still lacking. I am concluding with a valuable remark by Tseng (2006) regarding the aims, objective and the task of psychiatrists: "Historically, the study of culture-related specific syndromes prompted the development of transcultural psychiatry, and later, cultural psychiatry, as subfields of general psychiatry. However, clinically, instead of being overly concerned with how to consider and label more culture-related specific syndromes and debating how to categorize them diagnostically, we need to move ahead and concentrate on the understanding of the cultural implications of all forms of psychopathology and examine approaches to **culture relevant treatment**, that is, providing **culturally competent care for all patients**. This is a practical need that exists in contemporary societies, which are becoming increasingly multiethnic and polycultural." (emphasis by the present author).

7. References

AAA (1999). American Anthropological Association statement on race. *American Anthropologist*, 100, 712-713.

Abrums, M (2004). Faith and Feminism: How African American women from a forefront church resist oppression in health care. *Advances in Nursing Science*, 27, 187-201.

Alarcon, RD (2009). Culture, cultural factors and psychiatric diagnosis: review and projections. *World Psychiatry*, 8(3), 131-139.

Alarcon, RD, Foulks, EF & Vakkur, M (1998). *Personality Disorders and Culture: Clinical and Conceptual interactions*. John Wiley & Sons, ISBN: 978-0-471-14964-4, New York

Al-Issa, I (1995). *Handbook of Culture and Mental Illness: An International Perspective*. International University Press, ISBN 10-0823622886, Michigan, USA.

Anderson, LM, Scrimshaw, SC, Fullilove, MT, Fielding, JF, Normand, J & Task Force on Community Preventive Services (2003). Culturally competent healthcare system: A systematic review. *American Journal of Preventive Medicine*, 24 (3S), 68-79.

APA (1969). Position statement on the delineation of transcultural psychiatry as a specialized field of study. American Psychiatric Association. *American Journal of Psychiatry*, 126, 453-455.

APA (1994). *Diagnostic and Statistical Manual of Mental Disorders*. American Psychiatric Association. American Psychiatric Publishing, ISBN: 0-89042-062-9, Washington DC.

APA (2000). *Diagnostic and Statistical Manual of Mental Disorders,* 4th ed., Text Revision, American Psychiatric Publishing, ISBN 0-07-147898-1, Washington DC. pp. 897–903.

Arboleda, F, Sartorius, N (2008). *Understanding the Stigma of Mental Illness: Theory and Interventions* (World Psychiatric Association). Wiley-Blackwell, ISBN 13:978-0-470-723289, Sussex, England.

Argyle, M (1988). *Bodily Communication.* 2nd Ed. Methuen & Co Ltd, ISBN 0-416-67450, London.

Ata, A, Morrison, G (2005). Health care providers, bereavement anxieties and ethnocentric pedagogy: Towards a sense of otherness. *Advances in Mental Health,* 4(3), 175-178.

BBC (1999). *Mental health: Rights versus risk.* BBC News, 16.11.99: 03.57GMT. Accessed on 5.8.11 from: http://news.bbc.co.uk/1/hi/health/521660.stm

Banerjee, BG, Jalota, R (1988). *Folk Illness and Ethnomedicine.* Northern Book Centre, ISBN 81-85119-37-6, New Delhi.

Berlin, EA, Fowkes, WC (1983). A teaching framework for cross-cultural health care. *The Western Journal of Medicine,* 139, 934-938.

Berry, JW (1977). Immigration, acculturation and adaptation. *Applied Psychology: An International Review,* 46(1), 5-68.

Berry, JW, Sam, D (1980). Acculturation and adaptation. In, *Handbook of Cross-cultural Psychology: Social Beahvior and Application.* Vol. 3, Eds. J.W. Berry; M.H.Segal & C.Kagitcibasi, ISBN 0-205-16074-3, Allyn & Bacon, MA, USA. pp. 291-326.

Betancourt, JR, Green, AR, Carrillo, JE & Park, ER (2005). Cultural competence and health care disparities: Key perspectives and trends. *Health Affairs,* 24(2), 499-505

Bhopal, RS (2007). Racism in health and health care in Europe: reality or mirage? *European Journal of Public Health,* 17(3), 238-241.

Bhugra, D, Becker, MA (2005). Migration, cultural bereavement and cultural identity. *World Psychiatry,* 4(1), 18-24.

Bhugra, D, Bhui, K (1997) Cross-cultural psychiatric assessment. *Advances in Psychiatric Treatment,* 3, 103-110.

Bhugra, D, Osborne, T (2006). Cultural assessment and management. *Psychiatry,* 5(11), 379-382.

Bhui, K, Bhugra, D (2002a). Mental illness in Black and Asian ethnic minorities: pathways to care and outcomes. *Advances in Psychiatric Treatment,* 8, 26-33.

Bhui, K, Bhugra, D (2002b). Explanatory models for mental distress: implications for clinical practice and research. *British Journal of Psychiatry,* 181, 6-7.

Bhui, K, Stansfeld, S, Head, J, Haines, M, Hillier, S, Taylor, S, Viner, R & Booy, R (2005). Cultural identity, acculturation, and mental health among adolescents in east London's multiethnic community. *Journal of Epidemiology and Community Health,* 59, 296-302.

Boas, F (1887). Museums of ethnology and their classification. *Science,* 9, 589.

Borra, R (2008). Working with the cultural formulation in therapy. *European Psychiatry,* 23 (Supl.1), 43- 48.

Boyd, KM (2000). Disease, illness, sickness, health, healing and wholeness: exploring some elusive concepts. *Medical Humanities,* 26, 9-17.

Brody, EB (2001). Unity within diversity: Mental health in the global century. World Federation for Mental Health. *The Margaret Mead Memorial Lecture*, Vancouver BC. Canada. Accessed on 22.7.11from: www.critpsynet.freeuk.com/Brody.htm

Bronstein, P (1986). Self-Disclosure, paranoia and unaware racism: Another look at the Black client and the White therapist. *American Psychologist*, 41, 225-226.

Byrne, P (1999). Stigma of mental illness: Changing minds, changing behaviour. *British Journal of Psychiatry*, 174, 1-2.

Carey, GW (1970). Urban ecology, geography and health problems. *Bulletin of the New York Academy of Medicine*, 46(2), 73-82.

Charles, H, Manoramjitham, SD & Jacob, KS (1997). Stigma and explanatory models among people with schizophrenia and their relatives in Vellore, South India. *International Journal of Social Psychiatry*, 53(4), 325-332.

Cheetham, RW, Edwards, SD, Naidoo, LR, Griffiths, JA & Singh, VG (1983). Deculturation as a precipitant of parasuiside in an Asian group. *South African Medical Journal*, 63(24), 942-945.

Chowdhury, AN (1989). Biomedical potential for symptom choice in Koro. *International Journal of Social Psychiatry*, 35, 329-332.

Chowdhury, AN (1990). Trait anxiety profile of Koro patients. *Indian Journal of Psychiatry*, 32, 330-333.

Chowdhury, AN (1991). Medico-cultural cognition of Koro epidemic: An ethnographic study. *Journal of Indian Anthropological Society*, 26, 155-170.

Chowdhury, AN (1992a). Psychic infectivity: The role of positive illness cognition in psychiatric epidemic. *Journal of Personality and Clinical Studies*, 8, 125-128.

Chowdhury, AN (1992b). Clinical analysis of 101 Koro cases. *Indian Journal of Social Psychiatry*, 7, 67-70.

Chowdhury, AN (1994a). Koro in females: An analysis of 48 cases. *Transcultural Psychiatric Research Review*, 31, 369-380.

Chowdhury, AN (1994b). Heroin and HIV epidemic in India: A note on North-Eastern states. *Journal of Indian Anthropological Society*, 29, 287-302.

Chowdhury, AN (1996). Definition and classification of Koro. *Culture, Medicine and Psychiatry*, 20, 41- 65.

Chowdhury, AN (1998). Hundred years of Koro. *International Journal of Social Psychiatry*, 44, 182-189.

Chowdhury, AN (2002). Culture and suicide. *Journal of Indian Anthropological Society*, 37, 175-185.

Chowdhury, AN (2008). Ethnomedical concept of heat and cold in Koro: Study from Indian patients. *World Cultural Psychiatry Research Review*, 3, 146-158.

Chowdhury, AN, Dobson, TW (2002). Culture, psychiatry and New Zealand. *Indian Journal of Psychiatry*, 44(4), 356-361.

Chowdhury, AN, Sanyal, D., Bhattacharya, A., Dutta, ,SK., De, R, Banerjee, S, Bhattacharya, K, Palit, S, Bhattacharya, P, Mondal, R & Weiss, MG (2001). Prominence of symptoms and level of stigma among depressed patients in Calcutta. *Journal of Indian Medical Association*, 99, 20-23.

Chowdhury, AN, Rajbhandari, KC (1995). Koro with depression from Nepal. *Transcultural Psychiatric Research Review*, 32, 87-90.

Chowdhury, AN, Mukherjee, H, Ghosh, KK & Chowdhury, S (2003). Puppy pregnancy in humans: A culture-bound disorder in rural West Bengal, India. *International Journal of Social Psychiatry*, 49, 35-42.

Chowdhury, AN, Nath, AK & Chakraborty J (1993). An atypical hysteria epidemic in Tripura. *Transcultural Psychiatric Research Review*, 30, 143-151.

Chowdhury, AN, Ramkrishna, J, Chakraborty, A & Weiss, MG (2006). Cultural context and impact of alcohol use in Sundarban delta, West Bengal, India. *Social Science and Medicine*, 63, 722-731.

Cook, JA, Wright, ER (1995). Medical sociology and the study of severe mental illness: reflections on past accomplishments and directions for future research. *Journal of Health and Social Behaviour*, Spec No, 95-114.

Cooper-Patrick, L, Gallo, JJ, Gonzales, JJ, Vu, HT, Powe, NR, Nelson, C & Ford, DE (1999). Race, gender, and patient-physician relationship. *Journal of American Medical Association*, 282(6), 583-589.

Cort, MA (2004). Cultural mistrust and use of hospice care: Challenges and remedies. *Journal of Palliative Medicine*, 7(1), 63-71.

Cowen, M (2011) Cultural factors influence hallucination types in schizophrenia. *Comprehensive Psychiatry*, 52, 319-325.

Crisp, AH, Gelder, MG, Rix, S, Meltzer, HI & Rowlands, OJ (2000). Stigmatisation of people with mental illnesses. *British Journal of Psychiatry*, 177, 4 – 7.

Cross, T, Bazron, B, Dennis K., & Isaacs, M (1989). Towards a Culturally Competent System of Care, Volume 1. (Monograph) Georgetown University, National Center for Cultural Competence Center for Child and Human Development, Washington, DC. Acessed on 17.7.11 from: http://nccc.georgetown.edu/research/index.html

Dennis, GC (2001). Racism in medicine: planning for the future. *Journal of National Medical Association*, 93(3), Suppl. 1S- 5S.

Dong, Q, Day, KD & Collaco, CM (2008). Overcoming ethnocentrism through developing intercultural communication sensitivity and multiculturalism. *Human Communication*, 11(1), 27-38.

DuPraw, ME, Axner, M (1997). *Toward a more perfect union in an age of diversity*: Working on common cross-cultural communication challenges. Accessed on 7.5.11 from: http://www.pbs.org/ampu/crosscult.html

Edney, DR (2004) *Mass media and mental illness: A literature review*. Canadian Mental Health Association, Ontario. Accessed on 5.8.11 from: http://www.ontario.cmha.ca/docs/about/mass_media.pdf

Eisenberg, L (1977). Disease and illness: Distinctions between professional and popular ideas of sickness. *Culture, Medicine and Psychiatry*, 1(1), 9-23.

Emslie, C, Fuhrer, R, Hunt, K, Macintyre, S, Shipley, M & Stansfeld, S (2002). Gender differences in mental health: evidence from three organisations. *Social Science and Medicine*, 54, 621-624.

Fabrega, H Jr (2001). Culture and history in psychiatric diagnosis and practice. *Psychiatric Clinics of North America*, 24(3), 391-405.

Fabrega, H Jr. (1992). The role of culture in a theory of psychiatric illness. *Social Science and Medicine*, 35(1), 91-103.

Fernando, S (1991). *Mental Health, Race and Culture*. 3rd Ed. ISBN 9780230212718, Palgrave Macmillan,England.

Focus (2006): Cultural Formulation: From the APA practice guideline for the psychiatric evaluation of adults, 2nd edition. *Focus*, 4(1), 11

Gadit, AA (2009). Ecology and mental health: time to understand ecopsychiatry. *Journal of Pakistan Medical Association*, 59(1), 56-57.

Gaines, AD. (Ed.) (1992). *Ethnopsychiatry: The cultural construction of professional and folk psychiatries*. State University of New York Press, ISBN 0-7914-1022-6, Albany, NY.

GAP (2002). *Cultural assessment in psychiatry*. Report No. 145. Group for the Advancement of Psychiatry, Committee on Cultural Psychiatry. American Psychiatric Publishing, ISBN 0-87318-144-1, Washington DC.

Garland, EL, Howard, MO (2009). Neuroplasticity, psychosocial genomics and biopsychosocial paradigm in the 21st century. *Health and Social Work*, 34(3), 191-199.

Gask, L, Usherwood, T (2002). The consultation. *British Medical Journal*, 324, 7353, 1567.

Goffman, E (1990) *Stigma: Notes on the Management of Spoiled Identity*. Penguin Group, ISBN 978-0140124750, London.

Goldberg, DP, Bridges, K (1988). Somatic presentation of psychiatric illness in primary care setting. *Journal of Psychosomatic Research*, 32(2), 137-144.

Grier WH, Cobbs PM (1968). *Black Rage*. Basic Books, ISBN13: 9780465007035, New York.

Groen, S (2009). Recognizing cultural identity in mental health care: Rethinking the cultural formulation of a Somali patient. *Transcultural Psychiatry*, 46(3), 451-462.

Grusec, JE, Hastings, PD (2007). *Handbook of Socialization: Theory and Research*. Guilford Press, ISBN 9781593853327, New York, pp.547.

Guarnacca, PJ, Rogler, LH (1999). Research on culture-bound syndromes: New directions. *American Journal of Psychiatry*, 156, 1322-1327.

Guarnaccia, PJ, Canino, G, Rubio-Stipec, M & Bravo, M (1993). The prevalence of ataques de nervios in the Puerto Rico disaster study: the role of culture in psychiatric epidemiology. *Journal of Nervous and Mental Disorders*, 181, 157–165.

Hall, TM (2008). *Culture-bound syndromes in China*. Accessed on 22.6.11 from: http://homepage.mac.com/mccajor/cbs.html

Hallenbeck, J (2003). The explanatory model #26. *Journal of Palliative Medicine*, 6(6), 931.

Hardman, TC, Croft, P, Morrish, Z, Anto-Awoakye K & Lant AF (1998) Kinetic characteristics of the erythrocyte sodium-lithium countertransporter in black normotensive subjects compared with three other ethnic group. *Journal of Human Hypertension*, 12(1), 29-34.

Helman, CG (2007). *Culture, Health, and Illness*. 5th Ed., Hodder Arnold, ISBN 978-0-340-914-502, London.

Hofmann, HA. (2003). Functional genomics of neuronal and behavioural plasticity. *Journal of Neurobiology*, 54(1), 272-282.

Holley, HL (1998).Geography and mental health: a review. *Social Psychiatry and Psychiatric Epidemiology*, 33(11), 535-542.

Homer, U, Ashby, J (1986) Mislabelling the Black client: A reply to Ridley. *American Psychologist*, 41, 224-225.

Hwang, WC, Myers, HF, Abe-Kim, J & Ting, JY. (2008). A conceptual paradigm for understanding culture's impact on mental health: The cultural influences on mental health (CIMH) model. *Clinical Psychology Review*, 28(2), 211-227.

Jacobsen, FM (1994). Psychopharmacology. In, *Women of Color: Integrating Ethnic and Gender Identities in Psychotherapy.* Eds. L. Comas-Diaz & B. Greene, Guilford Press, ISBN 0-89862-371-5, New York. pp. 319-340.

Jadav, S. (2004). How culture bound is cultural psychiatry? *International Psychiatry,* 4, 6-8.

Jadav, S, Littlewood, R, Ryder, AG, Chakraborty, A, Jain, S & Barua, M (2007). Stigmatization of severe mental illness in India: Against the simple industrialization hypothesis. *Indian Journal of Psychiatry,* 49(3), 189-194.

James, S, Prilleltensky, I (2002). Cultural diversity and mental health. *Clinical Psychology Review,* 22(8), 1133-1154.

Jann, MW, Chang, WH, Davis, CM, Chen, TY, Deng, HC, Lung, FW, Ereshefsky, L, Saklad, SR & Richards, AL (1989). Haloperidol and reduced haloperidol levels in Chinese vs. non-Chinese psychiatric patients. *Psychiatry Research,* 30(1), 45-52.

Johnson, MRD, Cert, HE (2004). Cross-cultural communication in health. *Clinical Cornerstone,* 6(1), 50- 52.

Johnson, TM (1987). Premenstrual syndrome as a Western culture-specific disorder. *Culture, Medicine and Psychiatry,* 11(3), 337-356.

Josephson, AM, Peteet, JR (Eds.) (2004) *Handbook of Spirituality and Worldview in Clinical Practice.* American Psychiatric Publishing, ISBN 978-1-58562-104-0, Arlington, VA, USA.

Kai, J (2005). Cross-cultural; communication. *Ethics and Communication Skills,* 33(2), 31-34.

Kent, P, Bhui, K (2003). Cultural identity and mental health. *International Journal of Social Psychiatry,* 49(4), 243-246.

Kelly BD (2010). Globalization, psychiatry and human rights: new challenges for the 21st century. In, *Clinical Topics in Cultural Psychiatry,* Eds. R, Bhattacharya, S, Cross, D, Bhugra, Royal College of Psychiatrist, ISBN: 978-1-904671-82-4, London. pp. 3-14

Kirmayer, LJ (2001) Cultural variations in the clinical presentation of depression and anxiety. Implications for diagnosis and treatment. *Journal of Clinical Psychiatry,* 62 (Suppl 13), 22-28.

Kirmayer, LJ, Groleau, D, Guzder, J, Blake, C & Jarvis, E (2003). Cultural consultation: A model of mental health service for multicultural societies. *Canadian Journal of Psychiatry,* 48(3), 145-153

Kirmayer, LJ, Thombs, BD, Jurcil, T, Jarvis, GE & Guzder, J. (2008). Use of an expanded version of the DSM IV outline for cultural formulation on a cultural consultation service. *Psychiatric Service,* 59(6), 683-686.

Kirmayer, LJ, Young, A (1999). Culture and context in the evolutionary concept of mental disorder. *Journal of Abnormal Psychology,* 108, 446–452.

Kim, K (2006) Delusions and hallucinations in East Asians with schizophrenia. *World Cultural Psychiatry Research Review,* 1(1):37-42.

Kleinman, A (1988) *Rethinking in Psychiatry: From Cultural Category to Personal Experience.* Free Press, ISBN 0-02-917442-2, New York.

Kleinman, A (1992). *Patients and healers in the context of culture: an exploration of the borderland between anthropology, medicine, and psychiatry.* University of California Press, ISBN-978-0520045118, Berkeley, CA.

Kleinman, A., Eisenberg, L & Good, B. (1978). Culture, Illness, and Care: Clinical lessons from anthropological and cross-cultural research. *Annals of Internal Medicine,* 88:251-258

Kroeber, AL (1940). Stimulus diffusion. *American Anthropologist*, 42(1), 1–20.

Lancet (1999). Institutionalised racism in health care. *Lancet,* 353 (9155), 765.

Lauu, CJ (2000). Culturally competent health care. *Public Health Report*, 115, 25-33.

Levine, RE, Gaw, AC (1995). Culture-bound Syndromes. *Psychiatric Clinics of North America,* 18(3), 523- 536.

Lewis-Fernandez, R (1996). Cultural formulation of psychiatric diagnosis. Case No. 02. Diagnosis and treatment of nervios and ataques in a female Puerto Rican migrant. *Culture, Medicine and Psychiatry*, 20, 155–163.

Lewis-Fernandez, R, Diaz, N (2002). The cultural formulation: A method for assessing cultural factors affecting the clinical encounter. *Psychiatric Quarterly*, 73(4), 271-295.

Lieberman, JA, Yunis, J, Egea, E, Canoso, RT, Kane, JM & Yunis, EJ (1990). HLA-B38, DR4, DQw3 and clozapine-induced agranulocytosis in Jewish patients with schizophrenia. *Archive of General Psychiatry*, 47(10), 945-948.

Lim, R (2002). Cultural assessment in clinical psychiatry. *Psychiatric Service*, 53:1486.

Lin KM, Poland RE & Nakasaki G (Eds). (1993). Psychopharmacology *and Psychobiology of Ethnicity*. American Psychiatric Press, ISBN 88048-471-3, Washington DC.

Littlewood, R (1992). DSM-IV and culture: is the classification internationally valid? *Psychiatric Bulletin*, 16, 257-261.

Littlewood, R (1998). *The Butterfly and the Serpent: Essays in Psychiatry, Race and Religion.* Free Associations Press, ISBN 1-85343-400-0, London.

Littlewood, R (2002). *Pathologies of the West: An anthropology of mental illness in Europe and America.* Cornell University Press, ISBN 0-8014-8743-9, New York

Littlewood, R, Lipsedge, M (1988) Psychiatric illness among British Afro-Caribbeans. *British Medical Journal*, 296, 950-951.

Littlewood, R. & Lipsedge, M. (1997) *Aliens and Alienists: Ethnic Minorities and Psychiatry*, 3rd Ed., Taylor & Francis, ISBN 0-415-15725-0, London.

Locke, AL (1924). The concept of race as applied to social culture. *Howard Review*, 1: 290-299.

Lopez, SR, Guarnaccia, PJ (2000). Cultural psychopathology: Uncovering the social world of mental illness. *Annual Review of Psychology*, 51, 571-598.

Loudon, RF, Anderson, PM, Gill, PS & Greenfield, SM (1999). Educating medical students for work in culturally diverse societies. *Journal of American Medical Association*, 282(9), 875-880.

Lu, F (2006). DSM IV outline for Cultural Formulation: Bringing culture into the clinical encounter. *Focus*, 4, 9-10.

Lu, FG, Primm, A (2006). Mental health disparities, diversity and cultural competence in medical student education: How psychiatry can play a role. *Academic Psychiatry*, 30, 9-15.

Mann, CE, Himelein, MJ (2004). Factors associated with stigmatization of persons with mental illness. *Psychiatric Service*, 55(2), 185-187.

Maercker, A (2001). Association of cross-cultural differences in psychiatric morbidity with cultural values: A secondary data analysis. *German Journal of Psychiatry*, 4, 17-23.

Marano, L (1982). Windigo psychosis: The anatomy of an emic-etic confusion. *Current Anthropology*, 23(4), 385-412.

Marzan, M, McEvoy, M (2010). Innovative medical education: Opportunities for cross-cultural medical education. *Einstein Journal of Biology and Medicine*, 25-26(1), 15-18.

Matthews, HW (1995). Racial, ethnic and gender differences in response to medicines. *Drug Metabolism and Drug Interactions*, 12, 77-91.

Mayer, CR (1996). Medicine's melting pot. *Minnesota Medicine*, 79(5):5.

Mayer, JD (1996). The political ecology of diseases as one new focus for medical geography. *Progress in Human Geography*, 20(4), 441-456.

McCabe, R, Priebe, S (2004). Explanatory models of illness in schizophrenia: comparison of four ethnic groups. *British Journal of Psychiatry*, 185, 25-30.

Mckenzie, K, Bhui, K (2007). Institutional racism in mental health care. *British Medical Journal*, 334, 649- 650.

Mezzich, JE, Caracci, G, Fabrega, H Jr & Kirmayer, LJ (2009). Cultural formulation guidelines. *Transcultural Psychiatry*, 46(3), 383-405.

Mistry, M, Latoo, J (2009). Uncovering the face of racism in the workplace. *British Journal of Medical Practitioners*, 2(2), 20-24.

Moffic, HS (1983) Sociocultural guidelines for clinicians in multicultural settings. *Psychiatric Quarterly*, 55(1), 47-54.

Mull, JD (1993). Cross-cultural communication in the physician's office. *Western Journal of Medicine*, 159(5), 609-613.

Ng, CH, Lin, KM, Singh, BS & Chiu, E. (Eds) (2008). *Ethnopsychopharmacology: Advances in Current Practice*. Cambridge University Press, ISBN 978-0-521-87363-5, New York.

Nieva, VF, Sorra, J (2003). Safety culture assessment: a tool for improving patient safety in healthcare organizations. *Quality and Safety in Healthcare*, 12, ii17- ii23.

Nunez-Smith, M, Curry, LA, Bigby, JA, Krumholz, HM & Bradley, EH. (2007). Impact of race on the professional lives of physicians of African descent. *Annals of Internal Medicine*, 146, 45-51.

Oberg, K (1960). Culture shock: adjustment to new cultural environments. *Practical Anthropology*, 7, 177-182.

Olsen L, Bhattacharya J, Scharf A (2006) *Cultural Competence: What it is and why it matters*. California Tomorrow. Lucile Packard foundation for Children's Health. Accessed on 12.6.11 from: http://www.lpfch.org/informed/culturalcompetency.pdf

Palmer, GB (1996). *Toward a Theory of Cultural Linguistics*. University of Texas Press, ISBN 029276569X, Austin, TX. pp.114.

Papadopoulos, I, Tilki, M & Lees, S (2004). Promoting cultural competence in healthcare through a research-based intervention in the UK. *Diversity in Health and Social Care*, 1, 107-115

Payne, N (2004). *Ten tips for cross cultural communication*. Accessed on 22.6.11 from: http://www.culturosity.com/pdfs/TipsforCross-CulturalCommunication.pdf

Penn, DL, Couture, SM (2002). Strategies for reducing stigma toward persons with mental illness. *World Psychiatry*, 1(1), 20-21.

Pike KL (1967). *Language in relation to a unified theory of structure of human behaviour*. 2nd Ed., Mouton & Co., ISBN B0007ED6PU, Paris.

Puranik, A, Dunn, J (1995). Koro presenting after prostectomy in an elderly man. *British Journal of Urology*, 75(1):108-109.

Purnell, L (2005). The Purnell Model for Cultural Competence. *Journal of Multicultural Nursing and Health*, 11 (2), 7-15

Redfield, R, Linton, R & Herskovits, M.J (1936). Memorandum for the study of acculturation. *American Anthropologist*, 38(1), 149-152.

Report of the Surgeon General (1999). *Mental Health.* Accessed on 15.6.11 from: http://mentalhealth.samhsa.gov/cmhs/surgeongeneral/surgeongeneralrpt.asp

Ridley, C (1984). Clinical treatment of the non disclosing Black client: A therapeutic paradox. *American Psychologist,* 39(11), 1234-1244.

Ritenbaugh, C (1982). Obesity as a culture-bound syndrome. *Culture, Medicine and Psychiatry,* 6, 347-61.

Robertson, K (2005). Active listening- More than paying attention. *Australian Family Physician,* 34(12), 994-1061.

Rogers A, Pilgrim D (2010). *A Sociology of Mental Health and Illness.* 4th Ed. Open University Press, ISBN 978-0335-23665-7, Berkshire, England.

Rogler, LH (1993). Culture in psychiatric diagnosis: an issue of scientific accuracy. *Psychiatry,* 56(4): 324-327.

Ross, JL, Laston, SL, Pelto, PJ & Muna, L (2002). Exploring explanatory models of womens' reproductive health in rural Bangladesh. *Culture, Health and Sexuality,* 4(2), 173-190.

Rossi, E (2002a). *The Psychobiology of Gene Expression.*WW Norton & Company, ISBN 0393-70343-6, New York

Rossi, EL (2002b). Psychosocial genomics: gene expression, neurogenesis, and human experience in mind-body medicine. *Advances in Mind-Body Medicine,* 18(2), 22-30.

Rossi, EL (2004). Gene expression and brain plasticity in stroke rehabilitation: a personal memoir of mind-body healing dreams. *American journal of Clinical Hypnosis,* 46(3), 215-227.

Rudorfer, E, Lam, E, Chang, W, Zhang, MD, & Potter, WZ (1984) Desipramine pharmacokinetics in Chinese and Caucasian volunteers. *British Journal of Clinical Pharmacology,* 17:433-440.

Safran, W (1991). Diasporas in modern society: Myths of homeland and return. *Diaspora,* 1(1), 83-99.

Saha, S (2006). The relevance of cultural distance between patients and physicians to racial disparities in health care. *Journal of General Internal Medicine,* 21(2), 203-205.

Saldana, D (2001) Cultural competency: *A practical guide for mental health service providers.* Hogg Foundation for Mental Health, University of Texas: Austin.pp. 4. Accessed on 25.6.11 from:
http://www.hogg.utexas.edu/uploads/documents/cultural_competency_guide.pdf

Scheper-Hughes, N (1992). Hungry Bodies, Medicine, and the State: Toward a Critical Psychological Anthropology. In, *New Directions in Psychological Anthropology,* Eds. T. Schwartz, G. White, and C. Litz, Cambridhe Universtity Press, ISBN 0-521-41592-6, Cambridge, pp.221-250.

Sen, P, Chowdhury, AN (2006). Culture, ethnicity and paranoia. *Current Psychiatric Reports,* 8, 174-178.

Simons, RC, Hughes, CC (Eds.) (1985). *The Culture-Bound Syndromes: folk illnesses of psychiatric and anthropological interest.* D. Reidel Publishing Company, ISBN 978-9027718587, Dordrecht, The Netherlands.

Skelton, JR, Kai, J & Loudon, RF (2001). Cross-cultural communication in medicine: questions for educators. *Medical Education,* 35(4), 257-261.

Skultans, V, Cox, J (Eds) (2000). *Anthropological Approaches to Psychological Medicine: Crossing Bridges.* Jessica Kingsley Publishers, ISBN 1-85302-707, London.

Stumpf, SH, Bass, K (1992). Cross-cultural communication to help physician assistants provide unbiased health care. *Public Health Report*, 107(1), 113-115.

Sue, DW, Sue, D (1977). Barriers to effective cross-cultural counseling. *Journal of Counseling Psychology*, 24(5), 420-429.

Swaptz, L (1985). Anorexia nervosa as a culture-bound syndrome. *Transcultural Psychiatry*, 22(3), 205-207.

Taylor, SL, Lurie, N (2003). The role of cultural competent communication in reducing ethnic and racial healthcare disparities. *American Journal of Managed Care*, 10, 1-4.

Terrell, F, Terrell, SL (1981). An inventory to measure cultural mistrust among blacks. *Western Journal of Black Studies*, 5, 180–184.

Teutsch, C (2003). Patient-doctor communication. *Medical Clinics of North America*, 87, 1115-1145.

Thakker, J, Ward, T (1998). Culture and classification: The cross-cultural application of DSM IV. *Clinical Psychology Review*, 18(5), 501-529.

Ting-Toomey S (1999). *Communicating across Culture*. ISBN 1-57230-445-6, Guilford Press, New York.

Trujillo, M (2008). Multicultural aspect of mental health. *Primary Psychiatry*, 15(4), 65-71, 77-84.

Tseng WS (2001). *Handbook of cultural psychiatry*. Academic Press, ISBN 0-12-701632-5, San Diego.

Tseng, WS (2003). *Clinician's guide to Cultural Psychiatry*. Academic Press, ISBN 0-12-701633-3, California. pp. 46-51

Tseng, WS (2006). From peculiar psychiatric disorders through culture bound syndromes to culture-related specific syndromes. *Transcultural Psychiatry*, 43(4), 554-576.

Tseng, WS, Streltzer, J (2004). Introduction: Culture and psychiatry. In, *Cultural Competence in Clinical Psychiatry*, Eds. W.S Tseng & J. Streltzer, American Psychiatric Publishing, ISBN 1585621250, Washington D.C., pp.1-20

United Nations (1965). *International Convention on the Elimination of All Forms of Racial Discrimination*, 21 December 1965, United Nations General Assembly, Treaty Series, vol. 660, p. 195, Accessed on 12.7.11 from:
http://www.unhcr.org/refworld/docid/3ae6b3940.html

UNESCO (2001). *Universal Declaration of Cultural Diversity*, 2001. Paris. Accessed on 12.5.11 from: http://www.unesco.org/bpi/eng/unescopress/2001/01-120e.shtml

Vandevijver, F, Tanzer, NK (2004). Bias and equivalence in cross-cultural assessment: an overview. *Revue Europeenne de Psychologie Appliquee*, 54, 119-135.

Vigdor, JL (2008). *Measuring immigrant assimilation in the United States*. Civic Report 53, Manhattan Institute for Policy Research. Accessed on 12.5.11 from: http://www.manhattan-institute.org /html / cr_53.htm

Warner, R (1999). The emics and etics of quality of life assessment. *Social Psychiatry and Psychiatric Epidemiology*, 34(3), 117-121.

Weisner, TS (2002). Ecocultural understanding of children's developmental pathways. *Human Development*, 45, 275–281.

Weiss, MG (1997). Explanatory model interview catalogue (EMIC): Framework for comparative study of illness. *Transcultural Psychiatry*, 34(2), 235-263.

Weiss, MG (2001) Psychiatric diagnosis and illness experience. In, *Cultural Psychiatry: Euro-International Perspective*. Eds. A.T. Yilmaz; M.G. Weiss; A. Riecher-Rossler, No. 169, Karger, ISBN 3805570481, Basel. pp. 21-34.

Weisse, CS, Sorum, PC, Sanders, KN & Syat, BL (2001). Do gender and race affect decisions about pain management? *Journal of General Internal Medicine*, 16, 211-217.

Whaley, AL (2004). Ethnicity/race, paranoia, and hospitalization for mental health problems among men. *American Journal of Public Health*, 94(1), 78-81.

WHO   (2011) *Gender and women's mental health*. Accessed on 23.7.11 from: http://www.who.int/mental_health/prevention/genderwomen/en/

Yip, K (2003). Traditional Chinese religious beliefs and superstitions in delusions and hallucinations of Chinese schizophrenic patients. *International Journal of Social Psychiatry*, 49(2), 97-111.

Part 2

Understanding Etiological Factors

6

Phenotype in Psychiatric Genetic Research

Javier Contreras
University of Costa Rica
Costa Rica

1. Introduction

Mental illnesses differ from medical conditions in their lack of objectively assessable biological markers for the establishment of a diagnosis. In the absence of clear external validators such as laboratory tests or radiological examinations, accurate assessment of the clinical picture and phenomenology becomes crucial. Common diseases with successful genetic mapping studies are generally characterized by diagnostic assessments that are objective, have a clear biological basis, and measure phenotypic features shared relatively uniformly among affected individuals. For example, type 2 diabetes is diagnosed based on elevation in blood glucose above a generally accepted threshold, as assessed by a simple assay. This phenotypic feature is at the core of the diagnosis, even though other disease components may vary between affected individuals. For mental illness, however, no biological assays are currently available for diagnostic purposes; the phenotypic features are generally assessed by subjective ratings, and individuals are assigned a diagnosis based on report of symptoms, no one of which is present in all individuals assigned that diagnosis. There is now considerable interest in identifying quantitative assessments, which may provide a more objective means of rating psychopathology.

Many researchers on psychiatric genetics have given attention to populations that are more genetically homogeneous due to historical reasons. These isolated populations have been useful for the identification of genes for disorders in other medical fields. In addition to the genetic homogeneity, these unique groups may also help in the definition of the phenotype. Particularly, psychiatric disorders with psychosis such as schizophrenia (SZ), schizoaffective disorder (SCA) and bipolar disorder type I with psychosis (BPI) are major public health burdens and their biology is still largely unknown. It is unlikely that these disorders represent a single illness, however they overlap on many dimensions, including symptoms, neurocognition, and treatment. Families of individuals with SZ very often have other members with BPI and SCA (Kendler et al., 2010). Many authors argue that modifying genes may determine why one person develops SZ and another develops BPI or SCA (Van Erp et al., 2002). Nevertheless, the question whether or not phenotype uncertainty is responsible of the presumed genetic overlap remains unanswered.

The use of multiple sources of information in the diagnostic process is essential in genetic studies of mental illness. A best-estimation diagnostic approach ensures diagnostic precision and reduces misclassifications getting better phenotype characterization of the study subjects. Along with the clinical complexity and the assumed genetic heterogeneity, environmental factors play an important role in the final outcome of most psychiatric disorders. In this instance, stressful environmental factors have been clearly associated with increased risk for suicidal behaviour (Perez-Olmos et al., 2007). In this way, external factors interact with genetic predisposition in the occurrence of suicide. Likewise, subjects with chronic psychosis who experience a high number of adverse life events could be at particular risk to develop depression depending of their genetic susceptibility.

2. Psychiatric genetic research in the Central Valley of Costa Rica

The isolated Costa Rican Central Valley population (CRCV) was founded by approximately 86 Spanish families. These families colonized the area between 1569 and 1575 and intermarried with indigenous Amerindians. By the beginning of the 18th century, the population grew rapidly with little subsequent emigration for almost 200 years (Escamilla et al., 1996). Psychiatric genetic research in CVCR began on mid-1990s. Participants have been selected with regard to their ancestry by completing a genealogical search. Thus, the majority of the great-grandparents of each subject are descended from the original founding population of the CVCR. Documentation of the birthplace of the great-grandparents is possible due to the centralization of birth records. This yield to link up approximately half of these subjects to a founder couple who came into Costa Rica in the 17th century, which demonstrates the founder effects in this population.

At present, more studies are being conducted for SZ, SCA and BPI in the CVCR. It has been found that subjects recruited independently of each other within this population can be linked together once genealogies are studied. This suggests that accurate genealogical screening is crucial for selecting subjects whose ancestors are predominantly from the founder population. This research approach represents an advantage for fine mapping and the identification of susceptibility genes. Because both linkage and association approaches depend on the probability that affected individuals will share disease-susceptibility genetic variants and marker loci identical due to descent from a common ancestor, human geneticists have long been interested in identifying study samples characterized by relative genetic homogeneity.

3. The phenotype in psychiatric genetic studies

Segregation analyses, adoption studies and twin studies have consistently shown that regardless of the population studied, genetic factors play an important role in determining the risk of developing SZ, SCA and BPI. Evidence suggests that these disorders share common genes (Badner & Gershon, 2002). Although genetic studies of these disorders have made progress in recent years, the field lags behind other complex diseases in the identification of disease-related genes. SCA patients have increased familial risk of SZ and mood disorders. Relatives of SZ probands have increased risk for SCA and major depressive disorders. Many patients with SZ have concomitant major depression at some point in their illness, and the longitudinal course of this depression (which is difficult to accurately assess) is often the determining factor in assignation of a diagnosis of SCA versus SZ. A clinical characterization study from a Costa Rican sample reported that more than half of the patients with SZ have mood symptoms particularly depressive symptoms (Contreras et al., 2008). Conversely, many patients with BPI endorse lifetime history of psychotic symptoms. As illustrated in figure 1, SZ, SCA and BPI with psychosis share a common domain, psychosis. Another report from the same population found that 97.6% of the bipolar I patients have history of psychosis which might explain the clinical similarities found between patients with SZ versus BPI (Pacheco et al., 2009).

Their clinical complexity is not well considered in the current diagnostic system, which may explain some of the misclassification biases yielding to misleading research findings. Categorical diagnosis appears to be a poor predictor of correlation between the phenotype and the specific genotypic variants that contribute to an individual's risk of developing these mental disorders. In the absence of measurable biomarkers for most of these conditions, accurate assessment of the clinical picture and phenomenology of patients becomes even more crucial. It is now generally agreed that phenotypes (diagnoses) are best made by comprehensive characterization of lifetime clinical symptomatology based on information gathered from several sources (Maziade et al., 1992). The scientific rationale for such a recommendation is that systematic evaluation of all sources of information conduct to a best-estimate diagnosis that reduces diagnostic error (Merikangas et al., 1989).

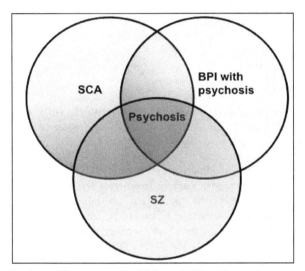

Fig. 1. Psychosis: the shared domain in SZ, SCA and BPI with psychosis.

3.1 Best estimation and consensus diagnostic process

The best estimation process uses a consensus-based approach to arrive at final diagnosis (Leckman et al., 1982). Clinical information is gathered from the Diagnostic Interview for Genetic Studies (DIGS), (Nurnberger et al., 1994), a Family Interview for Genetic Studies (FIGS) (Maxwell, 1992) and medical records.

The DIGS was developed by the National Institute of Mental Health (NIMH) in 1994. Its polydiagnostic capacity enables a detailed assessment of the course of the illness, chronology of the affective and psychotic disorders and comorbidity, as well as an additional description of symptoms including the possibility of an algorithmic scoring. The DIGS is an diagnostic instrument that allow psychiatrist form around the world to speak the same language; it includes a section describing the temporal relationships between affective disorders, anxiety disorders, psychosis and substance abuse disorders. It is reliable and valid instrument for genetic studies and has been used as a research instrument in other biological marker studies, given its diagnostic capacity for both the current and previous episodes. The direct interviews (DIGS) are conducted by trained psychiatrists and inter-rater reliability is evaluated to ensure consistency of the instrument. The psychiatrist is blind to family history, medical records, or any other information other than that they derived from the direct interview.

Final diagnoses is obtained through a consensus process where two independent psychiatrists review all available information, arrive at independent diagnoses, discuss the case and then arrive at consensus diagnoses. Each best estimate rater also score each affected subject for lifetime dimensions of psychosis using the Lifetime Dimensions of Psychosis Scale (LDPS) developed by Levinson et al; 2002. The LDPS creates a profile of the lifetime characteristics of each case based on retrospective ratings, encompassing dimensions of positive psychotic, depressive and manic symptoms, complicating factors and deterioration. Dimensional information allows researchers to capture subsyndromic symptoms used to define spectrum conditions like SZ, SCA, BPI. For instance, LDPS has been used to study disorganization and negative symptoms (dimension for hebephrenia) in a Costa Rican sample. It was found that prominent lifetime scores for disorganization and negative symptoms are associated with the cannabinoid receptor 1 gene (CNR1) (Chavarría-Siles et al., 2008). The defined dimension for hebephrenia resembles the chronic cannabinoid-induced psychosis.

In spite of a good research instrument such as the DIGS, additional sources of information are required to accurately capture the diagnosis of patients with psychotic disorders. A study comparing direct interview and consensus based multi-source methods found that the DIGS alone have low agreement for the diagnosis of SZ (Contreras et al., 2009). Disagreement is more commonly observed on those diagnoses involving mixed symptomatology (psychotic and affective symptoms). The lack of clarity in the DSM-IV criteria for SCA, the difficulty of accurately assessing the duration of mood symptoms and/or psychotic symptoms and their overlap may explain the poor agreement rate in this disorder. This finding provides more evidence on the importance of a final best-estimate and consensus diagnostic process for psychiatric genetic research.

4. Endophenotype

While psychiatric nosology defines SZ, SCA and BPI as unique illnesses with distinctive clinical characteristics, and presumably separated aetiologies, there is growing evidence that they share common susceptibility genes (Walss-Bass et al., 2005). Although it is unlikely that they are a single illness, there is an overlap on many dimensions, including symptoms, neurocognition, and effective treatment. To date, most genetic research has been focused on the categorical classification and few have explored quantitative phenotypes. Imprecision of psychiatric phenotyping might explain the failure of genetic research to identify susceptibility genes of these disorders where research diagnoses is attained by subjective assessments. Growing evidence supports the study of quantitative processes mediating between the genotype and gross clinical phenotype (endophenotype) (Preston et al., 2005).

Imprecision of psychiatric phenotyping might explain the failure of genetic research to identify genes that contribute to susceptibility of these disorders (Bearden et al., 2004). It is assumed that genes involved in endophenotypic variation are likely to represent more elementary phenomena than those involved in complex psychiatric diagnostic entities. It is also used interchangeably with the term 'intermediate trait,' describing a heritable quantitative phenotype believed to be closer in the chain of causality to the genes underlying the disease (Bearden & Freimer, 2006).

Clinical heterogeneity occurs when more than one clinical condition can be brought about by the same cause; causal heterogeneity occurs when two or more causes can, on their own, lead to the same clinical syndrome. Some individuals will have the "full disorder", which mean a clinical syndrome meets diagnostic criteria for a specific diagnosis. Others will not meet criteria for the full disorder yet will show the abnormalities that are called "spectrum conditions". There is a third group, cases of illness that mimic a genetic disorder but are not caused by genes, "phenocopies". It is likely that phenocopies account for many diagnostic errors whereby a patient is diagnosed with a genetic condition but actually has some other disorder. Hence, phenocopies are a dramatic form of causal heterogeneity where disease genes cause some cases and others are not. Most probably, the "other" cases are caused by some environmental event. Defining disorders as "genetic" and "nongenetic" can lead to controversial position. Some authors argue that it would make more sense to view the genetic and environmental contributions to illness as varying among people. By chance, some patients will have primarily genetic disorders and others will have primarily environmental disorders. Most of them are likely to have a mix of both types of causes as seen in clinical daily practice.

Gottesman proposed that SZ does not have a single cause but it is caused by the combination of many genes and environmental factors, each having a small additive effect on the expression of SZ. This view has been called "the multifactorial theory of SZ" because it proposes that multiple causes lead to illness. This theory posits that it is possible to separate patients into groups with greater and smaller genetic contributions to their disorder but most of them will fall between the two extremes of "primarily genetic" and "primarily environmental." This approach result of help for patients and their family members to better understand the causes of mental illness. It shows the role of environmental circumstances and how psychosocial therapies can help people with mental disorders even though many of these disorders are believe to be biologically based conditions reflecting the dysregulation of brain systems.

The "spectrum conditions" are used to describe mild psychopathology or other abnormalities of unknown clinical significance that occur among the otherwise well relatives of psychiatric patients. It supports the theory that most psychiatric disorders are not a discrete condition. Instead, it places many mental disorders within a continuum of psychopathology where genes and environmental insults determine the susceptibility to develop a psychiatric disorder. Figure 2 illustrates how this vulnerability is viewed as a quantitative or continuous trait. Many psychiatric disorders display a signature of complex inheritance. The liability to develop the disease is defined by a particular threshold of phenotypic severity. Milder forms of the illness are defined by less severe phenotypic features, and so there is familial aggregation of a spectrum of conditions that vary in severity. This pattern is consistent with models of inheritance that include multiple genes that interact with each other and environmental factor to confer susceptibility to illness.

An endophenotype is a heritable quantitative trait that is genetically correlated with disease liability, can be measured in affected and unaffected family-members and provides greater power to localize disease-related genes than affection status alone (Gottesman & Shields, 1973). They are less dependent on diagnostic certainty than more traditional genetic designs. Currently, an increasing number of researchers are using quantitative endophenotypes in extended pedigrees, which is considered the most powerful approach for localizing genes for affective and psychotic illnesses. Nevertheless, some geneticists argue against the endophenotype-based approach in psychiatry, noting the lack of evidence that such intermediate phenotypes are more closely related to risk genes than are the diseases themselves.

Personality traits and neurocognitive measures are inexpensive endophenotypes that can be collected in large-scale family-based studies. Many candidate endophenotypes for BPI (e.g. neurocognitive functions, behavioural traits, sleep abnormalities) have been proposed (Gottesman & Gould, 2003; Hasler et al., 2006). Research of candidate endophenotypes for SZ and BP has also been conducted in the population of the CVCR. It was observed that neurocognitive traits are strong candidate endophenotypes for SZ and BP separately. For instance, a processing speed measure (Digit-Symbol Coding) was a strong candidate endophenotype for both illnesses (Glahn et al., 2010) and closely related to genetic liability for SZ (Glahn et al., 2007).

A study of quantitative measure of anxiety as a candidate endophenotype for BPI in the CVCR was also performed. It was found that quantitative measurements of both, state and trait anxiety are highly heritable and share some genetic factors but only anxiety trait is associated with Costa Rican BPI (Contreras et al., 2010). Hence, quantitative trait of anxiety meets criteria for a candidate endophenotype in the studied sample. The relevance of this work can be summarized as follows: (1) Quantitative anxiety measures as an endophenotype may facilitate the identification of genes that predispose individuals to develop BPI. (2) Confirmation of this result will aid researchers to understand the essential pathophysiology underlying bipolar spectrum disorders. (3) If this trait is proven to be an endophenotype, it will be of help in diagnosing and treating BPI patients in a more reliable and biologically valid manner than our current classification allows. This will also have direct epidemiological implication on public health policies. (4) As for other bipolar endophenotypes, anxiety traits can be modelled in animal research. Several genetic, pharmacological, and behavioural animal models have long been used to establish animal anxiety-like phenotypes, as well as to assess their memory, learning, and other cognitive functions (Ennaceur et al., 2006; Kalueff & Murphy, 2007; Waikar & Craske, 1997; Wang et al., 2007; Yokoyama et al., 2009). Specifically, chronic oxytocin has been used to attenuate the high level of trait anxiety in rats (Slattery and Neumann, 2009). Some innate fear responses may also underlie the type of elevated anxiety levels found in the subjects with BPI.

Factor analysis of this trait in subjects with lifetime history of manic/hypomanic syndrome led to the classification of these individuals in two groups, worry and rumination, based on the nature of the symptoms (Contreras et al., 2011). Comorbid obsessive compulsive disorder in BP is characterized by episodic course, higher rates of certain obsessions (e.g. aggressive/impulsive, sexual, religious, and obsessional doubts) that require more frequent hospitalizations and complex pharmacological interventions (Perugi et al., 2002). A defining characteristic of obsessive compulsive disorder is unsuccessful suppression of unwanted thoughts. Obsessive symptoms have else been positively associated with rumination and inversely associated with perceived thought control ability (Grisham & Williams, 2009). Rumination involves repetitive thought about past events, current mood states, or failure to achieve goals (Martin & Tesser, 1996). Evidence suggests that rumination predicts the future occurrence of anxiety in anxious depressed comorbid conditions (Nolen-Hoeksema, 2000). In subjects with history of mania/hypomania, rumination may play an important role in triggering depressive episodes too. This analysis represents an important contribution to the understanding of underlying constructs in bipolar patients with sub-syndromic anxiety.

Further research will test whether these component factor scores are heritable, whether they share the same genetic factors, which (if they are not highly correlated) may further help define the components underlying BPI and other psychiatric disorders with a history of mania/hypomania.

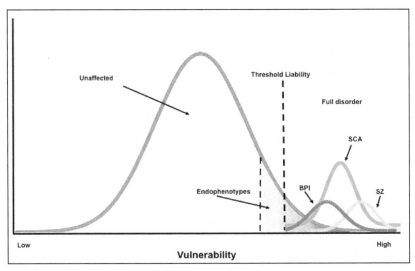

Fig. 2. Multifactorial vulnerability model for complex disorders.

5. Gene/environmental interaction

Gene-environment interactions result when genetic polymorphisms alter the ability of a specific region of the genome to be epigenetically altered in response to an environmental factor. Interaction between genes and environment plays an important role when studying the underlying etiological process of these psychiatric disorders (Kim et al., 2007). Many candidate genes have been studied, especially those directly implicated in the monoamines pathways. For example, allele- specific epigenetic modifications have been associated with "risk" polymorphisms in psychiatric candidate genes including the C/T(102) polymorphism in the serotonin receptor 2A gene (Polesskaya et al., 2006) and the Val66met polymorphism in the brain-derived neurotrophic factor gene (BDNF) (Mill et al., 2008). Increasing evidence suggests that epigenetic processes can be influenced by external environmental factors (Sutherland et al., 2003). Epigenetic events such as DNA methylation has been shown to vary as a function of nutritional, chemical, physical, and even psycho-social factors. As epigenetic changes are inherited mitotically in somatic cells, they provide a possible mechanism by which the effects of external environmental factors at specific stages in the life course can be propagated through development, producing long-term phenotypic changes. Epigenome seems to be particularly susceptible to disruption during rapid cell replication (Dolinoy et al., 2007).

In the same way, the polymorphism of the gene that codes for the serotonin transporter protein has been associated with specific clinical outcomes when interacting with environmental factors. This single gene (SLC6A4, Locus Link ID: 6532) has been mapped to chromosome 17q11.1-q12 (Murphy et al., 2004). This protein plays a crucial role in regulating the intensity and duration of serotonergic signalling at synapses and has been a target for many psychiatric drugs (Alessandro et al., 2008). There are at least two polymorphic variants that play a role in differential expression of the SLC6A4 gene. The short allele of these variants results in decreased expression of the serotonin transporter protein (Glatz et al., 2003). Several studies have analyzed the role of these variants in anxiety and depression (Uher et al., 2008). Depressive symptoms and suicidality have been associated with having one or two copies of the "s" allele, but only in the context of stressful life events (Caspi et al., 2003). Kendler and colleagues were able to replicate Caspi's finding showing in an independent sample that individuals with two "s" alleles showed an increased risk for depressive episodes in the context of stressful life events (Kendler et al., 2005).

Patients with SZ and SCA are at great risk for lifetime history of a full depressive syndrome or episode. One can hypothesize several potential pathways that might explain the high rates of depression in persons with a psychotic disorder. Lack of personal security, living conditions potentially harmful to the patients, psychological wellbeing, persecution and discrimination, bad peer relationships and unemployment are all potential consequences of interaction between the psychotic individual and his / her environment. For persons whose psychosis carries a paranoid element, the presumed threat from persecutors to the individuals' wellbeing may be sufficient to trigger depression and fear. For those patients who have sufficient insight to be aware of their illness and how it impacts their life, awareness of illness may be a direct trigger for a potentially dysphoric response. Postpsychotic depression, for instance, is a common occurrence in persons who are treated for first-break psychosis. By this mean, chronic psychosis might itself act as a "stressor" which interact with the "s/l" serotonin transporter variant to increase depression in persons with at least one copy of the "s" variant.

There is increasing evidence supporting the role of this gene in the course of mood symptoms in the context of psychosis (Contreras et al., 2008). A replication of the previous work was conducted using a narrower phenotype. Only subjects with SZ from the CVCR were included in the analysis. It was found that schizophrenic subjects carrying at least one short allele have higher risk for depressive syndromes (Contreras et al., 2010). Contrary to other scientific reports the authors did not find association between suicidal behaviour and the genetic variant.

6. Conclusion

Mental illnesses pose significant economic burdens, are associated with substantial morbidity and mortality rates and their etiological factors are poorly understood. Isolated populations such as the CVCR are essential for conducting studies of complex disorders. A centralized of health care; large family sizes and high rate of compliance of patients make this population ideal for genetic studies on mental illness. Within founder populations, genetic variants that are rare in other populations may also account for a greater proportion of the genetic cases, thus increasing the opportunity to identify predisposition genes of these common disorders.

Although genetic studies of SZ, SCA and BPI have made progress in recent years, the field lags behind other complex diseases in the identification of disease-related genes. The difficulty in finding genetic loci most likely derives from the complex nature of the illnesses.

The observed differences in social and functional decline among these psychiatric conditions support the original dichotomy described by Kraepelin based on chronicity and periodicity. By following this dichotomic concept some researchers have focused their work on a more severe and homogeneous phenotype. In this case, the categorical classification of the current diagnostic system has been utilized to define narrow phenotypes. Another group of researchers prefer to combine the traditional diagnostic approach with quantitative measurements. Thus, the measurement of more sophisticated dimensions such as neurocognitive endophenotypes and personality traits in multiplex multigenerational families have gained importance. Regardless of the diagnostic approach, a best estimation process is vital to avoid misclassification biases. The use of direct interview together with information from family members can help to identify problematic symptoms during diagnostic process. All efforts are oriented not only to the improvement of genotyping techniques and clinical classification but else to the understanding of the interaction of genes with environment. Some of the main limitations in this field of research are explain by the clinical and genetic complexity of psychiatric disorders, the lack of large sample sizes needed to detect associations at appropriate levels of statistical significance, the underlying stratification of study groups and the effect of medications on behavioural measurements. In order to overcome those obstacles, research is moving toward a more quantifiable and dimensional rating system. This will allow scientist to understanding the pathophysiology of mental illness that is of great public health significance. Identifying genes that contribute to risk of these diseases will provide critical information leading to the development of novel diagnostic and therapeutic strategies.

7. Acknowledgment

The author wishes to thank Henrriette Raventos and Michael Escamilla for their contribution to the psychiatric research field. We are also grateful to the families who have made this research possible.

8. References

American Psychiatric Association. (1994). *Diagnostic and statistical manual of mental disorders* (4th ed), American Psychiatric Press, Washington, DC.

Badner, J.A. & Gershon, E.S. (2002). Meta-analysis of whole-genome linkage scans of bipolar disorder and schizophrenia. *Mol. Psychiatry*, 7, pp. 405–411.

Bearden, C.E. & Freimer, N.B. (2006). Endophenotypes for psychiatric disorders: ready for primetime? *Trends Genet*, 22, 6, pp. 306–313.

Bearden, C.E., Reus, V.I. & Freimer, N.B. (2004). Why genetic investigation of psychiatric disorders is so difficult? *Curr. Opin. Genet. Dev.*, 14, 3, pp. 280–286.

Caspi, A., Sugden, K., Moffitt, T.E., Taylor, A., Craig, I.W., Harrington, H., McClay, J., Mill, J., Martin, J., Braithwaite, A. & Poulton, R. (2003). Influence of life stress on depression: Moderation by a polymorphism in the 5-HTT gene. *Science*, 301, pp. 386–389.

Chavarría-Siles, I., Contreras-Rojas, J., Hare, E., Walss-Bass, C., Quezada, P., Dassori, A., Contreras, S., Medina, R., Ramírez, M., Salazar, R., Raventos, H. & Escamilla, M.A. (2008). Cannabinoid receptor 1 gene (CNR1) and susceptibility to a quantitative phenotype for hebephrenic schizophrenia. *Am J Med Genet B Neuropsychiatr Genet,* 147, 3, pp. 279-84.

Contreras, J., Dassori, A., Medina, R., Raventós, H., Ontiveros, A., Nicolini, H., Munoz, R. & Escamilla, M. (2009). Diagnosis of schizophrenia in Latino populations: a comparison of direct interview and consensus based multi-source methods. *J. Nerv. Ment. Dis.,* 197, 7, pp. 530–535.

Contreras, J., Hare, E., Escamilla, M. & Raventos, H. (2011). Principal domains of quantitative anxiety trait in subjects with lifetime history of mania. *J Affect Disord,* In Press.

Contreras, J., Hare, L., Camarena, B., Glahn, D., Dassori, A., Medina, R., Contreras, S., Ramirez, M., Armas, R., Munoz, R., Mendoza, R.,   Raventos, H., Ontiveros, A., Nicolini, H., Palmer, R. & Escamilla, M. (2008). The Serotonin Transporter Gene and Depression in Chronic Psychotic Disorders. *Acta Psychiat Scand,* 119, 2, pp. 117-127.

Contreras, J., Hernández, S., Quezada, P., Dassori, A., Walss-Bass, C., Escamilla, M. & Raventos, H. (2010). Association of Serotonin Transporter Promoter Gene Polymorphism (5-HTTLPR) With Depression in Costa Rican Schizophrenic Patients. *J Neurogenet,* 24, 2, pp. 83-9.

Contreras, J., Montero, P., Dassori, A., Escamilla, M. & Raventos, H. (2008). Caracterización de un grupo de pacientes con esquizofrenia en el Valle Central de Costa Rica. *Acta Medica Costarricense,* 50, 3, 153-159.

Dolinoy, D.C., Weidman, J.R. & Jirtle, R.L. (2007). Epigenetic gene regulation: linking early developmental environment to adult disease. *Reprod Toxicol,* 23, pp. 297-307.

Ennaceur, A., Michalikova, S. & Chazot, P.L. (2006). Models of anxiety: responses of rats to novelty in an open space and an enclosed space. *Behav. Brain. Res.,* 171, 1, pp. 26-49.

Escamilla, M.A., Spesny, M., Reus, V.I., Gallegos, A., Sandkuijl, L.A., Fournier, E., Leon, P.E., Smith, L.B. & Freimer, N.B. (1996). Use of Linkage of Disequilibrium approaches to map genes for bipolar disorder in the Costa Rican population. *American journal of Medical Genetics,* 67, 3, pp. 244-253.

Glahn, D., Almasy, L., Barguil, M., Hare, E., Peralta, J., Kent, J.J., Dassori, A., Contreras, J., Pacheco, A., Lanzagorta, N., Nicolini, H., Raventós, H. & Escamilla, M. (2010). Neurocognitive endophenotypes for bipolar disorder identified in multiplex multigenerational families. *Arch Gen Psychiatry,* 67, 2, pp. 168-77.

Glahn, D.C., Almasy, L., Blangero, J., Burk, G.M., Estrada, J., Peralta, J.M., Meyenberg, N., Castro, M.P., Barrett, J., Nicolini, H., Raventos, H. & Escamilla, M.A. (2007). Adjudicating neurocognitive endophenotypes for schizophrenia. *Am J Med Genet B Neuropsychiatr Genet,* 144, 2, pp. 242-249.

Glatz, K., Messner, R., Heils, A., & Lesch, K.P. (2003). Glucocorticoid-regulated human serotonin transporter (5-HTT) expression is modulated by the 5-HTT gene promotor-linked polymorphic region. *J Neurochem,* 86, pp. 1072-1078.

Gottesman, I.I. & Gould, T.D. (2003). The endophenotype concept in psychiatry: etymology and strategic intentions. *Am. J. Psychiatry,* 160, pp. 636–645.

Gottesman, I.I. & Shields, J. (1973). Genetic theorizing and schizophrenia. *Br. J. Psychiatry,* 122, pp. 15–30.

Grisham, J.R. & Williams, A.D. (2009). Cognitive control of obsessional thoughts. *Behav Res Ther,* 47, pp. 395-402.

Hasler, G., Drevets, W., Gould, T., Gottesman, I. & Manji, H. (2006). Toward constructing an endophenotype strategy for bipolar disorders. *Biol. Psychiatry*, 60, 2, pp. 93–105.

Kalueff, A.V. & Murphy, D.L. (2007). The importance of cognitive phenotypes in experimental modeling of animal anxiety and depression. Neural Plast, 2007, pp. 1-7.

Kendler, K.S., Kuhn, J.W., Vittum, J., Prescott, C.A. & Riley, B. (2005). The interaction of stressful life events and a serotonin trans- porter polymorphism in the prediction of episodes of major depression: a replication. *Arch Gen Psychiatry*, 62, pp. 529–535.

Kendler, K.S., McGuire, M., Gruenberg, A.M., OHare, A., Spellman, M. & Walsh, D. (1993). The Roscommon Family Study I. Methods, diagnosis of probands, and risk of schizo- phrenia in relatives. *Arch Gen Psychiatry*, 50,7, pp. 527-540.

Kim, J.M., Stewart, R., Kim, S.W., Yang, S.J., Shin, I.S., Kim, Y.H. & Yoon, J.S. (2007). Interactions between life stressors and susceptibility genes (5-HTTLPR and BDNF) on depression in Korean elders. *Biol Psychiatry*, 62, pp. 423–428.

Leckman, J.F., Sholomskas, D., Thompson, W.D., Belanger, A., Weissman, M.M. (1982). Best estimate of lifetime psychiatric diagnosis: a methodological study. *Arch Gen Psychiatry*, 39, 8, pp. 879-883.

Levinson, D.F., Mowry, B.J., Escamilla, M.A. & Faraone, S.V. (2002). The Lifetime Dimensions of Psychosis Scale (LDPS): Description and interrater reliability. *Schizophr Bull*, 28, pp. 683–695.

Li, B., Xu, Y. & Choi, J. (1996). Applying Machine Learning Techniques, *Proceedings of ASME 2010 4th International Conference on Energy Sustainability*, ISBN 842-6508-23-3, Phoenix, Arizona, USA, May, 2010.

Martin, L.L. & Tesser, A. (1996). *Some ruminative thoughts*, R.S. Wyer, Editor, Advances in social cognition, Lawrence Erlbaum Associates, Hillsdale, NJ.

Maxwell, M.E. (1992). *Manual for the FIGS.* Bethesda, MD, National Institute of Mental Health.

Maziade, M., Roy, M.A., Fournier, J.P., Cliche, D., Merette, C., Caron, C., Garneau, Y., Montgrain, N., Shriqui, C. & Dion, C. (1992). Reliability of best-estimate diagnosis in genetic linkage studies of major psychoses: results from the Quebec pedigree studies. *Am J Psychiatry*, 149, pp. 1674–1686.

Merikangas, K.R., Spence, M.A. & Kupfer, D.J. (1989). Linkage studies of bipolar disorder: Methodologic and analytic issues. Report of MacArthur Foundation Workshop on Linkage and Clinical Features in Affective Disorders. *Arch Gen Psychiatry*, 46, pp. 1137–1141.

Mill, J., Tang, T. & Kaminsky, Z. (2008). Epigenomic profiling reveals DNA-methylation changes associated with major psychosis. *Am J Hum Genet*, 82, pp. 696–711.

Murphy, G.M., Hollander, S.B., Rodrigues, H.E., Kremer, C. & Schatzberg, A.F. (2004). Effects of the serotonin transporter gene promoter polymorphism on mirtazapine and paroxetine efficacy and adverse events in geriatric major depression. *Arch Gen Psychiatry*, 61, pp. 1163–1169.

Nolen-Hoeksema, S. (2000). The role of rumination in depressive disorders and mixed anxiety/ depressive symptoms. *J Abnorm Psychol*, 109, pp. 504-511.

Nurnberger, J.I., Blehar, M.C., Kaufmann, C.A., York-Cooler, C., Simpson, S.G., Harkavy-Friedman, J., Severe, J.B., Malaspina, D. & Reich, T. (1994). Diagnostic interview for genetic studies. Rationale, unique features, and training. NIMH Genetics Initiative. *Arch. Gen. Psychiatry*, 51, pp. 849-859.

Pacheco, A., Barguil, M., Contreras, J., Montero, P., Dassori, A., Escamilla, M. & Raventós, H. (2010). Social and clinical comparison between schizophrenia and bipolar disorder type I with psychosis in Costa Rica. *Soc Psychiatry Psychiatr Epidemiol*, 45, 6, pp. 675-680.

Perugi, G., Toni, C., Frare, F., Travierso, M.C., Hantouche, E. & Akiskal, H.S. (2002). Obsessive-compulsive-bipolar comorbidity: a systematic exploration of clinical features and treatment outcome. *J Clin Psychiatry*, 63, pp. 1129-1134.

Polesskaya, O.O., Aston, C. & Sokolov, B.P. (2006). Allele C-specific methylation of the 5-HT2A receptor gene: evidence for correlation with its expression and expression of DNA methylase DNMT1. *J Neurosci Res*, 83, pp. 362-373.

Preston, G.A. & Weinberger, D.R. Intermediate phenotypes in schizophrenia: a selective review. *Dialogues Clin Neurosci*, 7, pp. 165-179.

Serretti, A. & Kato, M. (1994). The serotonin transporter gene and effectiveness of SSRIs. *Expert Rev Neurother*, 8, pp. 111- 120.

Slattery, D.A. & Neumann, I.D. (2009). Chronic icv oxytocin attenuates the pathological high anxiety state in female high anxiety-related behaviour rats. *Neuropharmacology*, 58, 1, pp. 56-61.

Sutherland, J.E. & Costa, M. (2003). Epigenetics and the environment. *Ann N Y Acad Sci*, 983, pp. 151-160.

Uher, R. & McGuffin, P. (2008). The moderation by the serotonin transporter gene of environmental adversity in the aetiology of mental illness: review and methodological analysis. *Mol Psychiatry*, 13, pp. 131-146.

Van Erp, T.G., Saleh, P.A., Rosso, I.M., Huttunen, M., Lönnqvist, J., Pirkola, T., Salonen, O., Valanne, L., Poutanen, V.P., Standertskjöld-Nordenstam, C.G. & Cannon, T.D. (2002). Contributions of genetic risk and fetal hypoxia to hippocampal volume in patients with schizophrenia or schizoaffective disorder, their unaffected siblings, and healthy unrelated volunteers. *Am J Psychiatry*, 159, 9, pp. 1514-1520.

Waikar, S.V. & Craske, M.G. (1997). Cognitive correlates of anxious and depressive symptomatology: an examination of the Helplessness/Hopelessness model. *J. Anxiety. Disord.*, 11, 1, pp. 1-16.

Walss-Bass, C., Escamilla, M., Raventós, H., Montero, A., Armas, R., Dassori, A., Contreras, S., Liu, W., Medina, R., Balderas, T., Levinson, D., Pereira, R., Pereira, M., Atmetlla, I., NeSmith, L., Leach, R., & Almasy, L. (2005). Evidence of genetic overlap of schizophrenia and bipolar disorder: linkage disequilibrium analysis of chromosome 18 in the Costa Rican population. *Am. J. Med. Genet.*, 139, pp. 54-60.

Wang, D., Noda, Y., Tsunekawa, H., Zhou, Y., Miyazaki, M., Senzaki, K. & Nabeshima, T. (2007). Behavioural and neurochemical features of olfactory bulbectomized rats resembling depression with comorbid anxiety. *Behav. Brain. Res.*, 178, 2, pp. 262-273.

Yokoyama, F., Yamauchi, M., Oyama, M., Okuma, K., Onozawa, K., Nagayama, T., Shinei, R., Ishikawa, M., Sato, Y. & Kakui, N. (2009). Anxiolytic-like profiles of histamine H3 receptor agonists in animal models of anxiety: a comparative study with antidepressants and benzodiazepine anxiolytic. *Psychopharmacology*, 205, 2, pp. 177-187.

7

Abuse in Childhood and HPA Axis Functioning in Mentally Ill Patients

Śpila Bożena and Urbańska Anna
Department of Psychiatry Medical
University of Lublin
Poland

1. Introduction

In 1986 The European Council described family abuse as 'each activity or negligence of one of the family members that are life- threatening and can jeopardise physical and psychological integrity or freedom of another member of the same family or they seriously harm the development of his personality'. Ney et al. (1987)[1] ranked the types of violence and negligence according to the extent of destruction of an individual. The most traumatic forms of violence are:

- physical violence: hitting on the face, asphyxiation, striking with a belt, agitation, burns, bone fractures
- verbal violence: intimidation, blaming, embarrassing, discrimination
- sexual violence: gang rape, oral sex, forced masturbation, forced intercourse, forced participation in pornography

The epidemiological data point out the existence of the problem of abuse and using violence by parents towards children. It was stated that in the USA, from 11% to 62% of women (McCauley et al., 1997; Wyatt 1985)[2,3] and from 3% to 39% of men (Kercher et al., 1984)[4] were victims of sexual abuse in childhood. Different forms of abuse such as physical and emotional violence were believed to be an epidemic in the USA. What was researched were the traumatic experiences from childhood and later psychopathology. It was stated that sexual abuse in female children can later result in PTSD occurrence and concerns 10% of women in the USA (Kendler et al., 1995)[5].

[1] Ney, P.G. (1987). Does verbal abuse leave deeper scars: a study of children and parents. *Canadian Journal of Psychiatry* ,Vol. 32,pp. 371-377, ISSN 0706-7437.

[2] McCauley, J, Kern, D.E. et al. Clinical characteristics of woman with a history of childhood abuse: unhealed wounds. *JAMA*. 1997, 277; 1362- 1368, ISSN 0098-7484.

[3] Wyatt, G.E. (1985). The sexual abuse of Afro- American and white- American women in childhood. *Childhood Abuse Neglect*, vol.9, pp. 507- 519, ISSN 1097-6256.

[4] Kercher, R.C. & McShane M. (1984). The prevalence of child sexual abuse victimization in adult sample of Texas residents. *Childhood Abuse Neglect*, vol.8, pp. 495-502, ISSN 0145-2134.

[5] Kendler, K.S.; Kessler, R.C.; Walters E. et al. (1995). Stressful life events, genetic liability and onset of an episode of major depression. *American Journal of Psychiatry*, vol.152, pp. 833- 842, ISSN 0002-953X.

Cawson's research (Cawson et al., 2000; Cawson, 2002), which was carried out on a population of 2869 young British adults aged 18- 24 chosen randomly, found that maltreatment was experienced by 16 per cent of them[6]. Serious physical abuse by parents was experienced in the childhood of seven per cent of those researched, and six per cent of them experienced emotional maltreatment. Serious absence of care was experienced by six per cent of the sample; whereas five per cent of them suffered a serious absence of supervision. Childhood sexual abuse by parents was reported by 1 per cent of the sample. At the same time, 15 per cent experienced sexual abuse by other relatives or a known person, four per cent by a recently met stranger. Intermediate sexual abuse by parents affected 14 per cent of the sample in their childhood and intermediate absence of care- nine per cent, intermediate absence of supervision was experienced by 12 per cent (Cawson et al. 2000 & 2002). In the United States, it has been estimated that 11- 62% of women (Wyatt 1985; McCauley and Kern, 1997)[7],[8] and 3- 39% of men (Kercher & McShane, 1984)[9] have been victims of sexual abuse in childhood. Other forms of maltreatment such as physical and emotional abuse are regarded as widespread in the US.

While conducting research over various kinds of violence, Ney (1997) concluded that verbal violence, more than any other kind of it, influences the alteration of self- and world perception in the researched children. Verbal violence causes symptoms of fear of abandonment in children, mood disorders, difficulties in establishing and maintaining relationships, a feeling of guilt as well as auto- destructive behaviours. Children who are subject to physical violence are more aggressive, have a low self- esteem, impaired ability of achieving happiness in their lives, difficulties in expressing empathy, and - in case of a long-lasting violence - a connection can be noted between physical violence and the suppression of intellectual development, depression and aggressive behaviours (Heim et al., 2001; Ney, 1987; Ney, 1997; Rossman, 1985)[10],[11],[12],[13].

The outcomes of a variety of nowadays' scientific research indicate that there is a sound impact of some stressful events from childhood (trauma) on mental health (Ossowska 2002, Twardowska & Rybakowski 1996))[14],[15]. The research mainly concern sexual abuses,

---

[6] Cawson P., Wattam, C.; Brokers, S.& Kelly, G. (2000). *Child maltreatment in the United Kingdom*, NSPCC, ISBN 1-84228-006-6, London, United Kingdom.

[7] See 3

[8] See 2

[9] See 4

[10] Heim, Ch. & Nemeroff, Ch.(2001). The role of childhood trauma in the neurobiology of mood and anxiety disorders; preclinical and clinical studies. *Biological Psychiatry*, Vol.1, No. 49, pp. 1023-1039, ISNN 0006-3223.

[11] See 1

[12] Ney, P.G. & Peeters M.A. (1997). *The centurion's pathway*, Pioneer Publishing, ISBN 9780920952061, Victoria, USA.

[13] Rossman, P.G.(1985). The aftermath of abuse and abandonment: a treatment approach for ego disturbance in female adolescence. *Journal of American Academy of Child and Adolescent Psychiatry* , Vol.24, pp. 345-352, ISNN 0002-7138.

[14] Ossowska, G.(2002). *Poszukiwanie leków zapobiegających następstwom stresu przewlekłego. Nowy model „depresji" u szczurów*. Praca habilitacyjna, Akademia Medyczna w Lublinie, Zakład Poligraficzny BiS, Lublin, Poland.

[15] Twardowska, K. & Rybakowski J. (1996). Oś limbiczno – podwzgórzowo – przysadkowo – nadnerczowa w depresji (przegląd piśmiennictwa), *Psychiatria Polska*, Vol. 5, pp. 741 – 756, ISNN 0033-2674.

violence, lack of emotional support, loss of parents, separation, lack of parental warmth, familial conflicts, mental illnesses and psychoactive substance abuse by parents. The influence of sexual abuse and physical violence on a child's development has been put into a meticulous scrutiny here.

The experience of abuse in childhood is closely related to an increased number of traumatic experiences during a lifetime. The abuse may also enhance the susceptibility to the later development of PTSD through the change of psychological (e.g. the development of patterns of affection) and biological (the disruption of HPA axis functioning) developmental processes, including the interaction with genetic factors. In spite of the fact that different (except for abuse) types of traumatic experiences in childhood (e.g. a house burn-down or participation in a traffic accident), can force us to speculate that they will have an adverse effect on development, most of the current research points out childhood abuse and the linked stressful familial/ interpersonal events in life in the predictability of a wide range of later psychological and somatic problems.

The reasons for this state of matters are not yet fully understood, however, some of the potential explanations are the following:

1. In comparison to different types of traumatic events, childhood abuse happens more often in the context of the family ,

2. Every type of abuse in childhood is connected with an increased probability of exposure to another types of abuse and with an increased intensity of stressful situations connected with family/ parental dysfunctions (e.g. the psychoactive substance abuse by parents) , and

3. In comparison to some different types of exposure to trauma, childhood abuse is a frequently repeated experience, not only a single episode (e.g. multiple episodes of sexual abuse by the exact same tormentor for several years).

In McEven's work (2003)[16] it was described that one of the most important factors influencing a life- long health is the stability in the early period of life. Unstable parent-child relationships as well as an explicit abuse in childhood may lead to the development of behavioural and physical problems in childhood that also persist in the adult life. In people who experienced abuse in childhood, there was an increased mortality and morbidity of various diseases. On the other hand, however, the less extreme familial environmental features also cause an increased risk of somatic and mental disorders in children. As it was stressed in the current review of research, in families that are characterised by the lack of warmth and support or an insufficient supervision of the parents, there is an increased risk of somatic and mental disorders. The consequences of childhood abuse and familial dysfunction in an early period of life include a significant increase in substance abuse, depression and suicidal tendencies; promiscuity; an incidence of heart disease, cancer, chronic lung disease, extreme obesity, skeletal fractures and liver disease.

Abuse and negligence in early childhood is also connected with neuro- chemical imbalance which is related to low levels of serotonin as well as the development of hostility, aggression, substance abuse and suicide. Research on primate apes have shown than an early maternal deprivation lowers the levels of serotonin in the brain and it also enhances the tendency towards alcohol and aggressive behaviours. It also lowers affiliate behaviours.

---

[16] McEven,B.S. B.S.(2003). Early life influences on life-long patterns of behavior and health. *Mental Retardation and Developmental Disabilities Research Reviews,* Vol. 9, pp.149-154, ISSN 1080-4013.

Data from the research on humans point out similar patterns of an altered physiological function in children who were brought up in 'risky families' (i.e. families that are characterized by aggression, lack of parental warmth or an excessive/ insufficient regulation). Children from such families show irregular HPA axis activity, especially the increased levels of activity in this specific hormonal system.

In the Easton et al. research [17](2000) from Yale University School on the group of 105 addicts, a high incidence of abuse in childhood was observed. It was shown that 14% of the group were victims of family violence. The addicts that experienced this form of abuse showed a greater severity of depression symptoms that were estimated with the use of Beck's Depression Scale and more aggravated symptoms of addiction researched by Michigan Alcoholism Screening Test. They also required a more intensive individual therapy.

A lot of research was conducted that associated traumatic experiences from childhood with the later psychopathology.

Using violence towards children creates a possibility of occurrence in the adult life of the following: depression (Briere & Runtz, 1990; Wyatt 1985; Sweet et al. 1990)[18,19,20] anxiety disorders (Agid et al. 2000)[21], addictions (Agid et al. 2000, Kedler et al. 1995)[22,23] and personality disorders (Herman et al. 1989, Ogata et al. 1990)[24,25].

Analysing the impact of various kinds of stress on mental state, it is important to divide them into those taking place during the recent time and in the past, including childhood. In the light of the latest work of Heim et al., the trauma experienced in the early years of childhood can cause a preserved biological state that can be the risk factor for mental disorders development in the later life. For this reason, the ascertainment of childhood abuse should be considered as a crucial risk factor of the occurrence of mental disorder just as tobacco smoking is the risk factor of lung cancer[26].

2. Trauma as a chronic stress and its pathogenic role

The occurrence of a long- lasting activation of HPA axis, autonomic system and various executive centres during chronic stress causes many adverse effects of the organism, it

[17] Easton , C.J. (2000). Prevalence of family violence In clients entering substance abuse treatment. *Journal of Substance Abuse Treatment,* Vol.18, pp.23-28, ISSN 0740-5472.
[18] Briere ,J. & Runtz, M. (1990). Differential adult symptomatology associated with three types of abuse. *American Journal of Psychiatry ,* Vol. 14, pp. 357, ISNN 0145-2134.
[19] See 3 Wyatt
[20] Sweet, C.; Surrey, J.; Cohen, C. (1990). Sexual and physical abuse histories and psychiatric symptoms among male psychiatric patients. *American Journal of Psychiatry,* Vol. 147, pp 632, ISNN 0002-953X.
[21] Agid, O.; Kohn, Y.; Lere, B. (2000). Eviromental Sterss and psychiatric illness. *Biomedical Pharmacotherapy* vol. 54, pp. 135, ISSN 0753-3322.
[22] See 16.
[23] See 5.
[24] Herman, J.L; Perry, J.; Kolk B.A. (1989). Childhood trauma in borderline personality disorder. *American Journal of Psychiatry,* Vol. 146, pp. 490, ISNN 0002-953X
[25] Ogata, S.N.; Silk K. (1990). Childhood sexual and physical abuse in adult patients with borderline personality disorder. *American Journal of Psychiatry,* Vol. 147, pp. 1008, ISSN 0002-953X.
[26] Heim, Ch.; Newport, D.J.; Stacey, H.; Graham, Y.(2000). Pituitary-adrenal and autonomic response to stress in woman after sexual and physical abuse in children. *JAMA* Vol.,2, pp. 592-597, ISNN 0098-7484.

predisposes to the development of pathological processes that are mostly linked with chronic hypercortisonism and the activation of autonomic system. Stress activates many of the organism's systems, including the HPA axis and noradrenergic brain system, is also controls autonomic input. Chronic stress can lead to the development of numerous kinds of disorders. In the case of chronic stress, the number/ sensitivity of the corticosteroid G receptors decreases which maintains the existing stress reaction. This is how it comes to an eventual weakening of the vital mechanism that naturally reduces its severity- the negative feedback, due to which the increased cortisol inhibits the activity of superior stress centres. Chronic stress, therefore, in contrast to an acute stress, should be considered as a non-adaptive reaction. Thus, through the persistent hyperactivity of the HPA axis and its accompanying neuro- hormonal imbalance, it leads to the occurrence of disorders in organism functioning. The persistent hypercortisonism and hyperactivity of sympathetic system or its imbalance during chronic stress can lead to:

- Weakening of memory processes (most probably connected with the degeneration of CA_3 cells in hippocampus)
- Immunosuppression
- Inhibition of sex hormones production and osteoporosis
- Hypertension, tachycardia , decrease in the variability of heart rhythm/ cardiac dysrhythmia

The above processes favour the development of various diseases of the cardiovascular system, as well as metabolic, endocrine and neoplastic diseases. Chronic stress plays a major role in the pathogenesis of insulin resistance syndrome. It is characterised by:

- Hyperinsulinemia, glucose intolerance and hyperglycemia
- Hypertension
- Decrease of fraction HDL cholesterol density and increase of triglyceride concentration
- Abdominal obesity

Insulin resistance syndrome predisposes to various metabolic and cardiovascular diseases such as diabetes type II, atherosclerosis as well as ischemic heart disease (Lewandowski 2001)[27].

Persistent increased level of corticotrophin- releasing hormone (CRF), causes such symptoms as deterioration of mood and sexual drive, anxiety, sleep and eating disorders. The pathogenic action of chronic stress happens also on the level of genetic expression. After entering the cell, corticosteroids together with the receptors, create a complex that, after activation, enters the cell's nucleus and induces the genetic transcription through binding to the regulation site of specific genes. Under the influence of chronic stress, on a one hand, an increase in cortisol concentration appears , on the other, however, there is a decrease in the number/ sensitivity of corticosteroid receptors which is why it can contribute to the occurrence of disorders concerning these processes and the activation of genetic predisposition towards some diseases (Budziszewska & Lasoń,2003)[28]. The coincidence of subsequent stressful events in the adult life with the existing sensitivity of the HPA axis results in disorders of an enhanced production of cortisol and corticotrophin- releasing hormone (CRF) production reuptake in brain. CRF is a neuropeptide that influences the

---

[27] Landowski, J. (2001). Depresja jako przewlekły stres. *Dyskusje o Depresji*, Vol 17, pp.2.
[28] Budziszewska, B.; Lasoń W. (2003). *Neuroendokrynne mechanizmy działania leków przeciwdepresyjnych*, ISBN 83-917041-3-0, Wrocław, Poland.

production of ACTH through the pituitary gland, it is simultaneously a neuromodulator of many different neurotransmitter systems. It also has a significant influence on the brain adrenergic system through the locus coeruleus by altering the secretion of noradrenalin, serotonin and dopamine. The tonic activity of locus coeruleus changes into a fluctuating one, causing alterations in secretion of monoamines and subsequent anxiety symptoms (changes in 5- HT secretion), anhedonia as well as slowness and difficulties in concentration (changes of DA secretion) (Harro & Orleand 2001)[29]. Thus, a compilation of stresses in adult life on the childhood- originated sensitization in the range of the endocrine axis, Hypothalamus- Pituitary- Brain (HPA) can lead to a start of a cascade of abnormalities in monoaminergic systems which can be manifested by various clinical symptoms (Strickland et al. 2002)[30].

3. Hypothalamus- pituitary- adrenal axis

Monoaminergic neurotransmitters - noradrenalin (NA), serotonin (5-HT) and dopamine (DA) play an important role in various brain processes, including the limbic system functioning. The hypothalamus controls endocrine and vegetative systems. The Hypothalamus- Pituitary- Adrenal axis is a neuroendocrine system, in which there are mutual connections between the brain, hormones and various bodily organs. This system is engaged in the organism's reactions to stress. The activity of HPA axis shows 24 hour- long variations which are controlled by the central clock of suprachiasmatic nucleus, sending direct and indirect projections to the hypothalamus (Herbert J et al. 2006)[31].

Under the influence of stress and hence, various transmitters such as noradrenalin (NA), gamma- amino- butyric acid (GABA), serotonin (5- HT) as well as acetylcholine (ACH), hypothalamus produces, through the synthetic pathway, a hormone called Corticotrophin- Releasing Factor (CRF) that stimulates the anterior pituitary which leads to the synthesis and release of an adrenocorticotrophic hormone (ACTH). By the means of ACTH, there occurs secretion of hormones called corticosteroids in the adrenal gland. The main representative of this group of hormones in humans is cortisol (which is believed to be the main hormone of the sympathetic nervous system). The presence of cortisol in blood inhibits production of ACTH and corticotrophin- releasing hormone (CRF). The inevitable condition for an appropriate adjustment for stress is the termination of the stress reaction after the termination of the stimulus causing it. The defect of the stress reaction expiration or a situation of exposure to chronic stress may lead to pathological phenomena[32] (Parker et al. 2003). Naturally, homeostatic mechanisms in healthy people regulate an excessive physiological excitement. Abnormalities in HPA axis functioning may lead to prolongation

---

[29] Harro, J.; Oreland, L. (2001). Depression as a spreading adjustment disorder of monoaminergic neurons: a case for primary implication of the locus coeruleus. *Brain Research Review* , Vol. 38, pp. 79-128, ISNN 0165-0173.

[30] Stricland, P.; Dekin, W.; Percival C. (2002). Bio-social origins of depression in the community. Interactions between social adversity, cortisol, and serotonin neurotransmission. *British Journal of Psychiatry*, Vol. 180, pp.168, ISNN 0007-1250.

[31] Herbert ,J.; Goodyer, I.M.; Grossman ,A.B. (2006). Do corticosteroids damage the brain? *Journal of Neuroendocrinology* Vol.18, pp. 393-411, ISNN 0953-8194.

[32] Parker, K.; Schatzberg A.; Lyons D. (2003). Neuroendocrine aspects of hypercortisolism in major depression. *Hormones and Behavior* , Vol. 43, pp. 60-66 ,ISNN 0018-506X.

of stress; they also seem to play a vital role in the pathogenesis of some somatic diseases and mental disorders (e.g. affective disorders) (Ehlert et al. 2001 & Porter et al. 2006)[33],[34]. The dynamics of stress response in the HPA system consist of three phases:

1. Basal activity which reflects the non- stress- stimulated HPA activity
2. Stress activity in which the cortisol level increases above the basal level, indicating the beginning of the stressor activity.
3. Stress recovery in which the cortisol level returns to the basal level, indicating the expiration of the stressor (Burke et al. 2005)[35].

The consequences of stressful events in childhood are the disorders of neuroendocrine hypothalamus- pituitary- adrenal (HPA) axis' functioning manifested by its excessive activity (sensitisation) in an adult life.

In response to the stressor stimulus, an organism mobilises mechanisms of defence. The most important mechanism related to the organism reaction to stress is a proper functioning of the axis Limbic System- Hypothalamus- Pituitary- Adrenal (LHPA). Corticosteroids, which are produced by adrenal glands, inhibit the production and secretion of hormones by the superior centres: corticotrophin- releasing hormone (CRF) by the hypothalamus and adrenocorticotrophic hormone (ACTH) by the pituitary gland. This process takes place due to the corticosteroid receptors localized in the hypothalamus, pituitary or the limbic system, especially in the hippocampus. The most essential role in the control system is played by the prefrontal cerebral cortex as well as limbic system.

An increased concentration of corticosteroids may be also responsible for changes of a neurodegenerative nature in hippocampus as well as distortions in neuronal plasticity. In the research conducted on animals it was stated that corticosteroids in high concentrations:

- enhance neurodegenerative changes in hippocampus caused by various factors
- inhibit the formation of new cells (neurogenesis) in the Ammon's horn
- cause the decrease of the length and number of branching of apical dendrites of pyramidal cells of CA3 region in hippocampus (Lyons et al. 2001)[36].

The HPA axis enables an organism to adjust to the physiological and psychosocial changes in its environment. Both of the above systems were frequently examined in disorders associated with stress and depression. Scientific data suggest that those systems are inter- connected by the corticotrophin- releasing hormone (CRH). It is believed that anxiety disorders activate neuroendocrine systems in brain, however, it is not clear whether the situation is similar in case of depression .

On the basis of extensive basal and clinical results it was stated that the corticotrophin- releasing hormone and a group of related substances seem to play a key role in stress- related disorders, such as anxiety and depression.

[33] Ehlert, U.; Gaab, J.; Heinrichs, M. (2001). Psychoendocrinological contributions to the etiology of depression, posttraumatic stress disorder, and stress-related bodily disorders: the role of the hypothalamus-pituitary-adrenal axis. *Biological Psychology*, Vol. 57, pp.141-152, ISNN 0301-0511.

[34] Porter, R.J.; Gallagher, P. (2006). Abnormalities of the HPA axis in affective disorders: clinical subtypes and potential treatments. *Acta Neuropsychiatrica*, Vol. 18, pp. 193-209, ISNN 0924-2708.

[35] Burke, H.M.; Davis, M.C.;. Otte, C.; Mohr, D.C. (2005). Depression and cortisol responses to psychological stress: a meta-analysis. *Psychoneuroendocrinology*, Vol.30, No.9, pp. 846-56, ISNN 0306-4530.

[36] Lyons, D.M.; Yang, C; Sawyer-Glover, A.M.(2001). Early life stress and inherited variation in monkey hippocampal volumes.*Archives of General Psychiatry*, Vol. 58 pp.1145-1154, ISSN 0003-990X.

CRH is thought of as a brain fundamental mediator of stress response in relation to its participation in producing a neuroendocrine, autonomic and behavioral response to a stressful situation (Reul i in. 2005)[37].

Another hormone that participates in reaction to stress is dehydroepiandrosterone (DHEA) belonging to a group of steroid hormones and it is synthesized in the zona reticularis of the adrenal cortex from pregnenolon. Dehydroepiondrosterone is found in human blood plasma in the form of DHEA steroid of low plasma saturation stability and sulphate (DHEA- S) with half- life around 10- 12 hours.

The secretion of DHEA hormone is stimulated in similar way to the cortisol, i.e. by CRH and ACTH. In the brain, DHEA works as an agonist of the receptors of gamma- amino- butyric acid type A (GABA A), it protects neurons from the toxicity of glutamates and beta- amyloid peptides that secrete neurotoxic amino acids (Ritsner et al. 2004)[38] , blocks the excitability of neurons, having an anxiolytic, tranquilizing, sleep- inducing, mood- and cognition- improving effect.

DHEA- S, however, works antagonistically to the GABA A receptors through stimulation of the central nervous system, increasing its plasticity and susceptibility to convulsions. It also takes part in releasing pituitary and hypothalamic neuropeptides.

Another function of DHEA- S is enhancing the release of dopamine, noradrenalin and acetylcholine in the frontal lobes and limbic system what intensifies the memory and learning processes. DHEA- S works protectively in relation to the neurotoxicity of cortisol, especially in the hippocampus region (Goodyer et al. 2001, Załuska & Janota, 2009)[39],[40].

It is exactly the hippocampus as well as the limbic region where the concentration of DHEA is very high. However, it has not yet been agreed whether it is being produced there despite of the fact that there were quite a few reliable research reports completely devoted to its neurosteroidal genesis. Unfortunately, they also did not explain the mechanisms regulating the activity of cells producing neurosteroids (Holka- Pokorska 2005; Ritsner et al. 2004)[41],[42].

The research conducted both in the laboratorial and natural conditions, allow a conclusion to be formulated in the range of the meaning of DHEA- a hormone circulating not only in the blood, but also in the brain, that regulates the neurogenesis in the hippocampus as well as it modulates the lowering of elevation of corticosteroids, especially cortisol, thus influencing the formation of new neurons and increasing their survival (Herbert 2007).[43]

---

[37] Reul, J.M.& Holsoer, F.(2005). Corticotropin-releasing factor receptors 1 and 2 in anxiety and depression. Current Opinion in Pharmacology, Vol. 2, No.1, pp.23-33, ISSN 1471-4892.

[38] Ritsner, M.; Maayan, R.; Gibel, A.; Strous, R.D.; Modai, I.; Weizman, A. (2004). Elevation of the cortisol/dehydroepiandrosteron ratio in schizophrenia patients. European Neuropsychopharmacology, Vol. 14, pp.267-273, ISNN 0924-977X.

[39] Goodyer, I.M.; Park, R.J.; Netherton, C.M.; Herbert, J. (2001). Possible role of cortisol and dehydroepiandrosterone in human development and psychopathology. British Journal of Psychiatry, Vol. 179, pp..243-249, ISSN 0007-1250.

[40] Załuska, M.; Janota, B. (2009). Dehydroepiandrosteron (DHEA) w mechanizmach stresu i depresji. Psychiatria Polska , Vol.3. No.43, pp.263-274, ISSN 0033-2674.

[41] Holka-Pokorska,J. (2005).Dehydroepiandrosteron w leczeniu depresji. Wiadomości Psychiatryczne, Vol. 8, No.3, pp.149-155, ISSN 1505-7429.

[42] See 38

[43] Herbert, J. (2007). DHEA , In: Encyclopedia of stress, Eds. G. Fink (Ed.) 788-791,, Academic Press, ISBN 978-0-12-088503-9 ,London, United Kingdom.

Dehydroepiandrosterone serves a neuromodulating function as an agonist of GABA A receptors and an antagonist in relation to the action of cortisol, which is why the hypothesis of its vital importance in terminating the stress reaction and restoration of organism homeostasis is often supported. The hormone achieves it by the improvement of the strategy of handling stress (Załuska & Janota, 2009)[44].

The ratio of two steroid hormones (cortisol and DHEA) is an important indicator of their relative activity. A natural cortisol level and a lowered DHEA level can cause a harmful ratio for the brain's functioning. The ratio of hormones is described with the use of the term 'endocrine risk' with a greater probability of the occurrence of depression in a short period of time, more significantly in the afternoon measurements of cortisol levels than every single value considered separately.

The proportion of cortisol/ DHEA may be used as an indicator of the ability to maintain homeostasis when in stress. The available research results describe the influence of stress and the values of cortisol to DHEA ratio. In an acute stress, levels of both of the hormones (cortisol and DHEA) are subject to elevation and in chronic stress, a decrease of the concentration of cortisol, DHEA and DHEA- S can be observed, most probably as a sign of adaptive changes of an organism (Meewisse et al. 2007; Yehuda et al. 2006)[45],[46].

4. The influence of cortisol on the formation of fear symptoms

Fear arises as a result of a distortion of an interaction between the hippocampus system (conscious memory) and amygdale (emotional memory). Cortisol, being a stress hormone, leads to the decrease of the cohesion and density of hippocampus cells, impairing its function. This process is happening in the following way: a stressor that acts on individual and is emotionally recognised by the amygdale as a dangerous one, also stimulates both the hypothalamus and pituitary, leading to an elevation of the acetylcholine level, which subsequently increases the cortisol level. If a high cortisol level is maintained for a longer period of time (an induced one), it has an adverse effect on the hippocampus, interfering with the ability of conscious learning and memorising. The cortisol level, being an endocrine designatum of stress, lowers 'the possibility of creation in the hippocampus of a long-lasting strengthening of synapses, which is a metabolic substrate of conscious memorising'. In the research "the shrinkage of neuronal fibres in hippocampus during a forceful, even a short lived stress" was also proved (Herzyk 2003)[47].

What was described in the literature and research were the events of experiencing stress that positively influences the ability of conscious memorising, so called flash light effect, which is the result of the adrenalin action as a consequence of stress being rated by an individual as moderate. If, however, in the aftermath of a stressful event, the cortisol level is elevated, it

---

[44] See 37

[45] Meewisse, M.L.; Reitsma, J,B.; De Vries, G.J;, Gersons, B.P. & Olff, M. (2007). Cortisol and post-traumatic stress disorder in adults: systematic review and meta-analysis. British Journal Psychiatry, Vol. 191, pp.387-392, ISNN 0007-1250.

[46] Yehuda, R.; Brand, S.R.; Golier, J.A. & Yang R.K.(2006). Clinical correlates of DHEA associated with post-traumatic stress disorder. *Acta Psychiatrica Scandinavica*, Vol. 114 No.3, pp.187-193, ISNN 0001-690X.

[47] Herzyk, A.(2003). *Mózg, emocje i uczucia. Analiza neuropsychologiczna*. Wydawnictwo UMCS, ISBN 83-227-2152-8 ,Lublin, Poland

will subsequently amplify the activity of amygdala and the emotional subconscious memory, which influences destructively on the conscious memory. This is most probably the reason why the fear memory, encoded in the amygdala structure, remains for the whole life in human brain, being out of the reach of the consciousness. (Herzyk 2003)[48].

5. The genetics of stressor resistance

A hypothesis could be developed that any trauma experienced in childhood models the neuroplasticity of the brain, depending on the genetic basis (the genetic liability to stressors).

Some people have the ability of managing the most extreme kinds of stress, i.e. they have a high resilience to stress. In others, however, the influence of stressors from childhood and the piling up of another in the later adult life gives rise to a number of mental disorders such as PTSD, depression, anxiety disorders or others. The research concerning the gene liability to falling ill under the influence of chronic stressor factors can be of use while explaining personal differences. Polymorphisms of different genes were examined. The research of Binder and others (2008) concerning the polymorphisms of genes that regulate the activity of the glucocorticosteroid receptor (GR) gave very interesting results. The pre-clinical research point out that the FKBP5 gene localized on chromosome 6 modulates the binding of glucocorticosteroids with an appropriate GR receptor, thus regulating the response to stress. Protective alleles (RS 9296158 as well as RS 9470080) were found that have the ability to protect from falling ill. What was also found where the alleles of the risk of falling ill (RS 3800373 and RS 1360780) for this gene (4 from 8 SNP).

Different research suggests the role of a transcription factor (ΔFosB) which is induced by reward and stress in the nucleus accumbens (NAc). The activity of ΔFosB simplifies the creation of synaptic connections and adaptive behaviours by the reduction of an emotional load with NAc, thanks to the repression of excitement of the glutaminergic system. Experience induces the activity of the ΔFosB gene which leads to the increase of resilience to stress (Vialou 2010)[49].

6. Disturbances in reaction to stress in depression

Many research concerning the risk factors of depression was performed. The inheritance factors, gender and personality features have vast influences over the occurrence of depression. Except for the constitutional predisposing factors, an important role in the pathogenesis of depression is played by the environmental factors. Many works indicate a relationship between the psychosocial stress and the incidence of depression. Research proved that stress caused by some exceptional life events that happened in a specific, short period of time is of great importance for the development of depression (Bilikiewicz et al. 2002)[50]. It was also shown that there exists a connection between chronic stress (linked with e.g. work or marital problems) and the occurrence of depression.

---

[48] See 36

[49] . Vialou, V et al. (2010). ΔFosB in brain reward circuits mediates resilience to stress and antidepressant responses. Nature Neuroscience, Vol. 13, pp.745, ISSN 1097-6256.

[50] Bilikiewicz, A.; Pużyński, S.; Rybakowski, J.& Wciórka, J. (2002). *Psychiatria, tom I,* , Wydawnictwo Medyczne Urban & Partner, ISBN 83-87944-67-X,Wrocław, Poland.

A greater risk of major depression occurrence in adults that were molested in childhood was stated. For instance, in women who were victims of such abuse, the possibility of occurrence of major depression is 4 times as high and as for the risk of suicidal attempts, it is 44 times greater than in general population(Heim et al. 2001)[51].

What was also concluded was that the earlier in childhood the stress took place, the earlier the depression can occur in the adult life. In these particular cases the depression disorders have the tendency to be longer and the incidence of remmission is lower. On the basis of the research conducted in the United States, it can be drawn that various marital problems, parental divorce, abuse in the family, psychoactive substance abuse and many various mental disorders of parents are the result of a greater risk of falling victim of depression in the offspring (Nemeroff, 2002)[52]. According to other research there is a connection between the loss of parents and the development of depression in an adult age. There are research data suggesting that an increased susceptibility to depression in people who had lost their parents, occurs only in the case when they were left without a proper supervision in childhood. Also, a longer separation from parents might be the factor directly predisposing to becoming depressed. There is also a linkage between the lack of an appropriate mother care and the occurrence of depression (Twardowska & Rybakowski 1996, Nemeroff 2002)[53],[54].

A great number of data coming from different researches points out that traumatising experiences in childhood are strictly connected with a greater frequency of occurrence of depression in an adult life. Traumatising events before the 17th year of age include:

- lack of contact with mother for over a year
- staying in a hospital for over two weeks
- parents' divorce
- a long period of parent's unemployment
- experiences so traumatic that memories of them lasted for several years
- an abandonment without parental care because of one's bad behaviour
- alcohol or other psychoactive substances abuse by parents which caused problems in the family
- physical abuse (Bremner et al. 2000, Heim et al. 2001)[55],[56].

In comparison to children that were not exposed to maternal stress (especially depression in mother), children in the age of 4,5 year that were exposed to it showed a significantly higher cortisol concentration in saliva, but only in the case when the maternal stress was present in the infancy of the child, as well as in the period preceding the examination. In comparison to the 4,5- year old children with a lower cortisol concentration, the children with a higher level of it were subject to a greater risk of mental disorder occurrence, especially the

[51] Heim, Ch.; Owens, M. (2001). Znaczenie negatywnych wydarzeń z dzieciństwa w patogenezie depresji, In. *WPA Bulletin on Depression*, Vol.22, No.5, pp.3-7.

[52] Nemeroff, Ch., Wainwrigth, N.W.J; Surtees, P.G . (2002). Childhood adversity, gender and depression over the life-cours. *Journal of Affective Disorders*, Vol. 72, pp.33-44, ISSN 0165-0327.

[53] See 51

[54] See 15

[55] Bremner, J.D.; Vermetten, E.; Mazure, C.(2000). Development and preliminary psychometric properties of an instrument for the measurement of childhood trauma: The Early Trauma Inventory. *Depression and Anxiety*, Vol. 12, pp. 1-12, ISNN 1091-4269.

[56] See 26.

internalizing symptoms. These results show that the maternal stress is the factor that sensitises the infants that experience, in later life, the hyperactivity of the HPA axis during the exposition to a stressful situation from their mothers. An elevated concentration of cortisol in children with both: early- and later- occurring proneness to stress might be a marker of disorders in the stress response system that are clearly manifested in such developmental challenges as e.g. beginning school. It may lead to the increase of the risk of depression as well as anxiety disorders (Essex et al. 2000)[57].

In people with depression, signs of hyperactivity of the limbic system- hypothalamus- pituitary- adrenal axis (LHPA) can be observed, which is manifested by an elevated CRF level in the cerebrospinal fluid, an elevated cortisol level in blood, daily alterations in its secretion, lack of the cortisol response to the inhibiting action of dexamethasone (Ossowska 2002)[58] as well as a hypertrophy of the pituitary and adrenal glands. An autopsy research states the increase of CRF mRNA in the hypothalamus and a decrease of the number of CRF receptors; it also shows an elevation of mRNA encoding proopiomelanocortin in the pituitary. The persisting hyperactivity of the HPA axis in depression can result from a defect concerning the stress- activated mechanisms leading to the expiration of a stress reaction There are certain premises that claim that there is a virtual malfunction of the action of corticosteroid receptor in the limbic system that might be responsible for the inability of the stress reaction to expire. (Ossowska 2002, Heim 2002)[59],[60]. There was also a decrease of the number of these receptors on lymphocytes in people with depression. The distortion of action of the limbic system and hypothalamus by a chronic hypercortisonism leads (by a rule of vicious circle) to a further over- secretion of cortisol.

In the majority of cases of depression, one can find features of hyperactivity of the adrenal cortex, which are manifested by an excessive secretion of cortisol (hypercortisonism), changes in a daily cortisol secretion (longer and more frequent periods of secretion) as well as an increase urine eliminitation of the 17- hydroxysteroids and free corticosteroids. In recent years, in CT studies - structural signs of hyperactivity in the adrenal cortex were also noted in depression (an increase in the volume of the glands) (Heim et al. 2001, Twardowska & Rybakowski 1996)[61],[62].

7. HPA axis functioning disorders in depression

Psychosocial stress activates the HPA axis, however, it does not pose a mechanism of causing depression by stress. Depression occurs in the situation of the lack of a persisting hypercortisonism and the depressive patients usually have a lowered morning cortisol levels, which might be linked with a coexisting anxiety. The lead of 5- HT2 on the central level is strengthened in depression and is related to random events. It is compatible with the notion that the serotonergic system is responsible for the CUN level response to some unpleasant life events.

[57] Essex, M.J. et al. (2002) . Maternal stress beginning in infancy may sensitize children to later stress exposure: Effects on cortisol and behavior. *Biological Psychiatry* Vol.52, pp.776-784, ISNN 0006-3223
[58] See 14
[59] See Ossowska
[60] See heim
[61] See 26
[62] See 15

Strickland et al. (2002) study revealed an elevated cortisol level in the afternoon, after the action of some serious stress of the psychosocial kind in a current period of time; what is important, however, it was only observed in the female patients. It might mean that there is a primary disregulation in the HPA axis in some types of social depression which may result in an excessive reaction of cortisol secretion in a response to some stressful and solidified life difficulties. The primary disregulation of the axis might be responsible for the often reported elevated cortisol levels in the in- patients (hospitalized for depression), in whom the stress connected with the hospitalization might have co- existed with the HPA axis hyperactivity.

An increased activity of the HPA axis seems to have the most significant meaning in the pathogenesis of depression as well as in the mechanism of antidepressant drugs action. In the experimental research it was stated that corticosteroids and/ or the corticotrophin-releasing hormone may influence and intensify most of the changes observed in animals' models of depression.

In some of the depressed patients there is an elevated concentration of cortisol observed in the blood, urine and the cerebrospinal fluid, changes in the daily profile of cortisol secretion as well as an elevated corticotrophin- releasing hormone concentration in the cerebrospinal fluid. An increased activity of the HPA axis in depression is caused by hypersecretion of the corticotrophin- releasing hormone. In depression, there is a dysfunction of the HPA axis, which might have a genetic basis, however, the meaning of the past life events is also not excluded . The signs and symptoms that are characteristic for depression, include the changes in the HPA system, which in the majority of the patients, results in the alteration of corticotrophin (ACTH) regulation and a change in the secretive activity of cortisol. More detailed analyses of the HPA system have revealed that the signal of the corticosteroid receptor (CR) is distorted in severe depression, which leads, among all, to an increased production and secretion of corticotrophin- releasing hormone (CRH) in various regions of the brain, which is considered to be one of the main causes of depression (Holsboer, 2000)[63].

What also accompanies depression is the activation of the HPA axis and a lowered sensitivity to the negative feedback, when in the anxiety disorders it seems that the functioning of the HPA axis stays correct. (Young and others 1991, 1993, 2000, 2004; Abelson and Curtis, 1996).

8. Neuroendocrine mechanisms of antidepressive drugs action

What underlies the antidepressants' action are the adaptive changes in the neurotransmitter systems that occur under the influence of their constant administration. These changes include:

- decreased density and reactivity of β- adrenergic receptors
- increased density of α_1- adrenergic receptors
- decreased density of α_2- adrenergic receptors
- changes in density and reactivity of serotonin ($5HT_{1A}$, $5HT_{2A}$ and dopamine (D2/ D3) receptors, the calcium channels type I dependent on the voltage and glutaminergic receptors

---

[63] Holsboer, F. (2000). The cortycosteroid receptor hypothesis of depression. *Neuropsychopharmacology*, Vol. 23, pp. 477-501, ISSN 0893-133X .

A long- lasting period of antidepressant administration lowers the concentration of corticotrophin- releasing hormone in the hypothalamus, corticosterone and ACTH in blood (especially during stress), they also inhibit some of the corticosteroid and stress effects (7).

Tricyclic antidepressants, fluoxetin and tianeptin lower the hyperactivity of the HPA axis that is caused by the activation of the immune system (the administration of LPS, endotoxin of Gram- negative bacteria increasing the synthesis of proinflammatory cytokines).

The normalizing effect of antidepressants on the HPA axis activity has led to drawing a hypothesis that they can increase the density or functional activity of corticosteroid receptors engaged in the inhibition mechanism of the negative feedback. Two types of corticosteroid receptors were distinguished in the central nervous system:

1.   Type I (mineralocorticoids, MR)
2.   Type II (glucocorticosteroids, GR)

The MR receptors, with a high affinity for the natural glucocorticosteroids (cortisol and corticosterone) and a mineralocorticoid (aldosterone), are found in a high concentration in the hippocampus (a concentration similar to the GR one) and the prefrontal cortex (1/3 of the GR's concentration). In other regions of the brain, they are encountered in concentrations that are ten times lower if compared to the GR one. The type II receptors are relatively uniformly spaced in the brain.

The GR connection increases by about 10% in basic conditions (with a low blood concentration of corticosterone) to up to 70 - 90% during stress or in the period of maximal secretion of this steroid in the daily cycle. The MR stimulation (with the use of aldosterone or low concentrations of corticosterone) enhances the excitability of neurons, amplifies the stimulating activity of stimulant aminoacids and it lowers the inhibiting action of serotonin to the activity of neurons in the CA1 region of hippocampus proper. Conversely, the activation of GR inhibits the excitability of neurons as well as it weakens the stimulating action of the stimulant aminoacids and noradrenalin. While examining the participation of GR and MR in the regulation of the HPA axis' activity it was found that in its inhibition during stress there are engaged mainly the GR whose connection with corticosterone increases depending on the concentration of the steroid.

The observed weakening of the inhibition mechanism of the negative feedback in depression is explained by the lowering of the density or sensitivity of the GR. Damage in the hippocampus or the frontal part of the cerebral cortex causes hypercortisonism, whereas the implantation of corticosterone to these regions of brain lowers the ACTH concentration and corticosterone which are elevated during stress. The GR receptors located in the amygdala are engaged, on the other hand, in positive feedback reaction and they also enhance the activity of the HPA axis. In spite of the fact that the HPA axis hyperactivity might be the result of density changes of the receptors localized in different brain structures, the GR show their most intense activity in the hippocampus proper[64].

The majority of antidepressant normalize the activity of the HPA axis by:

-   increasing the density of the GR receptors in the hippocampus, thus strengthening the inhibition mechanism of the negative feedback
-   lowering the synthesis of proinflammatory cytokines which release CRF from the hypothalamus
-   directly repressing the gene encoding the CRF

---

[64] Yehuda, R. (1999). Linking the neuroendocrinology of post-traumatic stress disorder with recent neuroanatomic findings. *Seminars in Clinical Neuropsychiatry*, Vol 30, pp.1031-1048 ISSN 1084-3612..

9. Own research concerning the HPA axis disorders in depression and anxiety- depressive disorders

Numerous studies confirmed elevated cortisol and CRF levels in people suffering from depression if compared to the healthy ones. Next to the excessive secretion of this hormone, the researchers also observed distortions in its regulation. Many of the works regarded the Dexamethasone Suppression Test (DST). Originally, the researchers pointed out the test as being a useful diagnostic tool (Carrol & Feinberg, 1981; Holsboer, 2000)[65,66]. In patients with depression, there were changes in the secretion of cortisol and the pituitary- dependent hormones (Pfohl et al., 1985)[67]. The research suggests that the depressed patients have an elevated cortisol level for the whole day, not only in the morning, as it happens in the healthy controls. The recent studies have considerably widened the knowledge about the pathomechanism of stress and depression, especially in the range of the role of the hypothalamus- pituitary- adrenal (HPA) axis. It has been proved that as much as in the acute phase of depression an excessive secretion of CRH, ACTH and cortisol occurs, in the chronic depression, the secretion of ACTH decreases. It is most probably the result of a strong negative feedback inhibiting the influence of cortisol.

Own empirical research was performed concerning the connection of the HPA axis-functioning disorders with stressors and clinical symptoms in the depressed patients, if compared to the healthy ones.

9.1 The group under study

94 people were examined (66 women and 28 men), including 36 people with depression (according to ICD 10 F.32.), 22 of whom were treated due to the anxiety- depressive disorders (according to ICD 10- F. 41) and 36 healthy people, not treated at all as a control group.

The average age of the population was 34.9 (SD= 12.8). Patients with depression were, on average, 42.8 years old (SD=12.6), those with neurosis- 34.8 (SD=11.9) and the healthy ones-27.5 (SD=8.4) years old. In the subgroups of the healthy individuals and those with neurosis, prevailed singles (58.3% and 59.1%, respectively), whereas among the depressed ones 52.8% were married.

The cross- section of the education level varied in every group. In the group of the depressed, 1/3 of them was on pension, whereas the other 1/3 was vocationally active. In the subgroup of the people treated for neurosis, approximately ¼ constituting every of the following was respectively: employed, pensioners and unemployed.

9.2 Method

Blood samples were taken twice a day, at 08:00 (K1) and 16:00 (K2) in order to measure the cortisol level. On the next day, the Dexamethasone Suppression Test was made by administering orally 1 mg of dexamethasone (Dexamethasone tablets 1mg, Polfa Pabianice

[65] Caroll, B.J.; Feinberg, M.(1981). A specific laboratory test for the diagnosis of melancholia : Standardization, validation, and clinical utility. *Archives of General Psychiatry*. Vol. 38, pp. 15-22, ISNN 0003-990X.

[66] See 63

[67] Pfohl B.; Sherman B.; Schlechte. J.; Stone, R. (1985). Pituitary adrenal axis rhythm disturbances in psychiatric depression. *Archives of General Psychiatry*, Vol.42, pp.897-903, ISNN 0003-990X.

PL) at 23:00 hour. On the next day, the blood samples were taken again in order to measure the cortisol level, at 08:00 and 16:00 (K3 and K4). All of the patients considered were acquainted with the examination procedure and gave a written consent for it. The research was approved by the University Bioethical Committee. The marking of the concentration in the blood was made with the use of Elisa method.

The load of the stressful childhood events was examined with the use of the Early Trauma Inventory which was developed by the J.D. Bremner's group in the 2000[68]. The inventory examines 4 aspects of abuse in the childhood period:

General traumatic experiences (ETI I), Physical abuse (ETI II), Emotional abuse (ETI III), Sexual abuse (ETI IV).

Childhood Trauma Load Index was used for statistical calculations. The index is the sum of all the Indexes of all the above individual subscales (ETI S).

The level of anxiety and depression was assessed with the use of HADS Scale which was developed by Zigmond and Snaith. The Scale includes separate scores for anxiety- A (HADS A) and depression- D (HADS D). The severity of depression was measured with Beck's Scale for Measurement of Depression (BECK). The level of anxiety as a state (x- 1) and as a feature (x-2) was scaled with Spielberger's Inventory (STAI).

In order to assess the impact of stressors experienced in the last 12 months on the mental state, the PsychoSocial Stress Scale was used which was developed in 1967 by Holmes and Rahe. The Scale states that from 250 points there is an excessive stress load (STRES).

The obtained results of the research were subject to the statistical analysis, a U- Mann-Witney's test, a test of the validity of correlation coefficient of R Spearman, which was a non- parametric equivalent of a variation analysis test ANOVA of the Kruskal- Wallis' range.

9.3 Results and discussion

A naturalistic level of cortisol in blood at 08:00 should fall into the range of 60- 285 ng/ml (K1), whereas at 16:00 (K2) it should range from 40 to 150 ng/ml according to the laboratory norms.

An average morning cortisol concentration before the dexamethasone suppression proved to be the lowest for depression: K1= 185.7ng/ml, whereas the afternoon one for neurosis and depression: K2= 84.5 ng/ml. These results did not differ statistically in any significant way.

The threshold was agreed to be 40 ng/ml of the value of cortisol after the administration of dexamethasone, which was an indication of whether the suppression of cortisol secretion is correct or impaired; if the value was below the threshold, it meant a correct suppression.

The weakest suppression was found in the depressed patients with the K3 being 40.8 ng/ml and K4- 31.8 ng/ml. Therefore, an average morning cortisol level in depression patients after suppression (K3) was higher than the threshold value and indicates impaired cortisol suppression in the researched group. The strongest suppression occurred in the control group: K3= 12.1 ng/ml and K4= 18.1 ng/ml. The healthy people, with no clinical symptoms were characterized by a correct feedback inhibition of cortisol secretion after dexamethasone administration, which means an appropriate handling of an excessive supply of cortisol.

The anxiety- depressive patients achieved medium results that were similar to the results obtained by the healthy group. Only the morning cortisol level, before and after the administration of dexamethasone at 08:00, proved to be higher in anxiety- depressive

---

[68] See 55

patients than in the healthy ones. Thus, it seems that people with anxiety- depressive disorders might be characterized by less severe disorders of the HPA axis than the depressed ones. Nonetheless, there can also appear some abnormalities in functioning of the stress axis in this group.

The differences between the groups did not seem to be statistically significant (see: table 1).

Group		Number of results	Min.	Max.	Mean	Standard deviation
Control group	K1	35	79.40	358.00	198.1486	54.59455
	K2	35	10.55	187.00	84.9717	44.91104
	K3	32	3.37	122.00	12.0597	20.42394
	K4	28	4.53	105.87	18.0975	26.04248
Depression	K1	36	65.22	332.02	185.7139	64.87991
	K2	36	7.74	231.02	86.9161	44.02321
	K3	33	4.37	239.58	40.8391	61.36999
	K4	32	5.24	151.45	31.8594	39.31164
Neurosis	K1	20	90.52	329.35	217.0290	73.67715
	K2	18	13.13	200.31	84,5167	46.59056
	K3	20	4.13	208.08	20.6395	45.18454
	K4	15	3.72	162.97	19.0120	40.04291

Table 1. Average cortisol levels before (K1 and K2 and after dexamethasone suppression (K3 and K4) in individual groups of the people under examination in ng/ml.

A differentiating tendency in the morning cortisol concentration after suppression K3 ($p=0.06$) was observed in people with depression compared to the control group.

Statistical analyses were conducted in order to find differences in reactions to dexamethasone (DST) depending on the gender.

In table 2 results concerning the cortisol concentration in relation to the gender were shown. The feature of gender did not significantly statistically differ between the researched groups. The morning cortisol concentration (K1) was the highest in both men (K1=241.9 ng/ml) and women with anxiety- depressive disorders (217.6 ng/ml). Similarly, the afternoon cortisol concentration was the highest in men with anxiety- depressive disorders (K2= 104.1 ng/ml).

The cortisol suppression by dexamethasone influenced the cortisol levels quite differently depending on the gender of the researched. In women with depression there was the lowest suppression and thus the highest morning cortisol concentration K3=6.3ng/ml in comparison to the patients with anxiety- depressive disorders (K3=6.3 ng/ml) and the healthy ones (K3= 8.8ng/ml). The difference was statistically valid on the level of $p=0.03$. Those differences, however, were not observed in the male group.

The afternoon cortisol concentration after suppression in women with depression was also the highest (K4=34.7 ng/ml). In the male group, the patients with the anxiety- depressive disorders showed the lowest tendency towards cortisol suppression, where K3=39 ng/ml and K4=30.7 ng/ml, those differences, however, were not statistically valid.

It is therefore correct to state that the HPA axis functioning disorders in women with depression, in comparison to men, may have a different character. In the research on

Gender		Group	Mean	Standard deviation	N
Women	K1	Healthy	210.9000	53.25796	20
		Depression	189.0058	64.46846	26
		Neuroses	217.6429	87.80601	7
		General	201.0500	63.80486	53
	K2	Healthy	91.2750	38.30435	20
		Depression	89.0304	35.32379	26
		Neuroses	68.5600	37.10318	7
		General	87.1738	36.73782	53
	K3	Healthy	8.7970	4.62600	20
		Depression	43.4262	64.65060	26
		Neuroses	6.3486	2.08270	7
		General	25.4615	48.32329	53
	K4	Healthy	18.5310	28.63269	20
		Depression	34.7012	42.01123	26
		Neuroses	7.5986	4.86375	7
		General	25.0196	35.42213	53
Men	K1	Healthy	174.0667	66.76546	6
		Depression	179.1200	41.86135	6
		Neuroses	241.9071	61.88564	7
		General	200.6563	63.66812	19
	K2	Healthy	89.6500	52.28678	6
		Depression	75.6150	20.34181	6
		Neuroses	104.1071	49.93306	7
		General	90.5442	43.02977	19
	K3	Healthy	25.6100	47.24780	6
		Depression	31.5650	55.14208	6
		Neuroses	39.0771	74.78656	7
		General	32.4521	57.98278	19
	K4	Healthy	19.3483	22.75644	6
		Depression	19.5450	23.08311	6
		Neuroses	30.6971	58.35932	7
		General	23.5916	38.18667	19

Table 2. Cortisol concentration levels in the researched group with the division of gender

animals it was proved that the female gender predisposes to a greater reactivity and a longer time of the HPA axis' reaction to stress. These differences in people, however, would result from the influence of the gender- related steroids and the differences in the organisation of the brain structure (Kudelka et al.)[69]. In the research it was confirmed that in

---

[69] Kudelka, B.M. & Kirschbaum, C (2005). Sex differences In HPA axis responses to stress: a review. *Biological Psychology*, Vol.69, pp.113-132, ISSN 0301-0511.

comparison to men, women with depression had a weaker ability of self- regulation after the action of cortisol.

The assessment of the intensity of anxiety and depression with clinical scales (HADS, STAI, BECK) has shown increased, statistically valid intensifications of anxiety and depression in the group of patients with depression and the anxiety- depressive disorders in comparison with the healthy people from the control group, which is consistent with the clinical symptoms profile. The psycho- social stress level (STRES) proved to be the highest among the depressed- 158.3 points (SD=98.8) and it differed in a statistically significant way in comparison with the healthy individuals ($p<0.05$). Recurrences of depression in the course of affective unipolar disorders might be dependent on the triggering stress factors experienced in the last twelve months.

In table 3 average results of the childhood trauma load (ETI) in the studied subgroups were shown.

Group		N	Min.	Max.	Mean	Standard deviation
Healthy	ETI I	36	0	28	6.83	6.648
	ETI II	36	0	186	50.39	52.166
	ETI III	36	0	258	52.33	67.496
	ETI IV	36	0	30	2.33	6.770
	ETI SUM	36	1	484	111.61	115.867
Depression	ETI I	36	1	31	14.81	7.191
	ETI II	36	0	216	77.39	65.057
	ETI III	36	0	348	113.72	117.884
	ETI IV	36	0	126	12.50	25.632
	ETI SUM	36	1	538	218.31	180.604
Neuroses	ETI I	22	0	52	13.50	11.538
	ETI II	22	0	300	83.73	84.741
	ETI III	22	0	679	152.95	186.645
	ETI IV	22	0	182	19.45	45.654
	ETI SUM	22	12	880	269.64	280.553

Table 3. Childhood trauma load (ETI) in the studied subgroups.

It was stated that the statistical differences in the intensity of the childhood trauma load between people with depression and those suffering from anxiety- depressive disorders in the range of general traumatic events (ETI I), psychological violence (ETI III) and summary trauma (ETI SUMA) were on the level of $p< 0.05$. The highest wholesale intensities of childhood trauma load (ETI SUMA) were diagnosed in people with depression as well as with the anxiety- depressive disorders. Similarly, psychological abuse in childhood (ETI III) and general traumatic events (ETI I), afflicted patients from both groups significantly more often than healthy ones. These results are consistent with the results of other studies. Research suggests that exposing laboratory animals in their early period of life to stressor factors leads to lasting changes in the HPA axis activity and disturbances in functioning of the noradrenergic as well as serotoninergic systems (Manji et al. 2001)[70]. The disturbances in the functioning of the above systems are expressed as symptoms of anxiety and depression. Therefore, the dependencies between the HPA axis functioning and clinical symptoms were analysed.

In table 4 the dependencies of the cortisol concentration on other examined features are shown on the statistically valid level (Rho Spearman's) for the entire researched group (**Correlation is valid on the 0.01 level (bilaterally)

			K1	K2	K3	K4
Whole group	HAD A	Correlation coefficient	.037	-.083	.289(**)	.215
	HAD D	Correlation coefficient	-.014	-.095	.340(**)	.249(*)
	STAIX- 1	Correlation coefficient	.291(*)	-.026	.318(**)	.302(*)
	STAIX- 2	Correlation coefficient	.298(*)	.089	.254(*)	.194
	BECK	Correlation coefficient	.214	-.053	.299(*)	.192

Table 4. Statistically valid (Rho Spearman's) dependencies of the cortisol concentration on other examined features for the whole group.

The morning cortisol level before the suppression (K1) was positively correlated for the whole group with the feature and state of anxiety (STAI). We can therefore conclude that the actual experience of anxiety (STAI X-1) and the apprehensiveness' feature (STAI X- 2) are correlated with an increased release of morning cortisol from the adrenal glands in every person in the group.

What was also observed for the entire group were statistically significant positive correlations (p<0.05) of the level of depression (HADS D, BECK) and anxiety (HADS A, STAI) with the morning cortisol level after the dexamethasone suppression (K3). The afternoon cortisol concentration after suppression (K4) was essentially dependent on the intensity of depressiveness (HADS D) and the anxiety state (STAI X- 1) for the entire group. It was proved that the greater the depression and anxiety intensity, the greater the cortisol levels after dexamethasone suppression, which means a weaker suppression. This proves the connection of the anxiety symptoms and depression with the HPA axis functioning disorders and its feedback inhibition for the whole group.

In table 5 there are the dependencies of cortisol concentration from different examined features shown. They are statistically valid (Rho Spearman's) for the subgroups of the studied people.

In the control group it was stated that the greater the anxiety state (STAX- 1), the higher the afternoon cortisol concentration after suppression K4 (weaker suppression). A currently

---

[70] Manji, H.K.; Drevets, W.C.; Charney D.S.(2001)The cellular neurobiology of depression. *Nature Medicine*, Vol. 7, pp. 541–547, ISNN 1078-8956.

Group			K1	K2	K3	K4
Healthy	STAI X-1	Correlation coefficient	.142	.104	.168	.430(*)
Depression	STRES	Correlation coefficient	-.413(*)	-.318	-.287	.-299
	ETI IV	Correlation coefficient	-.023	-.177	-.451(**)	-.440(*)

*Correlation is valid on the 0.05 level (bilaterally), **Correlation is valid on the 0.01 level (bilaterally)

Table 5. Statistically valid (Rho Spearman's) dependencies of the cortisol concentration from different examined features for the whole group.

experienced feeling of anxiety or fear causes a distortion in the feedback inhibition of the HPA axis as well as its hyperactivity in the form of the persisting elevated cortisol level in healthy people.

The morning cortisol concentration before suppression (K1) was negatively connected with the level of psychosocial stress (STRES) in depression. It can be therefore concluded that the resilience to the current stressors (that occurred during the last 12 months) is lowered in people with depression. Usually, an appropriate reaction in stressful situations is the release of cortisol and its concentration increases in blood which is an adaptive reaction of an organism to fight the stressor. In people with depression, however, there is a lowering of the cortisol level under the influence of stressor factors which might be associated with an insufficiency in fighting any traumatic events. As it was given in the introduction, the HPA axis in people with depression is insufficient which may be the result of some developmental and plasticity disorders of the brain in some of the depressed, which is subsequently the result of trauma experienced during childhood. The piling up of another stressor factors in the adult life influences the intensity of depression symptoms. As the research reveals, especially sexual abuse (ETI IV) in childhood, had a significant impact on cortisol suppression (K3 and K4) in people suffering from depression (p<0.05). In the people with neuroses the dependencies that would be statistically valid were not found. The data concerning the influence of sexual abuse in childhood on the HPA axis are consistent with previous reports. The experience of sexual abuse in early childhood in people with affective disorders, increases the risk of an earlier occurrence of the symptoms, coexistence of different disorders (especially drugs and alcohol) as well as a more severe course of illnesses (Leverich et al. 2002)[71].

9.4 Conclusions from the research
1. The greater depressiveness and anxiousness, the weaker the cortisol suppression (higher K3 and K4 levels) for the whole studied group.
2. In people with depression, however, the current stress factors (STRES) and sexual abuse in childhood (ETI IV) worsened the suppression (higher results of K3 and K4).

[71] Leverich ,G.S.; McElroy, S.L.; Suppes, T, et al(2002).Early physical and sexual abuse associated with an adverse course of bipolar illness. *Biological Psychiatry,* Vol.51 No. 4, pp. 288-297, ISNN 0006-3223.

3.   The weakening of cortisol suppression in the DST test in women suffering from depression in comparison to the healthy ones seemed to be especially statistically valid (for K3, p=0.03)
4.   The results confirm the data regarding the association between the HPA axis disorders and stressors in people with depression and anxiety- depressive disorders if compared to the healthy people

10. Further research directions- different symptoms, common pathomechanism

What has been presented above is an attempt to find an aetiology that would fit into a broad trend of different research currently taking place over the influence of trauma on the incidence of mental disorders.

Literature concerning various traumatic events has documented a great variety of different symptoms that are often associated with an interpersonal abuse in the childhood and adult ages (e.g. an earlier sexual maltreatment of a child, rape or beating the spouse). The connection between these symptoms, which are less closely related with PTSD, and both of the traumatic persecutions (a childhood life- and adult life- related ones) have led to the fact that a lot of scientists have started to perceive the psycho- traumatic disorders, which include neither PTSD nor ASD as such (e.g. Herman, 1992) in a much broader way. More important in this case are: anger because of the persecution, depression, dissociation, sexual problems, interpersonal difficulties, self- mutilation and an excessive or disordered sexual activity. The research presented above fits into the range of influence of trauma on the occurrence of anxiety and depression symptoms in the adult life. Depressiveness is one of the symptoms of complex PTSD.

The term of 'Complex PTSD' was introduced in 1992 by J.L. Herman[72]. It includes PTSD, the diagnosis of which is present in ICD- 10 and DSM- IV classifications, accompanied by additional disorders such as: somatisation, dissociation, prolonged depression and personality disorder of broader- line type[73].

In American researches (Seng, 2005) the probability of Complex PTSD occurrence among children and female teenagers suffering from serious somatic illnesses was analysed. Increased frequency of Complex PTSD occurrence was found among young girls suffering from parasitic infections, endocrine, metabolic and immune system disorders. The presence of cardiovascular and skin diseases also increased the risk of complex PTSD occurrence[74].

Other American researches including women treated for mental disorders, both in ambulatory care and hospitalised indicated the occurrence of high levels of alexithymia among patients with PTSD coexisting with dysregulation, dissociation and somatisation

---

[72] Herman, L. (1992).Complex PTSD: A syndrome in survivors of prolonged and repeated trauma. *Journal of Traumatic Stress,* Vol. 5, pp. 377-391, ISSN 0894-9867.

[73] Allen, J.G. (2001). *Traumatic Relationships and serious mental disorders.* John Wiley & Sons, ISBN 0-471-49102-0, Chichester , England

[74] Seng, J.S.; Graham- Bermann, S.A. ; Clark, M.K.; MaCarthy, A.M.; Ronis, D.L. (2005). Posttraumatic stress disorder and physical comorbidity among female children and adolescents: results from service-use data. *Pediatrics,* Vol.116 , No.6, pp.767-76, ISNN 0031-4005.

(Complex PTSD) (McLean et al. 2006)[75]. German researches conducted on patients hospitalized in Psychiatric Ward for the accused revealed that 59% of them were neglected in their childhood, 75% were mentally and 52% physically abused. Complex PTSD developed among 44 per cent of the abused (Spitzer at al. 2006)[76]. PTSD patients during MRI examination appeared to characterize with a decreased volume of hippocampus, mostly its left side, subthalamic- pituitary- suprarenal axis disorders in the form of decreased cortisol concentration and increased night- and- day level of noradrenalin and adrenalin secretion. In comparison, endogenic depression patients have increased cortisol level in blood circulation system. Neurochemical examinations indicated an increased level of interleukins: IL- 1an IL- 6 among PTSD patients (Bilikiewicz 2002)[77].

The disorders in the range of humoral response and interleukins level were also observed in depression.

In some of the studied people with depression or anxiety- depressive disorders with childhood trauma load, there can be a comorbidity recognised, i.e. Complex PTSD symptoms, where the superior unit seems to be the Complex PTSD diagnosis. Depression in different patients may have a different profile of symptoms, yet it still is a 'bag' of such symptoms as pyrexia in contagious diseases. It is therefore vital that the aetiology of either depression, anxiety- depressive disorders or any other disorders, such as the dissociation ones is not yet known. It seems that in some of the patients with depressive symptoms, the aetiopathogenesis of illness after taking into account all the criteria and factors other than only the symptomatic ones, as in ICD- 10, can be established.

A common aetiopathogenetic path for a part of depressive, anxiety or even psychotic disorders could be:

1. Genetic liability
2. Early traumatic experiences tend to change the route of brain development under the influence of the neuroplasiticity alterations which are made by hormones secreted during the activity of chronic environmental factors in childhood
3. Lasting HPA axis functioning disorders in adulthood
4. The piling up of stressor factors in the adult life distorts the relative and delicate balance, causes the occurrence of an illness' symptoms and a growth of abnormalities in the HPA axis functioning.
5. Environmental factors modeling the aetiopathogenetic path leading to falling ill; with the negative piling up of stressors, they may protectively influence the development of mental disorders. According to current results these are:
   - an adequate care in childhood
   - social support

[75] Mclean, L.M.; Toner, B.; Jackson, J.; Desrocher, M.; Stuckless, N. (2006).The relationship between childhood sexual abuse, complex post-traumatic stress disorder and alexithymia in two outpatient samples: examination of women treated in community and institutional clinics. *Journal of Child Sexual Abuse*. Vol.15, No.3, pp.1-17, ISNN 1053-8712.

[76] Spitzer, C.; Chevalier, C.; Gillner, M.; Freyberger, H.J.; Barnow, S. (2006). Complex posttraumatic stress disorder and child maltreatment in forensic inpatients. Journal of Forensic Psychiatry &Psychol. Vol.17, No.2, pp.204-216, ISNN 1478-9949

[77] See 50

- psychotherapy and antidepressive drugs
- health- promoting personality factors such as the sense of coherence (developed by Antonovsky)

Antonovsky has developed the term of the sense of coherence which includes all three of the following: clearness, controllability (sense of resourcefulness) and reasonability. Clearness is associated with a cognitive aspect of a situation that a person is in. Controllability (sense of resourcefulness) is the sense of the disposal with abilities of handling life's challenges, an active influence on a situation in which one is found. Reasonability is a sense being expressed as a conviction that engaging into things is worth the attempt of investing energy in one's own life and challenges it brings. People differ among each other by the level of the sense of coherence. The greater sense of coherence, the greater the probability of fighting an likely illness, including depression[78].

In conclusion, it is high time to leave the routine thinking based on symptomatic classifications of mental illnesses and start searching aetiopathogenetic paths leading to the occurrence of an illness in a particular patient. It is postulated that it would be advisable to head towards a personalized medicine, which is already happening in case of oncology for instance. Going through the history of a patients' life, his/ her genotype and the actual symptoms will disallow the disrespectful classification of a patient as a disorder unit, moreover, it will make it possible to recognize the aetiology of his/ her illness and subsequently treat the patient in an adequate way.

11. References

Agid, O.; Kohn, Y.; Lere, B. (2000). Evironmental stress and psychiatric illness. *Biomedicine & Pharmacotherapy* vol. 54, pp. 135, ISSN 0753-3322.

Allen, J.G. (2001). *Traumatic relationships and serious mental disorders*. John Wiley & Sons, ISBN 0-471-49102-0, Chichester , England.

Antonovsky, A. (1995). *Rozwikłanie tajemnicy zdrowia. Jak radzić sobie ze stresem i nie zachorować*. Fundacja IPN, ISBN 83-85705-24-4, Warszawa, Poland

Bilikiewicz, A.; Pużyński, S.; Rybakowski, J.& Wciórka, J. (2002). *Psychiatria, t. 1.* Wydawnictwo Medyczne Urban & Partner, ISBN 83-87944-67-X, Wrocław, Poland.

Briere, J. & Runtz, M. (1990). Differential adult symptomatology associated with three types of abuse. *Child Abuse & Neglect* , Vol.14, pp. 357, ISSN 0145-2134.

Bremner, J.D.; Vermetten, E.; Mazure, C.(2000). Development and preliminary psychometric properties of an instrument for the measurement of childhood trauma: The Early Trauma Inventory. *Depression and Anxiety*, Vol. 12, pp. 1-12, ISSN 1091-4269.

Budziszewska, B.; Lason W. (2003). *Neuroendokrynne mechanizmy działania leków przeciwdepresyjnych*. ISBN 83-917041-3-0, Wrocław,Poland.

Burke, H.M.; Davis, M.C.; Otte, C.; Mohr, D.C. (2005). Depression and cortisol responses to psychological stress: a meta-analysis. *Psychoneuroendocrinology*, Vol. 30, No.9, pp. 846-56, ISSN 0306-4530.

---

[78] Antonovsky, A. (1995). *Rozwikłanie tajemnicy zdrowia. Jak radzić sobie ze stresem i nie zachorować*. Fundacja IPN, ISBN 83-85705-24-4, Warszawa, Poland.

Caroll, B.J.; Feinberg, M.(1981). A specific laboratory test for the diagnosis of melancholia : standardization, validation, and clinical utility. *Archives of General Psychiatry*, Vol. 38, pp. 15-22, ISSN 0003-990X.

Cawson, P.;Wattam, C.; Brookers, S.& Kelly, G. (2000). *Child maltreatment in the United Kingdom*, NSPCC, ISBN 1-84228-006-6, London, United Kingdom.

Easton, C.J. (2000). Prevalence of family violence in clients entering substance abuse treatment. *Journal of Substance Abuse Treatment*, Vol.18, pp.23-28, ISSN 0740-5472.

Ehlert, U.; Gaab, J.; Heinrichs, M. (2001). Psychoendocrinological contributions to the etiology of depression, posttraumatic stress disorder, and stress-related bodily disorders: the role of the hypothalamus-pituitary-adrenal axis. *Biological Psychology*, Vol. 57, pp.141-152, ISSN 0301-0511

Essex, M.J. et al. (2002). Maternal stress beginning in infancy may sensitize children to later stress exposure: effects on cortisol and behavior. *Biological Psychiatry* Vol.52, pp.776-784, ISSN 0006-3223.

Goodyer, I.M.; Park, R.J.; Netherton, C.M.; Herbert, J. (2001). Possible role of cortisol and dehydroepiandrosterone in human development and psychopathology. *British Journal of Psychiatry*, Vol. 179, pp.243-249, ISSN 0007-1250.

Harro, J.; Oreland, L. (2001). Depression as a spreading adjustment disorder of monoaminergic neurons: a case for primary implication of the locus coeruleus. *Brain Research Reviews*, Vol. 38, pp. 79-128, ISSN 0165-0173.

Heim, Ch.; Newport, D.J.; Stacey, H.; Graham, Y.(2000). Pituitary-adrenal and autonomic response to stress in woman after sexual and physical abuse in children. *JAMA* Vol. 2, pp. 592-597, ISSN 0098-7484

Heim, Ch. & Nemeroff, Ch.(2001). The role of childhood trauma in the neurobiology of mood and anxiety disorders; preclinical and clinical studies. *Biological Psychiatry*, Vol.1, pp. 1023-1039, ISSN 0006-3223.

Heim, Ch.; Owens, M. (2001). Znaczenie negatywnych wydarzeń z dzieciństwa w patogenezie depresji, In. *WPA Bulletin on Depression*, Vol.22, pp.3-7,

Herbert, J. (2007). DHEA, In: *Encyclopedia of stress*, Eds. G. Fink (Ed.) 788-791, Academic Press, ISBN 978-0-12-088503-9, London, United Kingdom.

Herbert ,J.; Goodyer, I.M.; Grossman ,A.B. (2006). Do corticosteroids damage the brain? *Journal of Neuroendocrinology* Vol.18, pp. 393-411, ISSN 0953-8194.

Herman , J.L; Perry, J.; Kolk B.A. (1989). Childhood trauma in borderline personality disorder. *American Journal of Psychiatry*, Vol. 146, pp. 490, ISSN 0002-953X.

Herman,.L. (1992). Complex PTSD: A syndrome in survivors of prolonged and repeated trauma. *Journal of Traumatic Stress*, Vol. 5, pp. 377-391, ISSN 0894-9867.

Herzyk, A.(2003). *Mózg, emocje i uczucia. Analiza neuropsychologiczna*. Wydawnictwo UMCS, ISBN 83-227-2152-8, Lublin, Poland.

Holka-Pokorska,J. (2005). Dehydroepiandrosteron w leczeniu depresji. *Wiadomości Psychiatryczne*, Vol. 8, pp.149-155, ISSN 1505-7429.

Holsboer, F. (2000). The corticosteroid receptor hypothesis of depression. *Neuropsychopharmacology*, Vol. 23, pp. 477-501, ISSN 0893-133X.

Kendler, K.S.; Kessler R.C., Walters E.(1995). Stressful life events, genetic liability and onset of an episode of major depression in women. *American Journal of Psychiatry,* Vol.152, pp. 833-842, ISSN 0002-953X.

Kercher, R.C. & McShane M. (1984). The prevalence of child sexual abuse victimization in adult sample of Texas residents. *Child Abuse & Neglect,* Vol.8, pp.495-502, ISSN 0145-2134.

Kudielka, B.M.& Kirschbaum, C. (2005). Sex diffreneces in HPA axis responses to stress: a review. *Biological Psychology,* Vol.69, pp.113-132, ISSN 0301-0511.

Landowski, J.; Radziwiłłowicz (red. nauk.) (2001). *Dyskusje o depresji : mechanizmy stresu w depresji nr 17.* "Servier", Warszawa, Poland

Leverich ,G.S.; McElroy, S.L.; Suppes, T, et al(2002). Early physical and sexual abuse associated with an adverse course of bipolar illness. *Biological Psychiatry,* Vol. 51 No. 4, pp. 288-297, ISSN 0006-3223.

Lyons, D.M.; Yang, C; Sawyer-Glover, A.M.(2001). Early life stress and inherited variation in monkey hippocampal volumes. *Archives of General Psychiatry,* Vol. 58 pp.1145-1154, ISSN 0003-990X.

Manji, H.K.; Drevets, W.C.; Charney D.S. (2001). The cellular neurobiology of depression. *Nature Medicine,* Vol. 7, pp. 541–547, ISSN 1078-8956.

McCauley, J; Kern, D.E. (1997). Clinical characteristics of woman with a history of childchood abuse: unhealed wounds. *JAMA,* Vol. 277, pp. 1362-1368, ISSN 0098-7484.

McEwen, B.S.(2003). Early life influences on life-long patterns of behavior and health. *Mental Retardation and Developmental Disabilities Research Reviews,* Vol. 9, pp.149-154, ISSN 1080-4013.

Mclean, L.M.; Toner, B.; Jackson, J.; Desrocher, M.; Stuckless, N. (2006). The relationship between childhood sexual abuse, complex post-traumatic stress disorder and alexithymia in two outpatient samples: examination of women treated in community and institutional clinics. *Journal of Child Sexual Abuse ,* Vol.15, pp.1-17, ISSN 1053-8712.

Meewisse, M.L.; Reitsma, J,B.; De Vries, G.J;, Gersons, B.P. & Olff, M. (2007). Cortisol and post-traumatic stress disorder in adults: systematic review and meta-analysis. *British Journal of Psychiatry,* Vol. 191, pp.387-392, ISSN 0007-1250.

Nemeroff, Ch., Wainwrigth, N.W.J; Surtees, P.G . (2002). Childhood adversity, gender and depression over the life-cours. *Journal of Affective Disorders,* Vol. 72, pp.33-44, ISSN 0165-0327.

Ney, P.G. (1987). Does verbal abuse leave deeper scars: a study of children and parents. *Canadian Journal of Psychiatry* ,Vol. 32,pp. 371-377, ISSN 0706-7437.

Ney, P.G. & Peeters M.A. (1997). *The centurion's pathway,* Pioneer Publishing, ISBN 9780920952061, Victoria, USA.

Ogata, S.N.; Silk K. (1990). Childhood sexual and physical abuse in adult patients with borderline personality disorder. *American Journal of Psychiatry,* Vol. 147, pp. 1008, ISSN 0002-953X.

Ossowska, G.(2002). *Poszukiwanie leków zapobiegających następstwom stresu przewlekłego. Nowy model „depresji" u szczurów.* Praca habilitacyjna, Akademia Medyczna w Lublinie, Zakład Poligraficzny BiS, Lublin, Poland.

Parker, K.; Schatzberg A.; Lyons D. (2003). Neuroendocrine aspects of hypercortisolism in major depression. *Hormones and Behavior*, Vol. 43, pp. 60–66, ISSN 0018-506X.

Pfohl B.; Sherman B.; Schlechte. J.; Stone, R. (1985). Pituitary adrenal axis rhythm disturbances in psychiatric depression. *Archives of General Psychiatry*, Vol. 42, pp.897-903, ISSN 0003-990X.

Porter, R.J.; Gallagher, P. (2006). Abnormalities of the HPA axis in affective disorders: clinical subtypes and potential treatments. *Acta Neuropsychiatrica*, Vol. 18, pp. 193-209, ISSN 0924-2708.

Reul, J.M.& Holsoer, F.(2005). Corticotropin-releasing factor receptors 1 and 2 in anxiety and depression. *Current Opinion in Pharmacology*, Vol. 2, No.1, pp.23-33, ISSN 1471-4892.

Ritsner, M.; Maayan, R.; Gibel, A.; Strous, R.D.; Modai, I.; Weizman, A. (2004). Elevation of the cortisol/dehydroepiandrosterone ratio in schizophrenia patients. *European Neuropsychopharmacology*, Vol. 14, pp.267-273, ISSN 0924-977X.

Rossman, P.G.(1985). The aftermath of abuse and abandonment: a treatment approach for ego disturbance in female adolescence. *Journal of the American Academy of Child and Adolescent Psychiatry*, Vol.24, pp. 345-352, ISSN 0002-7138.

Seng, J.S.; Graham- Bermann, S.A. ; Clark, M.K.; MaCarthy, A.M.; Ronis, D.L. (2005). Posttraumatic stress disorder and physical comorbidity among female children and adolescents: results from service-use data. *Pediatrics*, Vol.116 , pp.767-76, ISSN 0031-4005.

Spitzer, C.; Chevalier, C.; Gillner, M.; Freyberger, H.J.; Barnow, S. (2006). Complex posttraumatic stress disorder and child maltreatment in forensic inpatients. *Journal of Forensic Psychiatry & Psychology* Vol.17, pp.204-216, ISSN 1478-9949.

Stricland, P.; Dekin, W.; Percival C. (2002). Bio-social origins of depression in the community. Interactions between social adversity, cortisol, and serotonin neurotransmission. *British Journal of Psychiatry*, Vol. 180, pp.168-173, ISSN 0007-1250.

Sweet, C.; Surrey, J.; Cohen, C. (1990). Sexual and physical abuse histories and psychiatric symptoms among male psychiatric patients. *American Journal of Psychiatry*, Vol. 147, pp 632, ISSN 0002-953X.

Twardowska, K. & Rybakowski J. (1996). Oś limbiczno – podwzgórzowo – przysadkowo – nadnerczowa w depresji (przegląd piśmiennictwa), *Psychiatria Polska*, Vol. 5, pp. 741 – 756, ISSN 0033-2674.

Yehuda, R (1999). Linking the neuroendocrinology of post-traumatic stress disorder with recent neuroanatomic findings. *Seminars in Clinical Neuropsychiatry*, Vol 30, pp.1031-1048 ISSN 1084-3612.

Yehuda, R.; Brand, S.R.; Golier, J.A. & Yang R.K.(2006). Clinical correlates of DHEA associated with post-traumatic stress disorder. *Acta Psychiatrica Scandinavica*, Vol. 114 , pp.187-193, ISSN 0001-690X.

Vialou, V et al. (2010). ΔFosB in brain reward circuits mediates resilience to stress and antidepressant responses. Nature Neuroscience, Vol. 13, pp.745, ISSN 1097-6256.

Wyatt, G.E. (1985). The sexual abuse of Afro-American and white-American women in childhood. *Child Abuse & Neglect,* Vol.9, pp. 507-519, ISSN 0145-2134.

Załuska, M.; Janota, B. (2009). Dehydroepiandrosteron (DHEA) w mechanizmach stresu i depresji. *Psychiatria Polska* , Vol. 3. , pp.263-274, ISSN 0033-2674

8

Psychosis and Adhesion Molecules

Tsuyoshi Hattori, Shingo Miyata, Akira Ito,
Taiichi Katayama and Masaya Tohyama
Osaka University
Japan

1. Introduction

Schizophrenia is a chronic, severe, and disabling brain disorder that affects about 1% of the population worldwide. However the etiology and pathophysiology is poorly understood. It has been determined that schizophrenia is a multifactorial disorder influenced by genetic, neurodevelopmental and social factors (Mueser & McGurk, 2004; Weinberger, 1987). Numbers of linkage and association studies have shown that multiple susceptibility genes such as DISC1, Neureglin1, DTNBP1, RGS4, G72 were involved in the development of schizophrenia (Sibylle *et al.*, 2009). Moreover, accumulating evidence from recent studies suggests that environmental risk factors during fetal and perinatal life also contribute to the development of schizophrenia. The environmental risk factors of schizophrenia have been reported, such as infections, nutritional deficiencies, paternal age, fetal/neonatal hypoxic and obstetric insults and complications and maternal stress and other exposures (Brown AS, 2011). Postmortem human brain and developmental animal model of schizophrenia studies have shown abnormal neurodevelopment at sequential stages of brain development. Initial postmortem studies appeared to support the early neurodevelopmental model in neuronal migration and organization, considered fetal in origin (Jakob et al, 1986; Akbarian et al, 1993). Subsequent and more reproducible observations of reduced neuronal size and arborization, which could have developed later in life, indicated that the pathophysiological processed involved in schizophrenia need not be restricted to the pre- or perinatal period (Selemon et al, 1999). Candidate genes for schizophrenia are typically expressed across developmental periods, often in different brain regions.

Adhesion molecules are membrane-anchored molecules whose extracellular domains directly interact to help hold the membranes of two cells together. Adhesion might be a primary role of the interaction or it could be an epiphenomenon of ligand-receptor signals to the cell interior. The major families of adhesion molecules are cadherins, immunoglobulin superfamilies and integrins. Cadherins constitute a superfamily that is comprised of more than 100 members in vertebrates, grouped into subfamilies that are designated as classic cadherins, desmosomal cadherins, protocadherins, Flamingo/ CELSRs and FAT (Takeichi, 2006). Cadherins are calcium dependent, singlepass transmembrane molecules with five ectodomain repeats, which mediate mainly homophilic (more rarely heterophilic) adhesion

(Tepass *et al*, 2000). Strong cadherin adhesion is believed to be dependent on the formation of *cis* which the bind in *trans* to form adhesive `zippers` (Shan *et al*, 2000). The cytoplasmic domains of the cadherins contain binding sites for the catenins, which provide links to the cytoskeleton and mediate signaling (Yap *et al*, 2003). N-cadherin was one of the first adhesion molecules shown to be concentrated in the synaptic cleft (Yamagata et al, 1995), a localization subsequently shown for catenins and several other cadherins at several synaptic types. Immunogloblin superfamily molecules contain varying numbers of extracellular cysteine-looped domains first described in immunogloblins. Many have one or more fibronectin type III (FNIII) repeats between the immunoglobulin domains and the membrane (Rougon and Hobert, 2003). The integrin family of cell surface receptors is a major mediator of cell-cell and cell-extracellula matrix (ECM) interactions. Integrins can efficiently transducer signals to and from the external cell environment to the intracellular signaling and cytoskeletal compartments, while modulating signaling cascades initiated by other cellular receptors. Functional integrin receptors are formed by membrane spanning heterodimers of α and β subunits. There are at least 18 α and 8 β subunits that can form more than 20 different integrin receptors.

Major depressive disorder (MDD) is one of the mood disorders associated with significant morbidity. MDD is thought to be a multifactorial disease related to both environmental and genetic factors, though the genes responsible and the pathogenesis of major depression at the molecular level remain unclear. Among many environmental factors, repeated stressful events are associated with the onset of depression, and stress activates the hypothalamic–pituitary–adrenocortical (HPA) system (Gold et al., 1988a, b; Post, 1992; Bartanusz et al., 1993; Herman et al., 1995; Aguilera and Rabadan-Diehl, 2000; McEwen, 2004; Sala et al., 2004; Alfonso et al., 2005; Dallman et al., 2006). The negative feedback of corticosteroids on the HPA system occurs at the level of the hypothalamus and the anterior pituitary via the glucocorticoid receptors (Thomson and Craighead, 2008; Pariante and Lightman, 2008).

Dysregulation of this negative feedback mechanism is reported in patients with major depressive disease, which results in hyperactivity of the HPA system and higher basal levels of serum corticosterone (Carroll et al., 1976; Holsboer et al., 1984; Nemeroff et al., 1984; Halbreich et al., 1985a, b; Schatzberg et al., 1985; Gold et al., 1986a; Young et al., 1993). In addition, many clinical cases demonstrate that elevated corticosterone levels trigger depressive symptoms (Schatzberg et al., 1985; Gold et al., 1986b; Chu et al., 2001). These facts strongly indicate that sustained elevated levels of plasma corticosteroids are one of the causes of major depressive diseases.

Recent we showed that chronically elevated plasma corticosterone levels by exposing mice to repeated stress induced the upregulation of adhesion molecules such as N-cadherin, α-catenin, and β-catenin in the oligodendrocytes via the activation of phosphatidylinositol 3-kinase (PI3K)–3-phosphoinositide-dependent protein kinase (PDK1)–serum/glucocorticoid regulated kinase (SGK1)–N-myc downstream-regulated gene 1 (NDRG1) pathway, resulting in morphological changes in the oligodendrocytes (OLs) (Miyata et al., 2011). These findings show that SGK1 changes adhesion molecules expression levels and regulates the plasticity of the processes of the OLs under the stressful condition.

It has been known that adhesion molecules such as cadherins and integrins played important roles in neuronal development and function. Furthermore, in recent years, genetic association studies have been supporting the involvement of adhesion molecules in psychosis such as schizophrenia, bipolar disorder and autism. In this chapter, we will focus on the role of adhesion molecules in psychiatric disorders, especially schizophrenia and depression.

2. Schizophrenia and adhesion molecules

2.1 The major mental disorders related adhesion molecules

The major mental disorders such as schizophrenia, bipolar disorder and autism are substantially influenced by genetic factors. Recent genomic studies have identified a small number of common and rare risk genes contributing to these disorders and support epidemiological evidence that genetic susceptibility overlaps in these disorders (Lichtenstein et al, 2009). To date, a number of genetic association analyses have shown that genes coding adhesion molecules associated with schizophrenia, bipolar disorder and autism. A molecular pathway analysis applied to the 212 experimentally-derived pathways in the Kyoto encyclopedia of Genes and Genomics (KEGG) database identified significant association between the cell adhesion molecule (CAM) pathway and both schizophrenia and bipolar disorder susceptibility across three GWAS datasets (O'Dushlaine et al, 2011). Interestingly, a similar approach applied to an autistic spectrum disorders (ASDs) sample identified a similar pathway (Wang et al, 2009). Disruption of the NRXN1 gene has been reported in both schizophrenia and autism cases or families (Walsh et al, 2008; Szatmari et al, 2007). Axonal neurexins form trans-membrane complexes with neuroligin on dendrites and are required for the formation of synaptic contacts and for efficient neurotransmission-including maintaining postsynaptic NMDA receptor function. CDH4 is a classical cadherin thought to be involved in brain segmentation and neurite outgrowth. Total cerebral brain volume was the only genome-wide significant finding to emerge from a GWAS study of brain aging using MRI and cognitive assessment of 705 healthy participants from the Framingham study. Reduced brain volumes are a recognized feature of schizophrenia and this may point to a role in maintenance rather than formation of neuronal connections (Seshadri et al, 2007). A recent GWAS study in bipolar disorder and subsequent replication efforts have provided some support for association with CDH7 (Soronen et al, 2010). Another GWAS study in autistic spectrum disorders (ASDs) identified association with the chromosome 5q14.1 region containing other members of the cadherin superfamily, CDH9 and CDH10 (Wang et al, 2009). A number of microdeletion/microduplication syndromes have been identified that are associated with schizophrenia, ASDs, intellectual disability, specific language delay and other neurodevelopmental phenotypes. Many of these disrupt genes involved in CAM pathways. For instance, disruption of NRXN1 has been reported in cases of both autism and schizophrenia. CASK deletions are reported in individual with learning disability and brain malformation phenotypes. Disruption of CNTNAP1 has been reported in autism, language disorder and schizophrenia. A deletion between two cadherin (CDH12 and CDH18) genes on 5p14 was identified in a monozygotic twin pair discordant for schizophrenia. This 11kb deletion is present in the affected but not in the unaffected twin. Taken together, it is possible that susceptibility to schizophrenia, bipolar disorder and ASDs may involve common molecular aetiology where an accumulation of small effects from many common genetic risk variants or more highly penetrant mutations induce neuronal dysconnectivity by disrupting adhesion molecule function.

2.2 Involvement of N-cadherin and β1-integrin in neuronal development

Neural development and the organization of complex neuronal circuits involve a number of processed that require cell-cell and cell-matrix interaction. Vertebrate N-cadherin is expressed from the beginning of neural development, and its expression persists in differentiated neurons in various species (Hatta & Takeichi, 1986). Conventional knockout of the mouse N-cadherin gene causes early embryonic lethality, mainly because of heart defects (Radice *et al*, 1997). Therefore, the precise roles of N-cadherin in neuronal development at later developmental stages remain less clear. Nevertheless, some fragmental information on the specific role of N-cadherin in axon projection is available: studies using blocking antibodies against N-cadherin showed that this molecule is required for the correct innervations of specific laminae in the chicken tectum by retinal optic nerves (Inoue & Sanes, 1997). Some of the type II cadherins are involved in axon sorting and in the regulation of physiological function of the brain, such as long-term potentiation in the hippocampus. When a dominant-negative N-cadherin of which extracellular domain was deleted was expressed in the neural retina of *Xenopus* embryos, the extension of neurites from retinal ganglion cells was inhibited. Such N-cadherin mutant form was able to block the radial extension of horizontal cell dendrites, as well as their synaptic connections with photoreceptor cells in the retina. Furthermore, the mutant forms were used to show that cadherins are required for tangential migration of precerebellar neurons (Taniguchi et al, 2006). These results provide evidence that N-cadherin has important roles in neural cell-cell interactions and neurite extension in various systems.

As in the case of N-cadherin, β1-integrin also expresses at early developmental stage of the nervous system. Neural crest cells express many integrins and migrate through an extracellular matrix (ECM)-rich environment (Bronner-Fraser, 1994). In mice, genetic ablation of β1-integrin results in severe perturbations of the peripheral nervous system, including failure of normal nerve arborization, delay in Schwann cell migration, and defective neuromuscular junction differentiation, In addition to direct effects on migration, it has been shown that absence of specific integrin heterodimers compromises Schwann cell precursor survival, proliferation and differentiation (Pietri *et al*, 2004). Many of these observations are likely to reflect the roles of integrin receptors in regulating activation of MAP kinase, Rac, and other signaling pathways. In central nervous system, integrin deletion affects many aspects of forebrain and cerebellar development. Loss of β1-integrin results in disruptions of the basal lamina that separates the brain from the overlying mesenchyme. As a result, the migration of neurons is perturbed, resulting in abnormal lamination of the cortex and cerebellum. Although some evidence indicates that integrins modeulate neuronal interactions with radial glia which provide the substrate for the tangential migrations that establish the cortical lamination pattern (Sanada et al, 2004; Schmid et al, 2005), the major phenotype observed in β1-integrin defect models appears to stem form disruption of signaling pathways controlling neuronal migration that require integrity of the basal lamina. Although Localization studies indicate that integrins are present at synapses in the brain, genetic and pharmacological studies indicate that integrins are not required for synapse formation, but are required for normal synaptic plasticity. The presence of integrins in the mushroom body of the *Drosophila* brain was shown to be required for short-term memory. Studies in the murine hippocampus have demonstrated that β1-integrin were required for normal LTP (Chan *et al*, 2006; Huang *et al*, 2006)). Studies of mice with reduced expression of individual β1-integrin heterodimers have suggested that specific integrins have different functions at the synapse indicate that integrins are involved in regulation of both NMDA and AMPA receptor function and act through regulation of protein kinases and the actin cytoskeleton.

2.2.1 DISC1 is involved in neuronal development

Disrupted-in-schizophrenia 1 (DISC1) is a promising candidate susceptibility gene for major mental disorders, including schizophrenia. *DISC1* was originally identified at the break point of a balanced (1;11) (q42.1;q14.3) translocation that segregates with major mental illnesses in a large Scottish family (Millar *et al*, 2001). Recent linkage and association studies demonstrated association between DISC1 and schizophrenia in multiple populations, suggesting that DISC1 is a general risk factor for schizophrenia (Jaaro-Peled *et al*, 2009; Chubb *et al*, 2008; Hodgkinson *et al*, 2004; Cannon *et al*, 2005). To investigate the physiological roles of DISC1, a number of groups, including ours, have identified DISC1-interacting proteins, such as the fasciculation and elongation protein zeta-1 (FEZ1) (Miyoshi *et al*, 2003), DISC1-binding zinc-finger protein (DBZ) (Hattori *et al*, 2007), kendrin (Miyoshi *et al*, 2004), NudE-like (NDEL1/NUDEL) protein (Ozeki *et al*, 2003; Morris *et al*, 2003) and BBS1 (Ishizuka et al, 2011). Other relevant interacting proteins include GSK3b and PDE4B (Millar *et al*, 2005), which are involved in intracellular signaling pathways. The endogenous expression pattern of DISC1 is complex, and DISC1 co-localizes with centrosomal protein, mitochondria, and F-actin. DISC1 protein has conserved nuclear localization signals and has been found within the nuclei of certain cell types. Moreover, DISC1 is involved in cAMP, CREB, Notch, Wnt and MAPK signaling pathways. Recent studies have suggested that DISC1 plays various roles in cell proliferation, neural migration, dendritic development and synapse maintenance during neurodevelopment and influences adult brain functions.

2.2.2 DISC1 regulates N-cadherin expression

The strength of cell-cell adhesion is associated with the expression levels of cadherins at the cell surface (Steinberg & Takeichi, 1994). In neural cells, neural cell adhesion molecule (NCAM) and N-cadherin are two of the major adhesion molecules (Kiryushko *et al*, 2004). We have demonstrated that DISC1 induced cell adhesion through an increase in N-cadherin expression in PC12 cells (Fig. 1.a.c.d). Furthermore, the increased N-cadherin was concentrated at the cell-cell contact zone, showing that increased N-cadherin functions at cell-cell contact sites (Fig. 1.b). Our real-time PCR analysis showed up-regulation and down-regulation of N-cadherin mRNAs by DISC1 overexpression and knock-down in PC12 cells, respectively. Furthermore, the down-regulation of N-cadherin protein expression (at 72 hours after transfection) by DISC1 siRNA followed that of N-cadherin mRNA expression (at 48 hours after transfection). The expression levels of N-cadherin protein in DISC1-overexpressing cells were correlated with those of mRNA. The results using NLS1-deleted DISC1 (DISC1(46–854)-GFP) indicates that the expression of N-cadherin was regulated by nuclear DISC1. It is possible that nuclear DISC1 regulates level of N-cadherin mRNA , because a role for nuclear DISC1 in association with gene transcription was reported (Ma *et al*, 2002). Moreover, immunoprecipitation assays show that DISC1 does not interact with either N-cadherin suggesting that DISC1 does not regulate the expression of these molecules directly. In hippocampal neurons, DISC1 also enhanced N-cadherin, which accumulated at cell-cell contact sites, suggesting that the enhanced N-cadherin also functions at cell surfaces of neurons (Fig. 3.).

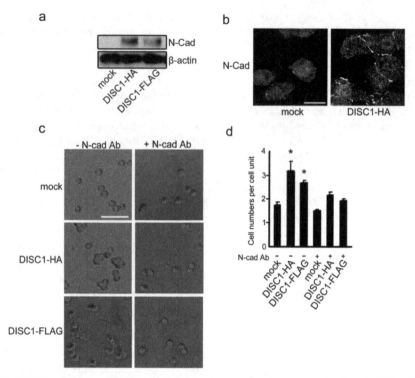

Fig. 1. DISC1 enhances cell-cell adhesion via increasing the expression level of N-cadherin. (a) Effect of DISC1 on the level of N-cadherin. PC12/mock, PC12/DISC1-HA and PC12/DISC1-FLAG stable cells were lysed and subjected to western blot analysis. (b) PC12/mock and PC12/DISC1-HA cells were fixed and immunostained with anti-N-cadherin antibody. (c) PC12 cells were dissociated with trypsin-EDTA and cultured on collagen-coated dishes for 2 hours in the presence of anti-N-cadherin antibody or rabbit IgG. Phase-contrast images are shown. Scale bar, 100 μm. (d) To quantify the results in (c), the average number of cells per unit, which consisted of a single cell or a cluster of two or more cells, was determined. Over 100 cells were examined in each case. Values are the means±s.e.m. of at least three independent experiments. *$p<0.05$ vs mock in the absence of anti-N-cadherin (Student's t-test).

2.2.3 DISC1 regulates β1-integrin expression

PC12 cells provide an excellent experimental system for studying the mechanisms of neurite outgrowth. It has been reported that DISC1 enhances neurite outgrowth of PC12 cells in the presence of nerve growth factor (NGF) (Miyoshi et al, 2003; Ozeki et al, 2003; Bozyczko et al, 1986). Neurite outgrowth of neuronal cells is directly mediated by integrin-ECM interactions in developing nervous systems, as well as in a PC12 neurite genesis model (Reichardt & Tomaselli, 1991; Tomaselli et al, 1987; Tomaselli et al, 1990). We have demonstrated that upregulation of β1-integrin expression by DISC1 enhanced neurite outgrowth by regulating cell-matrix adhesion in PC12 cells (Fig. 2.). This finding is based on the followting results (1) DISC1 overexpression enhanced NGF induced-neurite outgrowth (Fig. 2.b.c). (2) DISC1

overexpression increased β1-integrin expression, especially in the presence of NGF (Fig. 2.a).
(3) Inhibition of β1-integrin with anti-β1-integrin antibody suppressed the enhanced neurite
outgrowth induced by DISC1 to the control level (Fig. 2.b.c). (4) overexpression of β1-
integrin rescued the suppressed neurite outgrowth of DISC1-knockdown cells. (5) DISC1
overexpression enhanced cell-matrix adhesion. The increased expression of β1-integrin by
NGF and DISC1 was localized at the cell surface and growth cones of neurites, showting
that upregulated β1-integrin at the cell membrane and growth cones of differentiating PC12
cells participates in neurite extension. In support of this idea, integrins, including
β1-integrin, have been shown to mediate the promotion of neurite outgrowth. Unlike

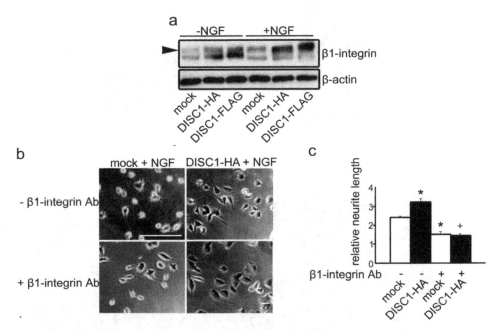

Fig. 2. DISC1 enhances neurite outgrowth via regulating the expression of β1-integrin. (a)
Effect of DISC1 on the level of β1-integrin expression in the absence or presence of NGF.
PC12/mock, PC12/DISC1-HA or PC12/DISC1-FLAG cells with or without NGF for 24
hours were lysed and subjected to western blot analysis. The arrow indicates the band
containing full-length β1-integrin. (a, b) PC12/mock or PC12/DISC1-HA cells treated with
anti-β1-integrin antibody were cultured in the presence of NGF for 24 hours. Shown are
phase-contrast images of the cells. The left panels show the results for PC12/mock cells with
NGF and the right panels results for PC12/DISC1-HA cells with NGF. The upper panels
present findings for cells not treated with anti-β1-integrin antibody and the lower panels
show findings for cells treated with anti-β1-integrin antibody. Scale bar, 200μm. (c)
Quantification of neurite lengths. The neurite length was analyzed on randomly selected
digital microscope images. Data are expressed as the means±s.e.m. of at least three
independent experiments. At least 100 cells were counted in each case and analyzed in a
blinded manner. $*p < 0.05$ vs. mock withoutβ1-integrin antibody, $+p < 0.05$ vs. DISC1-HA
without β1-integrin antibody (Student's t-test).

N- cadherin, the regulation of β1-integrin expression by DISC1 is not transcriptional. The results using NLS1-deleted DISC1 indicate that the expression of β1-integrin was not regulated by nuclear DISC1. In hippocampal neurons, DISC1 also enhanced the expression of β1-integrin protein at the cell membrane of cell bodies and neurites (Fig. 3.). Therefore, it is possible that upregulation of β1-integrin expression by DISC1 enhances neurite outgrowth by regulating cell-matrix adhesion in primary neurons.

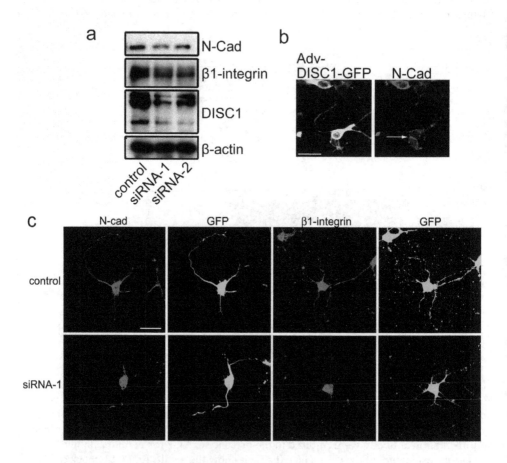

Fig. 3. (a) siRNAs targeting specific DISC1 sequences (siRNA-1 and siRNA-2) or scramble siRNA (control) was transfected into rat primary neurons at 1 DIV and cells were harvested at 4 DIV. The expression of DISC1, N-cadherin and β1-integrin was assayed by western blotting. (b) Adv-DISC1-GFP-infected neurons (1DIV) were fixed (4DIV) and immunostained with anti-N-cadherin. Arrow indicates enhanced N-cadherin expression at cell-cell contact. (c) Scramble or siRNA-1 with GFP-expressing vector-transfected neurons (1 DIV) were fixed (4 DIV) and immunostained with anti-N-cadherin or anti-β1-integrin antibody. Scale bars, 20 μm.

3. Depression and adhesion molecules

Repeated stressful events are known to be closely associated with the onset of depression (Gold et al., 1988a, b; Post, 1992; McEwen, 2004; Sala et al., 2004; Alfonso et al., 2005). Furthermore, chronic stress activates the HPA system chronically by elevation of plasma corticosterone levels (Bartanusz et al., 1993; Herman et al., 1995; Aguilera and Rabadan-Diehl, 2000; Dallman et al., 2006). However, the molecular pathway in the brain caused by the excess level of plasma corticosteroids is hardly elucidated. Here we will show that chronically stressed mice indicates depression-like symptoms and the functional implications of changes in adhesion molecules in the mice brain exposed to chronic stresses.

3.1 Repeated WIRS exposed mice are suitable model of depression-like symptoms

The HPA system is initiated by the activation of the paraventricular nucleus (PVN) of the hypothalamus, leading to the secretion of corticotropin-releasing hormone (CRH) from the neuron terminals of the PVN neurons. CRH triggers the release of adrenocorticotropic hormone (ACTH) from the anterior pituitary. ACTH subsequently stimulates the release of cortisol or corticosterone in humans and rodents, respectively (Thomson and Craighead, 2008; Pariante and Lightman, 2008). However, the molecular pathway in the brain affected by excess levels of plasma corticosteroids is not known. We firstly established a suitable model of depression-like symptoms wherein the HPA system plays an important role.

The mice exposed to repeated water-immersion restraint stress (WIRS) (chronic stress exposure) demonstrated chronically elevated plasma corticosterone levels. Furthermore, these chronic stress exposed mice showed significant longer immobility times than control mice, indicating increased despair. In addition, exposing mice to chronic stress resulted in a significant decrease in neurogenesis in the hippocampus (Miyata et al., 2011). As demonstrated in the mice exposed to chronic stress, continuous upregulation of plasma corticosterone levels, increased immobility time, and neurogenesis inhibition in the hippocampus are well known to occur in patients with depression.

3.2 Elevation of SGK1 and phosphorylated SGK1 in the OLs after chronic stress exposure

The microarray technique was showed that *Sgk1* consistently altered expression in the medial prefrontal cortex of chronically stressed mice. Furthermore, we recently reported the first *in vivo* and *in vitro* demonstration of chronic stress increases SGK1 expression and SGK1 activation (Miyata et al., 2011). It was previously reported that subcutaneous injection of corticosterone causes the upregulation of SGK1 in OLs (van Gemert et al., 2006), suggesting that various stressors that induce increases in plasma corticosterone levels possibly upregulate SGK1 expression in OLs. Although mechanism that up-regulated corticosterone regulates Sgk1 expression is still obscure (Webster et al., 1993a, b), it is probable that up-regulated corticosterone binds to Sgk1 gene directly to elevate its expression in the OLs, because glucocorticoide responsible element is present at the promoter region of *Sgk1* gene (Maiyar et al., 1996, 1997).

The first step of the activation of SGK1 is phosphorylation at Ser422 by mTOR and other protein kinase (Feng et al., 2004; Hong et al., 2008). The form of posphorylation of SGK1 Ser422 is substrate for the PDK1 which phosphorylates SGK1 at Thr256 in the SGK1 activation loop to cause the activation of SGK1 (Kobayashi et al., 1999; Biondi et al., 2001). In fact, chronic stress exposure resulted in an increase of phosphorylated SGK1 at Thr256 in OLs (Miyata et al., 2011).

3.3 Activated SGK1 up-regulates the expression of the adhesion molecules in OLs *via* elevation of the NDRG1 phosphorylation after chronic stress exposure

Several molecules interacting with Sgk1 in the brain are reported. For example, they are NDRG1, NDRG2, Tau, Huntingtin, IκB kinase α (IKKα) and p300 (Murray et al., 2004; Rungone et al., 2004; Chun et al., 2004; Tai et al., 2009). Among them, NDRG1 has been shown to be localized in OLs in the brain (Okuda et al., 2008) and NDRG1 has shown as the substrate of SGK1 (Murray et al., 2004). The SGK1 and NDRG1 interact in OLs and chronic stress increased both SGK1 and NDRG1 phosphorylation levels (Fig. 4.). We reported that chronic stress elevates the expression of SGK1 and increased SGK1 is phosphorylated SGK1 by the activated PDK1 via PI3K signal pathway (Miyata et al., 2011). However, molecular

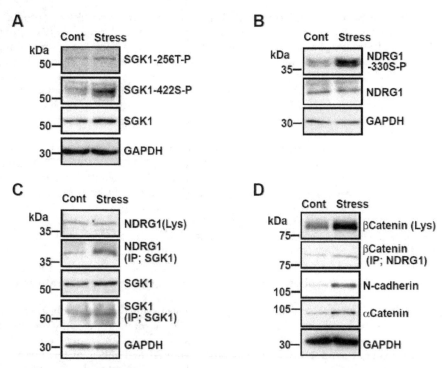

Fig. 4. Activated SGK1-NDRG1 pathway by repeated exposure to WIRS (chronic stress exposure) upregulates adhesion molecules expression levels in oligodendrocytes.
(A) Western blot analysis shows SGK1 protein, its phosphorylation at positions T-256 (SGK1-256T-P) and S-422 (SGK1-422S-P) in the oligodendrocytes of the corpus callosum after chronic stress exposure. (B) Western blot analysis shows that repeated exposure to WIRS elevated phosphorylated NDRG1 levels in the corpus callosum. (C) Immunoprecipitation and western blot analysis show that chronic stress exposure elevated the interaction between SGK1 and NDRG1 (second column). However, NDRG1 expression did not increase in the corpus callosum (first column). (D) Immunoprecipitation and western blot analysis show that repeated exposure to WIRS elevated the interaction between NDRG1 and β-catenin (second panel), and that the expression levels of β-catenin, N-cadherin, and α-catenin were elevated in the corpus callosum. (Adapted with permission from Miyata et al. 2011.)

mechanism of the activation of PI3K signal pathway by enhanced plasma corticosterone level after chronic stress exposure remains unknown.

Recently, NDRG1 has been shown to play a key roll in stabilizing the adherens junctions by up-regulation of recycle of E-cadherin in the prostate cancer cells (Kachhap et al., 2007; Song et al., 2010). We further reported that expression of adhesion molecules such as N-cadherin, α-catenin and β-catenin was increased in the corpus callosum after chronic stress exposure and interaction between NDRG1 and β-catenin (Fig. 4.).

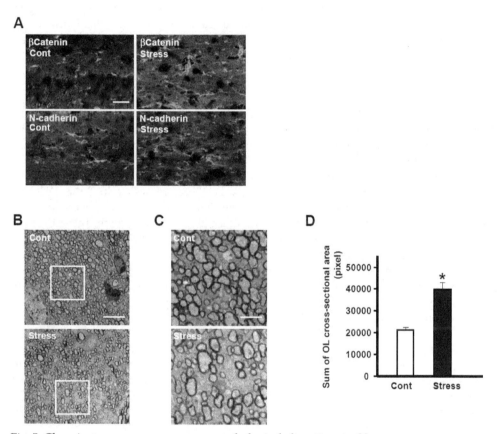

Fig. 5. Chronic stress exposure causes morphological alterations in OLs.
(A) Immunohistochemical analysis of β-catenin and N-cadherin in the corpus callosum demonstrates increased labeling of the processes of the oligodendrocytes (i.e., greater number and intensity) in mice exposed to repeated WIRS. Scale bar = 50 μm. (B, C) Representative transverse electron micrographs of the corpus callosum from control (upper panels of B and C) and chronic stress exposed mice (lower panels of B and C). Scale bars = 5 μm. (E) The higher magnification of the square region of (D). Scale bar = 2 μm. (F) Results of the quantification of the sum of oligodendrocytes in the cross-sectional area. The results are expressed as the mean ± SEM of 3 independent experiments. *p < 0.05, t-test. (Adapted with permission from Miyata et al. 2011.)

3.4 Up-regulation of the adhesion molecules expression in OLs causes the morphological changes of OLs and MDD

Adhesion molecules such as N-cadherin, α-catenin and β-catenin are key molecules composing the adherent junction (Aberle et al., 1996). Therefore, increase of the expression of these molecules suggests the extension of the site where OLs are adjacent to other elements. Cellular membrane of OLs and their processes labeled by the N-cadherin and β-catenin after chronic stress exposure increased markedly, showing that chronic stress exposure induces the morphological change of OLs (Fig. 5.). The volume of OL processes occupying the intrafibrial space increased markedly in the corpus callosum of the chronic stress exposure mice comparing with that found in the normal mice (Fig. 5.). Furthermore, the abnormal arborization of OLs and depression-like symptoms returned to the control levels after mice recovered from the chronic stress (Miyata et al., 2011).

4. Conclusion

To date, genetic association studies have been showing that adhesion molecules such as cadherins strongly associated with the development of psychosis including schizophrenia, bipolar disorder and autism, because these disorders have common abnormalities in molecular pathways. Adhesion molecules play important roles in neurodevelopmental events such as neuronal migration, neurite extension, syanptogenesis and synaptic plasticity from early embryo to postnatal stages. Furthermore, we clarified that DISC1, a candidate susceptibility gene for major mental illness, regulates the expressions of adhesion molecules, which affect cellular adhesion and neurite outgrowth. Taken together these results, abnormality of adhesion molecules caused by genetic susceptibility in genes encoding adhesion molecules and DISC1 may result in impairment of brain development. Our data has shown that DISC1 expressed in the developing cerebral cortex, hippocampus and cerebellum of rat brain. N-cadherin and β1-integrin also express in the developing cerebral cortex and hippocampus, which suggesting that DISC1 might be involved in neuronal migration, formation of axon, dendrite and spine and synaptic plasticity by regulating these adhesion molecules in such areas. To clarify this possibility, investigating the alteration of the expression and functions of adhesion molecules in DISC1 transgenic or knockout mice is necessary. In addition, N-cadherin and β1-integrin express not only in neurons but also in glial cells and regulate the differentiation of radial glial cells and oligodendrocytes. In recent report, DISC1 also expresses in these glial cells. Further studies are needed to clarify the role of DISC1 and adhesion molecules in glial cells in brain development.

Recent several studies have reported that MDD impair OLs function, for example, decrease of myelin basic protein (Honer et al., 1999), reduction of corpus callosum of female depression patients (Lacerda et al., 2005), the low density of total glia and OLs in amygdala (Hamidi et al. 2004), and the reduction of the expression of OL-related genes in the temporal cortex (Aston et al., 2005). Furthermore, recent our study indicated that the SGK1–NDRG1–adhesion molecules activation causes excess arborization of OL processes and this abnormality in the OL is related to depression-like symptoms (Fig. 6.). Elucidating the functional roles of the SGK1-NDRG1-adhesion molecules pathway in the OLs is a primary goal of future study for the pathogenesis of MDD.

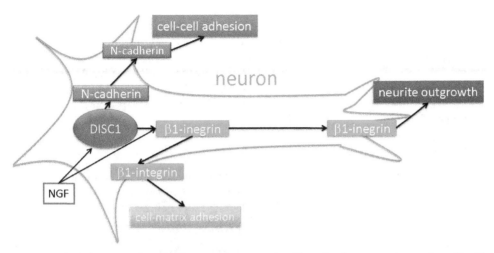

Fig. 6. DISC1 enhances cell-cell adhesion via increasing N-cadherin expression at the cell-cell contact. DISC1 also increases the expression of β1-integrin at the cell surface, which enhances cell-matrix adhesion and neurite outgrowth. Both DISC1 and β1-integrin are positively regulated by Nerve Growth Factor (NGF).

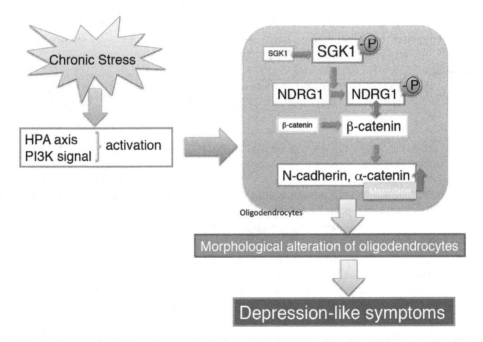

Fig. 7. Elevation of corticosterone induced by chronic stress induce the adherent molecules and morphological change in the oligodendrocytes of corpus callosum via the activation of SGK1-NDRG1 pathway. (Adapted with permission from Miyata et al. 2011.)

5. Acknowledgement

This work has been supported in part by the Osaka Medical Research Foundation for Incurable Diseases, a Grant-in-Aid for Scientific research from Japan Society for the Promotion of Science, a Grant-in-Aid for Scientific Research on Innovative Areas "Neural Diversity and Neocortical Organization" and the Global COE Program from the Ministry of Education, Culture, Sports, Science, and Technology (MEXT) of Japan and a grant from Dainippon Sumitomo Pharma Co. Ltd.

6. References

Aberle, H.; Schwartz, H. & Kemler, R. (1996) Cadherin-catenin complex: protein interactions and their implications for cadherin function. *J. Cell Biochem.*, 61, 514-523.

Aguilera, G.; & Rabadan-Diehl, C. (2000) Vasopressinergic regulation of the hypothalamic-pituitary- adrenal axis: Implications for stress adaptation. *Regul. Pept.*, 96, 23–29.

Akbarian, S., W. E. Bunney, Jr., S. G. Potkin, S. B. Wigal, J. O. Hagman, C. A. Sandman & E. G. Jones, (1993) Altered distribution of nicotinamide-adenine dinucleotide phosphate-diaphorase cells in frontal lobe of schizophrenics implies disturbances of cortical development. *Archives of general psychiatry* 50: 169-177.

Alfonso, J.; Frasch, A.C. & Flugge, G. (2005) Chronic stress, depression and antidepressants: effects on gene transcription in the hippocampus. *Rev. Neurosci.*, 16, 43-56.

Aston, C.; Jiang, L. & Sokolov, B.P. (2005) Transcriptional profiling reveals evidence for signaling and oligodendroglial   abnormalities in the temporal cortex from patients with major depressive   disorder. *Mol. Psychiatry*, 10, 309-322.

Bartanusz, V.; Jezova, D.; Bertini, L.T.; Tilders, F.J.; Aubry, J.M. & Kiss, J.Z. (1993) Stress-induced increase in vasopressin and corticotropin-releasing factor expression in hypophysiotrophic paraventricular neurons. *Endocrinology*, 132, 895–902.

Biondi, R.M.; Kieloch, A.; Currie, R.A.; Deak, M. & Alessi, D.R. (2001) The PIF-binding pocket in PDK1 is essential for activation of S6K and SGK, but not PKB. *EMBO J.*, 20, 4380-4390.

Bronner-Fraser, M., M. Sieber-Blum & A. M. Cohen, (1980) Clonal analysis of the avian neural crest: migration and maturation of mixed neural crest clones injected into host chicken embryos. *The Journal of comparative neurology* 193: 423-434.

Brown, A. S., The environment and susceptibility to schizophrenia. *Progress in neurobiology* 93: 23-58.

Carroll, B.J.; Curtis, G.C.; Davies, B.M.; Mendels, J. & Sugerman, A.A. (1976) Urinary free cortisol excretion in depression. *Psychol. Med.*, 6, 43–50.

Chan, C. S., E. J. Weeber, L. Zong, E. Fuchs, J. D. Sweatt & R. L. Davis, (2006) Beta 1-integrins are required for hippocampal AMPA receptor-dependent synaptic transmission, synaptic plasticity, and working memory. *J Neurosci* 26: 223-232.

Chu, J.W.; Matthias, D.F.; Belanoff, J.; Schatzberg, A.; Hoffman, A.R. & Feldman, D. (2001) Successful long-term treatment of refractory Cushing's disease with high-dose mifepristone (RU 486). *J. Clin. Endocrinol. Metab.*, 86, 3568-3573.

Chun, J.; Kwon, T.; Lee, E.J.; Kim, C.H.; Han, Y.S.; Hong, S.K.; Hyun, S. & Kang, S.S. (2004) 14-3-3 Protein mediates phosphorylation of microtubule-associated protein tau by serum- and glucocorticoid-induced protein kinase 1. *Mol. Cells*, 18, 360-368.

Dallman, M.F.; Pecoraro, N.C.; La Fleur, S.E.; Warne, J.P.; Ginsberg, A.B.; Akana, S.F.; Laugero, K.C.; Houshyar, H.; Strack, A.M.; Bhatnagar, S. & Bell, M.E. (2006) Glucocorticoids, chronic stress, and obesity. *Prog. Brain Res.*, 153, 75-105.

Feng, J.; Park, J.; Cron, P.; Hess, D. & Hemmings, B.A. (2004) Identification of a PKB/Akt hydrophobic motif Ser-473 kinase as DNA-dependent protein kinase. *J. Biol. Chem.*, 279, 41189-41196.

Gold, P.W.; Loriaux, D.L.; Roy, A.; Kling, M.A.; Calabrese, J.R.; Kellner, C.H.; Nieman, L.K.; Post, R.M.; Pickar, D. & Gallucci, W. (1986a) Responses to corticotropin-releasing hormone in the hypercortisolism of depression and Cushing's disease. Pathophysiologic and diagnostic implications. *N. Engl. J. Med.*, 314, 1329–1335.

Gold, P.W.; Calabrese, J.R.; Kling, M.A.; Avgerinos, P.; Khan, I.; Gallucci, W.T.; Tomai, T.P. & Chrousos, G.P. (1986b) Abnormal ACTH and cortisol responses to ovine corticotropin releasing factor in patients with primary affective disorder. *Prog. Neuropsychopharmacol. Biol. Psychiatry*, 110, 57-65.

Gold, P.W.; Goodwin, F.K. & Chrousos, G.P. (1988a) Clinical and biochemical manifestations of depression. Relation to the neurobiology of stress (1). *N. Engl. J. Med.*, 319, 348–353.

Gold, P.W.; Goodwin, F.K. & Chrousos, G.P. (1988b) Clinical and biochemical manifestations of depression. Relation to the neurobiology of stress (2). *N. Engl. J. Med.*, 319, 413–420.

Halbreich, U.; Asnis, G.M.; Shindledecker, R.; Zumoff, B. & Nathan, R.S. (1985a) Cortisol secretion in endogenous depression. I. Basal plasma levels. *Arch. Gen. Psychiatry*, 42, 904–908.

Halbreich, U.; Asnis, G.M.; Shindledecker, R.; Zumoff, B. & Nathan, R.S. (1985b) Cortisol secretion in endogenous depression. II. Time-related functions. *Arch. Gen. Psychiatry* 42, 909–914.

Hamidi, M.; Drevets, W.C. & Price, J.L. (2004) Glial reduction in amygdala in major depressive disorder is due to oligodendrocytes. *Biol. Psychiatry*, 55, 563-569.

Hatta, K. & M. Takeichi, (1986) Expression of N-cadherin adhesion molecules associated with early morphogenetic events in chick development. *Nature* 320: 447-449.

Hattori, T., K. Baba, S. Matsuzaki, A. Honda, K. Miyoshi, K. Inoue, M. Taniguchi, H. Hashimoto, N. Shintani, A. Baba, S. Shimizu, F. Yukioka, N. Kumamoto, A. Yamaguchi, M. Tohyama & T. Katayama, (2007) A novel DISC1-interacting partner DISC1-Binding Zinc-finger protein: implication in the modulation of DISC1-dependent neurite outgrowth. *Molecular psychiatry* 12: 398-407.

Hattori, T., S. Shimizu, Y. Koyama, K. Yamada, R. Kuwahara, N. Kumamoto, S. Matsuzaki, A. Ito, T. Katayama & M. Tohyama, DISC1 regulates cell-cell adhesion, cell-matrix adhesion and neurite outgrowth. *Molecular psychiatry* 15: 778, 798-809.

Herman, J.P.; Adams, D. & Prewitt, C. (1995). Regulatory changes in neuroendocrine stress-integrative circuitry produced by a variable stress paradigm. *Neuroendocrinology*, 61, 180– 190.

Holsboer, F.; Von Bardeleben, U.; Gerken, A.; Stalla, G.K. & Muller, O.A. (1984) Blunted corticotropin and normal cortisol response to human corticotropin-releasing factor in depression. *N. Engl. J. Med.*, 311, 1127.

Honda, A., K. Miyoshi, K. Baba, M. Taniguchi, Y. Koyama, S. Kuroda, T. Katayama & M. Tohyama, (2004) Expression of fasciculation and elongation protein zeta-1 (FEZ1) in the developing rat brain. *Brain research* 122: 89-92.

Honer, W.G.; Falkai, P.; Chen, C.; Arango, V.; Mann, J.J. & Dwork, A.J. (1999) Synaptic and plasticity-associated proteins in anterior frontal cortex in severe mental illness. *Neuroscience*, 91, 1247-1255.

Hong, F.; Larrea, M.D.; Doughty, C.; Kwiatkowski, D.J.; Squillace, R. & Slingerland, J.M. (2008) mTOR-raptor binds and activates SGK1 to regulate p27 phosphorylation. *Mol. Cell*, 30, 701-711.

Huang, Z., K. Shimazu, N. H. Woo, K. Zang, U. Muller, B. Lu & L. F. Reichardt, (2006) Distinct roles of the beta 1-class integrins at the developing and the mature hippocampal excitatory synapse. *J Neurosci* 26: 11208-11219.

Inoue, A. & J. R. Sanes, (1997) Lamina-specific connectivity in the brain: regulation by N-cadherin, neurotrophins, and glycoconjugates. *Science (New York, N.Y* 276: 1428-1431.

Jakob, H. & H. Beckmann, (1986) Prenatal developmental disturbances in the limbic allocortex in schizophrenics. *Journal of neural transmission* 65: 303-326.

Kobayashi, T. & Cohen, P. (1999a) Activation of serum- and glucocorticoid-regulated protein kinase by agonists that activate phosphatidylinositide 3-kinase is mediated by 3-phosphoinositide-dependent protein kinase-1 (PDK1) and PDK2. *Biochem. J.*, 339, 319-328.

Kobayashi, T.; Deak, M.; Morrice, N. & Cohen, P. (1999b) Characterization of the structure and regulation of two novel isoforms of serum- and glucocorticoid-induced protein kinase. *Biochem. J.*, 344, 189-197.

Kachhap, S.K.; Faith, D.; Qian, D.Z.; Shabbeer, S.; Galloway, N.L.; Pili, R.; Denmeade, S.R.; DeMarzo, A.M. & Carducci, M.A. (2007) The N-Myc down regulated Gene1 (NDRG1) Is a Rab4a effector involved in vesicular recycling of E-cadherin. *PLoS One*, 2, e844.

Lacerda, A.L.; Brambilla, P.; Sassi, R.B.; Nicoletti, M.A.; Mallinger, A.G.; Frank, E.; Kupfer, D.J.; Keshavan, M.S. & Soares, J.C. (2005) Anatomical MRI study of corpus callosum in unipolar depression. *J. Psychiatr. Res.*, 39, 347-354.

Lichtenstein, P., B. H. Yip, C. Bjork, Y. Pawitan, T. D. Cannon, P. F. Sullivan & C. M. Hultman, (2009) Common genetic determinants of schizophrenia and bipolar disorder in Swedish families: a population-based study. *Lancet* 373: 234-239.

Maiyar, A.C.; Huang, A.J.; Phu, P.T.; Cha, H.H. & Firestone, G.L. (1996) p53 stimulates promoter activity of the sgk serum/glucocorticoid-inducible serine/threonine protein kinase gene in rodent mammary epithelial cells. *J. Biol. Chem.*, 271, 12414-12422.

Maiyar, A.C.; Phu, P.T.; Huang, A.J. & Firestone, G.L. (1997) Repression of glucocorticoid receptor transactivation and DNA binding of a glucocorticoid response element within the serum/glucocorticoid-inducible protein kinase (sgk) gene promoter by the p53 tumor suppressor protein. *Mol. Endocrinol.*, 11, 312-329.

McEwen, B.S. (2004) Protection and damage from acute and chronic stress: allostasis and allostatic overload and relevance to the pathophysiology of psychiatric disorders. *Ann. N.Y. Acad. Sci.*, 1032, 1-7.

Millar, J. K., S. Christie, S. Anderson, D. Lawson, D. Hsiao-Wei Loh, R. S. Devon, B. Arveiler, W. J. Muir, D. H. Blackwood & D. J. Porteous, (2001) Genomic structure and localisation within a linkage hotspot of Disrupted In Schizophrenia 1, a gene disrupted by a translocation segregating with schizophrenia. *Molecular psychiatry* 6: 173-178.

Miyata, S.; Koyama, Y.; Takemoto, K.; Yoshikawa, K.; Ishikawa, T.; Taniguchi, M.; Inoue, K.; Aoki, M.; Hori, O.; Katayama, T. & Tohyama, M. (2011) Plasma corticosterone activates SGK1 and induces morphological changes in oligodendrocytes in corpus callosum. *PLoS One*, 6, e19859.

Miyoshi, K., M. Asanuma, I. Miyazaki, F. J. Diaz-Corrales, T. Katayama, M. Tohyama & N. Ogawa, (2004) DISC1 localizes to the centrosome by binding to kendrin. *Biochemical and biophysical research communications* 317: 1195-1199.

Miyoshi, K., A. Honda, K. Baba, M. Taniguchi, K. Oono, T. Fujita, S. Kuroda, T. Katayama & M. Tohyama, (2003) Disrupted-In-Schizophrenia 1, a candidate gene for schizophrenia, participates in neurite outgrowth. *Molecular psychiatry* 8: 685-694.

Murray, J.T.; Campbell, D.G.; Morrice, N.; Auld, G.C.; Shpiro, N.; Marquez, R.; Peggie, M.; Bain, J.; Bloomberg, G.B.; Grahammer, F.; Lang, F.; Wulff, P.; Kuhl, D. & Cohen, P. (2004) Exploitation of KESTREL to identify NDRG family members as physiological substrates for SGK1 and GSK3. *Biochem. J.*, 384, 477-488.

Mueser, K. T. & S. R. McGurk, (2004) Schizophrenia. *Lancet* 363: 2063-2072.

Nemeroff, C.B.; Widerlov, E.; Bissette, G.; Walleus, H.; Karlsson, I.; Eklund, K.; Kilts, C.D.; Loosen, P.T. & Vale, W. (1984) Elevated concentrations of CSF corticotropin-releasing factor-like immunoreactivity in depressed patients. *Science*, 226, 1342-1344.

Okuda, T.; Kokame, K. & Miyata, T. (2008) Differential expression patterns of NDRG family proteins in the central nervous system. *J. Histochem. Cytochem.*, 56, 175-182.

Pariante, C.M. & Lightman, S.L. (2008) The HPA axis in major depression: classical theories and new developments. *Trends Neurosci.*, 31, 464-468.

Post, R.M. (1992) Transduction of psychosocial stress into the neurobiology of recurrent affective disorder. *Am. J. Psychiatry*, 149, 999-1010.

Radice, G. L., H. Rayburn, H. Matsunami, K. A. Knudsen, M. Takeichi & R. O. Hynes, (1997) Developmental defects in mouse embryos lacking N-cadherin. *Developmental biology* 181: 64-78.

Rangone, H.; Poizat, G.; Troncoso, J.; Ross, C.A.; MacDonald, M.E.; Saudou, F. & Humbert, S. (2004) The serum- and glucocorticoid-induced kinase SGK inhibits mutant huntingtin-induced toxicity by phosphorylating serine 421 of huntingtin. *Eur. J. Neurosci.*, 19, 273-279.

Rougon, G. & O. Hobert, (2003) New insights into the diversity and function of neuronal immunoglobulin superfamily molecules. *Annual review of neuroscience* 26: 207-238.

Sala, M.; Perez, J.; Soloff, P.; Ucelli, di Nemi, S.; Caverzasi, E.; Soares, J.C. & Brambilla, P. (2004) Stress and hippocampal abnormalities in psychiatric disorders. *Eur. Neuropsychopharmacol.*, 14, 393-405.

Sanada, K., A. Gupta & L. H. Tsai, (2004) Disabled-1-regulated adhesion of migrating neurons to radial glial fiber contributes to neuronal positioning during early corticogenesis. *Neuron* 42: 197-211.

Schatzberg, A.F.; Rothschild, A.J.; Langlais, P.J.; Langlais, P.J.; Bird, E.D. & Cole, J.O. (1985) A corticosteroid/dopamine hypothesis for psychotic depression and related states. *J. Psychiatr. Res.*, 19, 57–64.

Schmid, R. S., R. Jo, S. Shelton, J. A. Kreidberg & E. S. Anton, (2005) Reelin, integrin and DAB1 interactions during embryonic cerebral cortical development. *Cereb Cortex* 15: 1632-1636.

Schwab, S. G. & D. B. Wildenauer, (2009) Update on key previously proposed candidate genes for schizophrenia. *Current opinion in psychiatry* 22: 147-153.

Selemon, L. D. & P. S. Goldman-Rakic, (1999) The reduced neuropil hypothesis: a circuit based model of schizophrenia. *Biological psychiatry* 45: 17-25.

Seshadri, S., A. L. DeStefano, R. Au, J. M. Massaro, A. S. Beiser, M. Kelly-Hayes, C. S. Kase, R. B. D'Agostino, Sr., C. Decarli, L. D. Atwood & P. A. Wolf, (2007) Genetic correlates of brain aging on MRI and cognitive test measures: a genome-wide association and linkage analysis in the Framingham Study. *BMC medical genetics* 8 Suppl 1: S15.

Shan, W. S., H. Tanaka, G. R. Phillips, K. Arndt, M. Yoshida, D. R. Colman & L. Shapiro, (2000) Functional cis-heterodimers of N- and R-cadherins. *The Journal of cell biology* 148: 579-590.

Shimizu, S., S. Matsuzaki, T. Hattori, N. Kumamoto, K. Miyoshi, T. Katayama & M. Tohyama, (2008) DISC1-kendrin interaction is involved in centrosomal microtubule network formation. *Biochemical and biophysical research communications* 377: 1051-1056.

Song, Y.; Oda, Y.; Hori, M.; Kuroiwa, K.; Ono, M.; Hosoi, F.; Basaki, Y.; Tokunaga, S.; Kuwano, M.; Naito, S. & Tsuneyoshi, M. (2010) N-myc downstream regulated gene-1/Cap43 may play an important role in malignant progression of prostate cancer, in its close association with E-cadherin. *Hum. Pathol.*, 41, 214-222.

Soronen, P., H. M. Ollila, M. Antila, K. Silander, O. M. Palo, T. Kieseppa, J. Lonnqvist, L. Peltonen, A. Tuulio-Henriksson, T. Partonen & T. Paunio, Replication of GWAS of bipolar disorder: association of SNPs near CDH7 with bipolar disorder and visual processing. *Molecular psychiatry* 15: 4-6.

Tai, D.J.; Su, C.C.; Ma, Y.L. & Lee, E.H. (2009) SGK1 phosphorylation of IkappaB Kinase alpha and p300 Up-regulates NF-kappaB activity and increases N-Methyl-D-aspartate receptor NR2A and NR2B expression. *J. Biol. Chem.*, 284, 4073-4089.

Takeichi, M., (2007) The cadherin superfamily in neuronal connections and interactions. *Nature reviews* 8: 11-20.

Taniguchi, H., D. Kawauchi, K. Nishida & F. Murakami, (2006) Classic cadherins regulate tangential migration of precerebellar neurons in the caudal hindbrain. *Development (Cambridge, England)* 133: 1923-1931.

Tepass, U., K. Truong, D. Godt, M. Ikura & M. Peifer, (2000) Cadherins in embryonic and neural morphogenesis. *Nat Rev Mol Cell Biol* 1: 91-100.

Thomson, F. & Craighead, M. (2008) Innovative approaches for the treatment of depression: targeting the HPA axis. *Neurochem. Res.*, 33, 691-707.

van Gemert, N.G.; Meijer, O.C.; Morsink, M.C. & Joëls, M. (2006) Effect of brief corticosterone administration on SGK1 and RGS4 mRNA expression in rat hippocampus. *Stress*, 9, 165-170.

Walsh, T., J. M. McClellan, S. E. McCarthy, A. M. Addington, S. B. Pierce, G. M. Cooper, A. S. Nord, M. Kusenda, D. Malhotra, A. Bhandari, S. M. Stray, C. F. Rippey, P. Roccanova, V. Makarov, B. Lakshmi, R. L. Findling, L. Sikich, T. Stromberg, B. Merriman, N. Gogtay, P. Butler, K. Eckstrand, L. Noory, P. Gochman, R. Long, Z. Chen, S. Davis, C. Baker, E. E. Eichler, P. S. Meltzer, S. F. Nelson, A. B. Singleton, M. K. Lee, J. L. Rapoport, M. C. King & J. Sebat, (2008) Rare structural variants disrupt multiple genes in neurodevelopmental pathways in schizophrenia. *Science (New York, N.Y* 320: 539-543.

Wang, K., H. Zhang, D. Ma, M. Bucan, J. T. Glessner, B. S. Abrahams, D. Salyakina, M. Imielinski, J. P. Bradfield, P. M. Sleiman, C. E. Kim, C. Hou, E. Frackelton, R. Chiavacci, N. Takahashi, T. Sakurai, E. Rappaport, C. M. Lajonchere, J. Munson, A. Estes, O. Korvatska, J. Piven, L. I. Sonnenblick, A. I. Alvarez Retuerto, E. I. Herman, H. Dong, T. Hutman, M. Sigman, S. Ozonoff, Λ. Klin, T. Owley, J. A. Sweeney, C. W. Brune, R. M. Cantor, R. Bernier, J. R. Gilbert, M. L. Cuccaro, W. M. McMahon, J. Miller, M. W. State, T. H. Wassink, H. Coon, S. E. Levy, R. T. Schultz, J. I. Nurnberger, J. L. Haines, J. S. Sutcliffe, E. H. Cook, N. J. Minshew, J. D. Buxbaum, G. Dawson, S. F. Grant, D. H. Geschwind, M. A. Pericak-Vance, G. D. Schellenberg & H. Hakonarson, (2009) Common genetic variants on 5p14.1 associate with autism spectrum disorders. *Nature* 459: 528-533.

Webster, M.K.; Goya, L.; Ge, Y.; Maiyar, A.C. & Firestone, G.L. (1993a) Characterization of sgk, a novel member of the serine/threonine protein kinase gene family which is transcriptionally induced by glucocorticoids and serum. *Mol. Cell Biol.*, 13, 2031-2040.

Webster, M.K.; Goya, L. & Firestone, G.L. (1993b) Immediate-early transcriptional regulation and rapid mRNA turnover of a putative serine/threonine protein kinase. *J. Biol. Chem.*, 268, 11482-11485.

Weinberger, D. R., (1987) Implications of normal brain development for the pathogenesis of schizophrenia. *Archives of general psychiatry* 44: 660-669.

Yamagata, M., J. P. Herman & J. R. Sanes, (1995) Lamina-specific expression of adhesion molecules in developing chick optic tectum. *J Neurosci* 15: 4556-4571.

Yap, A. S. & E. M. Kovacs, (2003) Direct cadherin-activated cell signaling: a view from the plasma membrane. *The Journal of cell biology* 160: 11-16.

Young, E.A.; Kotun, J.; Haskett, R.F.; Grunhaus, L.; Greden, J.F.; Watson, S.J. & Akil, H.
(1993) Dissociation between pituitary and adrenal suppression to dexamethasone
in depression. *Arch. Gen. Psychiatry*, 50, 395–403.

9

Breaking a Diagnosis of Dementia

M. Dalvi
William Harvey Hospital, Ashford Kent
Kent &Medway NHS& Social Care Partnership Trust, Kent,
UK

1. Introduction

There are 700,000 people in the UK living with Dementia (Knapp etal, Dementia UK: The full Report Alzheimer's Society2007). This has prompted the government to publish the first National Dementia Strategy which has made dementia a national priority. Dementia has a huge impact on physical, psychological and social aspects of care and also poses ethical challenges. One major ethical challenge which looms large, is the difficulty faced by clinicians in disclosing the diagnosis of dementia. The National Dementia strategy acknowledges this. 61% General practitioners routinely withhold diagnosis (Vassilas C& Donaldson J, 1998) and 60% Old Age Psychiatrists do not always disclose diagnosis as 20% do not see any benefit (Downs et al, 2002). This is similar to disclosure practices with cancer patients in the 1960's whereby 90% of physicians did not disclose the diagnosis of cancer to their patients (Oken etal 1961). This however saw a fundamental shift in the seventies when only 10% of physicians withheld the diagnosis of cancer (Novack etal, 1979). This may be related to new cancer medications and patient rights. There are many reasons for not disclosing a diagnosis of dementia. Physicians fear causing harm to their patients. (Pinner G& Bouman W, 2002). Some medical practitioners find it hard to share a diagnosis of dementia(Illife,S etal,03) and others report explaining a diagnosis of dementia is more difficult than for other diseases(Glosser etal,1985). This can lead to variability in diagnostic disclosure which I will address here. Since the last decade great progress has been made in identifying biomarkers and molecular changes in the brain associated with Alzheimer's disease. With various disease modifying medications like Bapineuzumab in phase III trials showing promising results, diagnostic disclosure is finding itself in the limelight for ethical and scientific reasons.

2. Problems with diagnosis of dementia

There are inherent problems with diagnosing dementia itself due to the insidious nature of the condition and difficulty in detecting transition between normal ageing and the onset of dementia. Diagnosis is based on clinical criteria and takes into account history, physical and neurological examination along with appropriate laboratory investigations. Due to the lack of a single and definitive tool for diagnosing Alzheimer's disease and other forms of dementias, one can easily miss out on early diagnosis. A definitive diagnosis of dementia is only possible at post-mortem. Several diagnostic tools are available with their own unique problems. The widely used Mini-mental state exam had demonstrated less sensitivity to mild dementia in highly educated people and those with non-cortical dementias. (Rothlind & Brondt, 1993). The NINCD-ADRDA criteria (McKhann etal, 1984) have a high degree of sensitivity but low specificity for the diagnosis of possible Alzheimer's disease (Knopman etal, 2001). This may lead to over diagnosis of some patients without dementia. All this can lead to diagnostic uncertainty and when coupled with therapeutic nihilism may lead to resistance in the disclosure of diagnosis. Although there is a substantial body of evidence which favours diagnostic disclosure there is a huge variability in all the aspects of disclosure (Carpenter& Dave, 2004). Bamford and colleagues concluded from their meta-analysis that the process of disclosure is not easy. People with dementia are less often told of their diagnosis than their family members. There is widespread use of euphemisms and family members generally prefer not to inform the diagnosis to their relatives.

3. Ethical principles in diagnostic disclosure

According to duty based ethics developed by the German philosopher Emmanuel Kant, it is morally wrong not to disclose the diagnosis even if it has harmful consequence. This may directly contradict the ethical principle of non-maleficence i.e. avoiding harm. So there is an ethical dilemma as to whether all treatments and interventions which may lead to harm whether psychological or in the form of side-effects should be avoided on the grounds that "avoiding harm always takes priority over doing good".

Autonomy: Patients have the right to think, decide, and act on the basis of such thoughts, freely and independently. Clinicians are faced with a dilemma of respecting patients' autonomy on one hand and concerns of carers at the same time. This has now been clarified by the Nuffield Council of Bioethics in its report Dementia: Ethical issues (Nuffield Council of Bioethics .Dementia: Ethical issues, Oct 2009). It suggests a broad concept of autonomy called "Relational autonomy" for patients suffering from dementia. (Nuffield Council of Bioethics. Dementia: ethical issues.2009). It suggests that as patient's sense of self is grounded in their social network, the whole family should be helped to support the autonomous wishes of the patient. This concept in my view is very helpful as on one hand it helps to maximise patients' freedom and on the other hand helps to minimise risk. It also recommends that clinicians should actively encourage patients to share details about their illness with their family.

General Medical Council recommends that doctors must give their patients information they request for. In practice, patients with dementia rarely ask for information, so should we hide the diagnosis if they don't ask for it? Is this ethical?

4. Current practice

Views of consultants, patients and family members in sharing the diagnosis are different (McWilliams, 1998) Patients prefer to be told of their diagnosis (George& Gove, 2007) however in reality things are different. Only half of geriatricians openly discuss the diagnosis with their patients (Carpenter&Dave, 2004). Family members generally prefer not to inform people with dementia, despite agreeing that they would want to know the diagnosis if they were in that situation. (Bamfordetal, 2004).

Keady& Gilleard (2002) report that the experience of patients about assessment and disclosure is negative. Patients' perceived it as a controlling, insensitive process with feelings of insecurity, uncertainty and anxiety. Delays in assessments in the memory clinic was unsettling and patients felt stigmatised to the diagnosis and location of the memory clinic. (Pratt& Wilkinson, 2001) report that patients had feelings of shock, anger and denial after receiving the diagnosis. They felt pressured to perform well on the memory tests because of drug therapy. Patients were concerned about late disclosure of diagnosis and lack of information on prognosis.

Reasons against diagnostic disclosure: are largely based on the principle of non-maleficence (Drickamer etal, 1992). This is due to the following reasons

1.   concerns for causing harm, distress to patients i.e. Therapeutic lying (Bakhurst,1992)
2.   lack of definitive diagnosis
3.   No curative treatment.
4.   Concerns about ability to understand information in advanced dementia.
5.   No benefits, costs outweigh benefits.
6.   Stigma associated with dementia.

Reasons for diagnostic disclosure are based on the ethical principle of autonomy.

1.   Patient has the right to honest information, to know about their diagnosis according to the above principle. Hiding diagnosis will breach autonomy.
2.   Several studies confirm that patients with dementia prefer to be informed of the diagnosis of dementia(Erde etal,1988 Maranski,2000.,Clare,2003.,Van Hout etal,2006)
3.   Non disclosure can upset, confuse patients and break trust(Bamford etal,2004)
4.   Patients feel relieved after diagnosis(Derksen etal,2006)
5.   It helps patients plan for the future.
6.   For travel and vacation purposes.
7.   Obtaining a second opinion.

There is more evidence base for diagnostic disclosure as opposed to non- disclosure. Patients prefer to be informed of the diagnosis and are distressed if they arc not informed of their diagnosis (Clare, 2003; Pratt& Wilkinson, 2003). The work done by (Jha etal, 2001) emphasises that there is no evidence that disclosing diagnosis leads to harm in the form of stigma, depression or suicide.

Criticisms of the studies. Most of the above studies are surveys of convenience samples which compromise validity of results. The questionnaires may not be valid and reliable and can lead to social desirability effect. The study done by Erde and colleagues has recruited younger mostly cognitively intact patients which is not a representative sample.

There are various models of diagnostic disclosure but one should embrace a person-family centred approach based on breaking bad news. It should be a gradual educative process involving discussions with both the patient and family maintaining the dignity of the patient.

4.1 Impact of new medical technology on diagnostic disclosure

There is a growing evidence base for use of MRI, CSF amyloid, tau assays in Early Diagnosis of Dementia Duara and colleagues (Duara etal, 2008) highlights the role of structural MRI in the early diagnosis of AD. Medial temporal atrophy has consistently been shown to represent an early imaging feature of AD and to predict conversion from MCI to AD. (DeCarli etal, 2007) CSF assays and PET amyloid tracer uptake are sensitive at the earliest stage of Alzheimer's disease. 18F PET and MRI are sensitive at the Mild cognitive impairment stage and continue to change well into the dementia stage. This will greatly improve accuracy of early diagnosis and hence will have an impact on diagnostic disclosure .This will end uncertainty of diagnosis especially at the Mild cognitive impairment stage and clinicians will become more confident in diagnostic disclosure.

4.2 Preparation for a diagnostic assessment

Factors influencing diagnosis. (Bamford etal, 2004)

1. Disease factors
   a. Severity of cognitive impairment.
   b. Diagnostic uncertainty.
2. Clinician Factors
   a. Beliefs and type of clinician
   b. Age and time since clinician qualified.
   c. Clinician's attitude to early diagnosis.
3. Patient Factors
   1. Age of patient.
   2. Patient's desire to be told.
   3. Insight of patient
   4. Personality of the patient
   5. Emotional stability of patient
   6. Comorbidity of patient.
4. IV) Carer Factors
   a. Age of carer
   b. Carer's desire for patient to be told of the diagnosis.

More research is needed as to which of the above factors strongly influences the clinician during diagnostic disclosure. There is an emerging body of evidence on how cultural and religious beliefs of doctors influence End of Life care decisions and similar studies regarding personal values, religious and cultural beliefs influencing diagnostic disclosure are necessary.

5. Outcomes of disclosure for patient's with dementia

1. Positive Outcomes.
   a. End to uncertainty
   b. Confirmation of suspicions
   c. Increased understanding of problems
   d. Access to support
   e. Helps to develop positive coping strategies
   f. Planning and short term goals
2. Negative Outcomes
   a. Negative effects on self esteem and personhood
   b. Preoccupation with Diagnosis
   c. Anxiety about increasing disability.
   d. Restricted activities
   e. Crisis after diagnosis
   f. Hyper vigilant state after diagnosis

These outcomes need to be discussed with patients following which there needs to be sufficient space for patient's emotions. Clinicians may find it particularly challenging to disclose diagnosis in uncertain cases with comorbid psychiatric disorders. or for patient's who have normal tests. Patients with premorbid high IQ may score within the normal range on neuropsychological assessments and this may prove challenging for the clinician breaking the diagnosis.

6. Pre assessment Counselling framework

a. Consent & Choice
b. Collaboration& Control
c. The person and their context

a. Consent- The patient should be informed about the reasons for the referral, process of assessment and beyond, outcomes of their assessment, implications of receiving a diagnosis of dementia as one of the possible outcomes of assessment. Every competent patient is considered to be autonomous and hence has the right of control over his body and hence we should obtain consent for diagnostic disclosure. An important step here is to give all the information to the patient before the disclosure. Not giving sufficient information before and after the diagnosis is not ethical. Also if the patient is not offered enough information to make their decision, their consent may not be valid. Ability to give consent may depend on context and patients should be given a choice.

b. Promoting Control and Collaboration: Patients should know that they have a choice regarding diagnostic disclosure. Their preference regarding type of feedback and location of the feedback should be honoured to prevent distress. Patients should be encouraged to share their diagnosis with their family members keeping in line with the new concept of "Relational Autonomy".

c. The Person and their context- Current life difficulties and their own ideas about their difficulties should be explored. Things that are going well should also be looked into. Coping strategies should be looked into and past crisis and response to it need to be explored. Their support networks and perceptions of significant others should be explored. Prior experiences of people they know with memory problems should be discussed. Past experiences of psychiatric services should be explored.

Post Diagnostic information

1. Emotions should be explored. Depression, denial, Anxiety are common. Earlier emotional experiences may be experienced again.
2. Cognitive changes and its impact should be addressed. Information about general loss of information processing, loss of function of recognition which may trigger emotions like anxiety and fear should be explained.
3. Losses e.g. loss of identity, loss of social role should be explored.
4. Future impact on relationships and attachments should be explained- Importance of bonds and relationships for support should be explained.
5. Environment and its impact- Loss of sense of familiar places should be explained.
6. Information about services like cognitive stimulation groups, support groups, Alzheimer's Society café, Admiral Nurses, Intermediate care team should be provided.

6.1 Case Study 1

Andrew who is a retired engineer lives with his wife Joan who suffered from memory lapses for several years. They have an outpatient clinic appointment in hospital for assessment of her memory problems. Joan was assessed by the doctor and asked to wait in another room. John who was outside in the waiting area was called in all by himself and the news that his wife has Alzheimer's disease was broken to him and the symptoms were confirmed.

Andrew was in the room with 3 strangers who sat looking at him waiting for his reaction. He was asked whether his wife Joan should be informed of her diagnosis. Andrew asked for

**Establish Early Diagnosis& Encourage patients to involve their family in the disclosure
Understand attitudes of patient& Family towards cognitive loss
Discuss diagnostic uncertainty if any
Address fears,concerns and their beliefs about dementia**

During Diagnosis

**Discuss it in a manner consistent with the patients' wishes
Use language which patient easily understands
Keep space for emotions, reflection & tackle denial.
Additional information on Further tests, Finances, driving
Individual prognosis, Type of dementia and medications.**

Patient centered approach

**Use individualised approach taking into account cultural background.
Look into patients expectations
Assess immediate psychological impact.
Post diagnostic counselling should focus on remaining capabilities, coping strategies.**

Fig. 1. Evidence based approach for diagnostic disclosure of Dementia.

advice from the doctor who informed him that it was ultimately his decision. Andrew decided to call Joan in the clinic room as he thought that Joan was a mature lady and would understand and adapt to the situation. Andrew felt he could perhaps help her realise that she did have a progressive memory problem. Andrew was informed of the diagnosis and she sat motionless, disbelieving in the diagnosis. For a while after the diagnosis was disclosed Joan was calm. She however had frequent appointments in the memory clinic with further tests due to which she began to rebel. Andrew helped her to go to a local day centre which worked for a while after which she refused to go. Joan started developing verbally aggressive behaviour towards Andrew and he bore the brunt of it. He was hence put in touch with the admiral nurse service for carer distress and is trying very hard to cope.

Case study 1 highlights several ethical problems, examples of bad clinical practice and is not the best example of patient centred care. Early diagnosis is beneficial and helpful (Milne& Wilkinson, 2002). It helps patients to prepare and plan for the future. People with dementia want early disclosure of the diagnosis (Jha etal, 2001). People have the right to be informed of their diagnosis and this should not be withheld on the grounds that patient has dementia or memory problems. In the case study 1 the patient Joan suffered from lapses of memory for several years which went unnoticed. Early or even timely diagnosis would have helped the patient to plan for her future care and treatment. Patients' autonomy should be respected and patient should be informed of the diagnosis and then at the same time encouraged to share the diagnosis with their family and carer. In Case 1 Joan's autonomy was not respected and instead the patient's husband was informed of the diagnosis first and asked if the diagnosis can be broken to Joan when in fact Joan was capable of understanding the information. This also amounts to breach in confidentiality. In any memory service, patients' right to be informed of their diagnosis should be respected and diagnosis should not be withheld solely on grounds that it may provoke anxiety and suffering. Confidentiality should be maintained and if the patient clearly refuses for a disclosure this should be respected. Diagnosis should be a process, a series of steps (Aminzadeh etal, 2007) which was not the case in Case study1 where it was a sudden event. Diagnosis should be disclosed in a compassionate manner and should involve the patient maintaining dignity and a sense of hope (Connel C etal, 2004). This did not happen in case study1 where the disclosure was insensitive and not person-centred. Dignity and solidarity were not maintained. Since the users and carers are quite vulnerable during this process, it is quite important to have space for emotions and reflection (Derksen E et al, 2006). Information on the illness, prognosis and necessary services was not provided in Case study 1 which is morally wrong. Giving clear and factual information to the patient in different forms is necessary. Post diagnostic counselling to focus on the remaining capability of the patient was not in place. This needs to be tailored specifically to the needs of the patient. (Derksen E etal, 2006).

Ethical issues.

Several ethical issues stand out in Case 1 however the second point is quite important.
1. Early diagnosis was not made
2. Patient's autonomy was not respected as carer was informed of the diagnosis prior to patient.
3. Confidentiality was breached.
4. Disclosure was sudden, insensitive and not person-centred.
5. No information and support was given after diagnostic disclosure to both patient and carer.

In Case study 1 it was ethically wrong that the carer was informed of the diagnosis first and asked if the diagnosis should be disclosed to the patient. Ethics dictates that a doctor should give an honest response about the diagnosis, even if it is uncertain to respect the patient's wellbeing and autonomy. Joan appears to have capacity to absorb the relevant information and hence is autonomous. The doctor should have respected Joan's autonomy and should have disclosed the diagnosis to her. After this disclosure the doctor should have taken Joan's consent to disclose the diagnosis to her husband. This ethical dilemma is commonplace in clinical practice and should be considered carefully. Clinicians are faced with a dilemma of respecting patient's autonomy on one hand and concerns of carers on the other hand. Nuffield Council of bioethics suggests a broad concept of autonomy called "Relational Autonomy" for patients suffering from Dementia. It suggests that as patient's sense of self is grounded in their social network, the whole family should be helped to support the autonomous wishes of the patient. This is a very useful concept and should be practiced.

6.2 Case Study 2

Elizabeth is a married lady in her early sixties who lives with her husband . Elizabeth works as a school teacher and teaches classical languages. Her work colleagues recently noticed some minor word finding problems which they found unusual taking into account her command on languages. Her husband noticed this too but put it down to anxiety as their son recently met with an accident and was in hospital due to which she has become somewhat distractable. They hence went to see the G.P. on insistence of their daughter . Her husband confirms that her word finding problems have not deteriorated but has noticed that Elizabeth avoids using the phone. Her husband also noticed that she can drift off from conversations but tends to get back to the original point. She on occasions can go to the kitchen and forget the very purpose of it and at times can mislay her personal belongings.

Her G.P carried out blood investigations and CT scan which were normal. She scored 28/30 on the MMSE. Her G.P. made a referral to Old Age Psychiatric services as he was unsure if Elizabeth was developing memory problems or if this was related to anxiety due to her son's accident.

The G.P referral was discussed in the Old age Psychiatry referral meeting and was allocated to be seen by the Neuropsychologist. An MRI with a medial temporal view was also ordered by the Consultant. The MRI sequences were discussed with the Neuroradiologist and agreed by him.

Elizabeth saw the Neuropsychologist in 2 weeks time for a Neuropsychological assessment which revealed early signs of cognitive impairment .She also had a MRI scan the same week which showed advanced involutional changes with both central and peripheral atrophy along with moderate bilateral hippocampal atrophy. She saw the Consultant the following week in his clinic. Elizabeth and her husband were called in together in the clinic. They were made comfortable and the purpose of the consultation was discussed. Elizabeth was asked if she wanted to know of her diagnosis and if she was happy to share it with her husband. After obtaining her consent , she was asked what she thought about her word-finding problems and what did she put it down to. She was given space to voice her concerns and her thoughts on the matter. She was then given a detailed feedback of the neuropsychological test she had last week and the findings were explained to her. She was then asked if she would like to see the MRI images on the computer and after taking her consent . The MRI scan findings were explained to her visually on the computer. Following this the diagnosis of dementia was broken in a very sensitive manner giving reasons as to why this was a disease process rather than normal ageing or a anxiety disorder. Elizabeth was given space for her emotions following which she was given a choice about the available medications. She was given patient information leaflets about local services . Patient was asked if she would like the letter copied to her and was given a choice about attending the post diagnostic counselling group and the Living Well Programme.

Discussion: This is a very good example of diagnostic disclosure and also how medical technology assists in speedy and early diagnosis. The G.P was quite candid that he was not able to come to grips of what was going on as so often is the case for Mild cognitive impairment and hence referred Elizabeth to old age psychiatric services. The expertise of the Consultant was very valuable as this patient required higher investigations ie MRI scan with specific sequences and also a Neuropsychological assessment.

The patient pathway was effective and the waiting time was reasonable. This did not cause undue distress to the patient or her family. The consultation was good and it was clear that he clinician breaking the diagnosis was experienced and did the diagnostic disclosure in a patient centred manner.

His communication skills were good and he did give space for emotions which is very important. MRI Brain images were shown which is a very powerful tool useful in diagnostic disclosure and also for tackling denial if any.

7. Conclusion

Disclosure of diagnosis of dementia is not straightforward. It involves not only the patient but multiple people, professionals and family members. There is robust evidence which favours diagnostic disclosure. Most studies indicate that patients would like to be told of their diagnosis and would like their carers to be informed as well. Patients who are autonomous have the right to be informed of their diagnosis and doctors should try to involve family members. The new concept of Relational Autonomy is quite useful and hence should be practiced widely. In my view each case should be considered individually, choices should be respected irrespective of the dementia stage and disclosure should be an ongoing process. Questions still remain as to how much information should be disclosed in patients with advanced dementia who are not capable to understand the information. How do we balance autonomy on one hand and carers wishes not to disclose the diagnosis? Is disclosure an absolute right or a relative one?

8. References

Aminzadeh, F., Byszewski, A.,Molnar, F; Eisner ,M. Emotional impact of dementia diagnosis (2007) Exploring patients with dementia and caregivers' perspective *Ageing Mental Health* ;11:281-90

Bamford, C., Lamont, S., Eccles .M., Robinson L., May C., Bond, J. Disclosing a diagnosis of dementia: a systematic review (2004) *Int J Geriatric Psychiatry*.Feb; 19(2):151-69.

Carpenter, B., Dave, J. *Gerontologist*. 2004 Disclosing a dementia diagnosis: a review of opinion and practice, and a proposed research agenda Apr; 44(2):149-58.

Connell, C., Boise, L., Stuckey, J., Holmes, S., Hudson, M. Attitudes towards diagnosis and disclosure of dementia among family caregivers and primary care physicians Gerontologist 2004, 44: 500-7

DeCarli,C. et al.Qualitative estimates of medial temporal atrophy as a predictor of progression from mild cognitive impairment to dementia.*Arch.Neurol*.64,108-115(2007)

Derksen. E., Vernooij-Dassen, M., Gillissen, F., Olde Rikkert, M., Scheltens, P. *Aging Ment Health*. (2006) Impact of diagnostic disclosure in dementia on patients and carers: qualitative case series analysis. September; 10

Downs, M., Clibbens, R., Rae, C. What do general practitioners tell people with dementia and their families about the condition? (2002)A survey of experiences in Scotland. Dementia*: The International J. Soc. Res. Prac.* 1: 47- 58

Drickamer, M., Lachs, M., (1992) should patients with Alzheimer's disease be told of their diagnosis? *New England Journal of Medicine* 1992; 326:947-51.

Duara,R. et al.Medial temporal lobe atrophy on MRI scans and the diagnosis of Alzheimer's disease .*Neurology* 71,1986-1992(2008

Georges J& Gove D(2007) Disclosing a diagnosis; The Alzheimer's Europe View, Journal of Dementia Care, 15(6) Nov-Dec 28-30.

Glosser, G., Wexler, D., Balmelli, M., (1985*) J Am Geriatric Soc.* Physicians' and families' perspectives on the medical management of dementia. Jun; 33(6):383-91.

Gordon, M., Goldstein, D., *Canadian Family Physician*. (2001) Alzheimer's disease. To tell or not to tell. Sep; 47:1803-6, 1809

Beady & Gilleard (2002) The Person with Alzhemier's disease ,Pathways to understanding the experience Editor Harris, Braudy, Johns Hopkins University Press ,USA page 3-28

Knapp, M., Prince, M., Albanese ,E., Banerjee ,S., Dhanasiri ,S., Fernandez ,JL., Ferri ,C., McCrone,P .,Snell, T., Stewart,,R (2007), Dementia UK, The full report Alzhiemer's Society London

Pinner, G., Bouman, W (2002) to tell or not to tell: on disclosing the diagnosis of dementia. *Int Psychogeriatrics* 14:127-37

Pratt R& Wilkinson H, (2001) Tell me the truth, The effect of being told the diagnosis of dementia from the perspective of the person with dementia. Mental Health foundation www.mentalhealth.org.uk

Jha, A., Tabet, N., Orrell, M. *Int J Geriatr Psychiatry.* (2001)To tell or not to tell-comparison of older patients' reaction to their diagnosis of dementia and depression Sep; 16(9):879-85

Maranski M. would you like to know what is wrong with you? (2000) on telling the truth to patients with dementia. *Journal of medical ethics* 26: 108-13

McKhann, G., Drachman, D., Folstein, M Neurology. (1984) Clinical diagnosis of Alzheimer's disease: Report of the NINCDS-ADRDA Work Group under the auspices of Department of Health and Human Services Task Force on Alzheimer's Disease

Novack, DH., Plumer, R., Smith R, L., Ochitill, H., Morrow G, R., Bennett, JM. *JAMA.* (1979) Changes in physicians' attitudes toward telling the cancer patient. Mar 2; 241(9):897-900.

Oken, D (1961) what to tell cancer patients. *Journal of the American Medical Association*, 175, 1120-1128

Rothlind, J & Brandt J, Journal of Neuropsychiatry & Clinical Neurosciences (1993) A brief assessment of frontal and subcortical functions in Dementia. 5: 73-77

Van Hout, HP. Vernooij-Dassen, MJ., Jansen DA., Stalman, WA. Aging Ment Health. (2006) Do general practitioners disclose correct information to their patients suspected of dementia and their caregivers? A prospective observational study. Mar; 10(2):151-5

Vassilas, C, Donaldson J (1998) Telling the truth: What General Practitioners say to patients with Dementia or terminal Cancer?   British Journal of general practice March 48(428) 1081-1082

Childhood Maltreatment and County-Level Deprivation Jointly Modify the Effect of Serotonin Transporter Promoter Genotype on Depressive Symptoms in Adolescent Girls

Monica Uddin[1], Erin Bakshis[2] and Regina de los Santos[2]
[1]Center for Molecular Medicine and Genetics and Department of Psychiatry and Behavioral Neurosciences, Wayne State University, Detroit, MI
[2]Department of Epidemiology, University of Michigan School of Public Health, Ann Arbor, MI
USA

1. Introduction

Depression is a commonly occurring mood disorder defined by the presence of persistent sad feelings, low energy, loss of interest in activities that were once pleasurable, feelings of guilt or low self-worth, disturbed sleep or appetite, and poor concentration, among other symptoms (American Psychiatric Association, 1994). Among adults 18 and older in the United States, the prevalence of major depressive disorder (MDD) is higher than that of any other commonly occurring DSM-IV mental disorder in the U.S., with a lifetime prevalence of 16.6%, and 12-month prevalence estimated at 6.7% (Kessler & Wang, 2008). The World Health Organization estimates that depression will rank second among the leading contributors of disease burden by the year 2020 (WHO, 2009). MDD is associated with enormous costs to both the individual and society, with the economic burden of depression estimated to be $83 billion per year as of 2000 (Greenberg et al., 2003), and the impairment in proper role functioning due to MDD known to be significantly worse when compared to a number of commonly occurring chronic medical disorders (Druss et al., 2009). The large public health burden of MDD is due, at least in part, to its onset relatively early in life: at least 25% of lifetime MDD cases start before age 19 (Kessler et al., 2005).

Despite substantial research, our understanding of the factors that contribute to the etiology of depression remain incomplete. Genetic factors account for an estimated 35-45 percent of the variance in risk for depressive symptoms (Shih et al., 2004). In addition, meta-analysis supports an association between polymorphisms in six different candidate genes and MDD (Lopez-Leon et al., 2008). Nevertheless, there is growing recognition that genetic influences on depression may only be evident under certain environmental conditions – i.e. that there may be gene X environment (G X E) interactions, such that individuals of the same genotype may express different phenotypes depending on their environmental contexts (Moffitt et al., 2005). In particular, a growing body of work indicates that genetic variation, in combination with adverse experiences early in life, shape risk for mental illness.

Seminal work by Caspi et al (Caspi et al., 2003) was the first to demonstrate that genetic variation at the promoter (5-HTTLPR) region of the serotonin transporter (SCL6A4) locus interacted with the experience of childhood maltreatment, including physical and sexual abuse, such that childhood maltreatment predicted adult depression only among individuals carrying an s allele but not among l/l homozygotes (Caspi et al., 2003). These findings were replicated by subsequent studies (Scheid et al., 2007), and detected not only in adults but also adolescents and children (Eley et al., 2004; Kaufman et al., 2004; Sjoberg et al., 2006). Nevertheless, some studies have either failed to detect any significant findings with respect to 5-HTTLPR x maltreatment interactions in depression (Chipman et al., 2007; Surtees et al., 2006) or have detected significant interactions, but for other 5-HTTLPR genotypes/alleles (Laucht et al., 2009). In addition, two recent meta-analyses have called into question the weight of evidence of G x E associations reported for the 5-HTTLPR locus (Munafo et al., 2009; Risch et al., 2009). These meta-analyses, however, have been criticized on a variety of levels, including (but not limited to) the heterogeneity in measurement of both environment and outcome (Lotrich & Lenze, 2009), the use of a dichotomized outcome for studies that were originally assessed with dimensional outcomes (Schwahn & Grabe, 2009), and a failure to consider the biological plausibility of G x E interactions at the 5-HTTLPR locus in light of animal and clinical data (Koenen & Galea, 2009; Rutter et al., 2009). Furthermore, an additional, more recent meta-analysis, including a greater number of studies, confirmed previous findings of an association between increased risk of depression under stressful conditions among carriers of the s allele (Karg et al., 2011); notably, this association was particularly pronounced when analyses were restricted to studies that assessed childhood maltreatment as the stressor of interest (Karg et al., 2011).

Importantly for the present study, we have also suggested that an additional consideration is the failure of the current literature to consider measurement of relevant social environmental variables that may interact with underlying genetic variability and vulnerability to produce increased risk for, or resilience to, mental illness. (Koenen & Galea, 2009; Koenen et al., 2010) Recent work suggests that macrosocial contextual influences, in conjunction with genetic variation at the 5-HTTLPR locus, contribute to risk of mental illness (Koenen et al., 2009; Uddin et al., 2010); and as outlined above, there is clear evidence that genetic variation moderates the effect of childhood maltreatment on risk of depression. Nevertheless, there has, to date, been little consideration of the joint and/or interacting effects of how these risk factors, operating at multiple levels, shape risk for mental illness. To address this gap in the literature, here we assess whether 5-HTTLPR genetic variation, childhood maltreatment, and macrosocial context interact to shape risk for depressive symptoms in a U.S. adolescent population. Consistent with recent recommendations regarding G X E studies involving the 5-HTTLPR locus (Uher & McGuffin, 2008), and depression more generally (Lupien et al., 2009), we conducted this investigation separately for males and females, and report results separately for each genotype.

2. Methods

2.1 Sample

The data source for our analysis is drawn from the National Longitudinal Study of Adolescent Health (AddHealth), a nationally representative, school-based sample of over 90,000 adolescents in grades 7 – 12, initially sampled in 1994 – 1995 in the United States and followed for three subsequent waves. A subsample (N=20,745) of participants from the in-school portion of the study was selected to participate in an additional, 90-minute in-home interview during Wave I, which provided the primary data source for the analyses reported here. In 2002, during Wave III, DNA samples were collected from a subsample of siblings (n=2,574) who had participated in the in-home interview portion of the study. The in-home and genetic data are part of the restricted use/contractual AddHealth dataset (Harris, 2008) and IRB approval to work with this dataset was secured prior to undertaking any of the below-described analyses. More detail regarding the design and data availability for the genetic component of AddHealth is available elsewhere (Harris et al., 2006).

The sample for our primary analysis is comprised of 1,097 individuals from the sibling subsample who provided DNA, belonged to a same sex sibling cluster, and for whom there was a complete set of data available for each sibling in the cluster for each of the measures included in our models. The analytic sample did not differ from the excluded sample with respect to genotype, childhood maltreatment, county-level deprivation or depressive symptoms, i.e. the main variables in the study.

2.2 Measures
2.2.1 Individual- and family-level health indicators

Depressive symptom scores were obtained using a shortened, 17-item version of the Center for Epidemiological Studies Depression Scale (CES-D) (Radloff, 1977), based on the CES-D questions that were posed in the AddHealth *Feelings Scale* during the in-home interviews conducted during Wave I (Apr. – Dec. 1995) and II (Apr. – Aug. 1996). Responses to the 17 questions were ordinal, ranging from 0 (never or rarely) to 3 (most or all of the time) and were summed for use as the outcome variable in all analyses, with higher scores indicative of more depressive symptoms. Respondents were required to answer all 17 questions in Waves I and II in order to be included in our analyzed sample. The final current depression index was standardized to the mean in order to facilitate model interpretation. Shortened versions of the CES-D have previously been found to have very high sensitivity and specificity for detecting depressive symptoms (Kohout et al., 1993).

Siblings were classified as monozygotic twins (MZ), dizygotic twins (DZ), full siblings (FS), half siblings (HS), or cousins (CO), as indicated in the AddHealth data files.

Genotype: The 5-HTTLPR locus is characterized by a variable number of tandem repeat (VNTR) polymorphism with two predominant alleles: the long (*l*) allele with 16 repeats and the short (*s*) allele with 14 repeats, the latter of which corresponds to a ~44bp deletion in reference to the long allele (Heils et al., 1996). Respondents were assigned one of three possible 5-HTTLPR genotypes: homozygote long (*ll*; referent category), homozygote short (*ss*), and heterozygote (*sl*).

Age and race/ethnicity: Age was calculated using date of birth and date of interview and left as a continuous variable in the model. Race/ethnicity was self-reported using the following categories: White (reference), African-American, Hispanic, Asian, and other race.

Family structure assessed the number of household resident parent(s) and categorized respondents as belonging to a two-biological parent family (referent category), a one-biological parent family (i.e. single biological parent or one biological parent and a stepparent) or "other family structure."

Family-level socioeconomic position (SEP) was assessed via whether at least one resident parent was receiving public assistance (PA).

Social support was measured by averaging the responses to eight questions that represent respondents' perceived value and support from family members, friends and teachers;

responses ranged from 1 (not at all) to 5 (very much). If respondents missed one or more of the 8 questions, the average was determined from the remaining, answered questions.

Childhood maltreatment was assessed retrospectively in Wave III of the AddHealth study, conducted in August 2001 to April 2002, when participants were between 18 and 26 years old. Participants were asked "By the time you started sixth grade, how often had your parents or other adult care-givers slapped, hit, or kicked you?" and "how often had one of your parents or other adult care-givers touched you in a sexual way, forced you to touch him or her in a sexual way, or forced you to have sexual relations?" These questions thus assessed participants' exposure to maltreatment by an age that captured the youngest age of AddHealth participants at Wave I. Although additional measures assessing the occurrence of supervision neglect and physical neglect were also available in the AddHealth dataset, we focused on exposure to physical and/or sexual maltreatment due to its more robust association with depression (Brown et al., 1999). Exposure to maltreatment was coded 1 if a participant had been exposed one or more times to physical and/or sexual abuse, and 0 otherwise. If a participant was missing data for either physical or sexual maltreatment (or both), they were excluded from analyses.

2.2.2 County-level health indicator

Consistent with previous work (Robert, 1998), county-level public assistance (PA) was selected as a measure of exposure to poor social environments, i.e. a proxy for county-level deprivation. The proportion of households receiving PA income in each county for each respondent was assessed using U.S. Census data from 1990, geocoded to respondents' interview data via the AddHealth contextual database. We calculated the median proportion of PA based on the counties represented by respondents in our dataset and a dummy variable was then created indicating 1 if the value was greater than the median and 0 otherwise. Individuals who relocated to a different county between Waves I and II were removed from the dataset.

2.3 Statistical analysis
2.3.1 Hardy Weinberg Equilibrium

Genotype frequencies were assessed for Hardy-Weinberg Equilibrium (HWE) using Rodriguez et al.'s (Rodriguez et al., 2009) online HWE Chi Square calculator by randomly sampling one sibling per family cluster. Calculations were performed separately for each gender.

2.3.2 Analytic models

A repeated multi-level modeling approach using mixed models was employed in our study. Mixed models have proven to be useful when dealing with nested and clustered data (Searle et al., 1992). In our analysis, level 1 refers to the repeated measurements of individuals' depressive symptom scores, level 2 refers to the individual respondent, and level 3 refers to the family cluster to which the respondent belongs. Equation one (Eqn1) below describes the basic mixed model used in our analysis:

$$\text{CESD}_{ij(s)} = \beta_0'X_{ij} + \beta_1'\text{5-HTTLPR}_{ij} + \beta_2'\text{family structure}_{ij} + \beta_3'\text{SEP}_{ij} + \beta_4\text{support}_{ij} + \beta_5\text{maltreatment}_{ij} + \beta_6\text{county level predictor}_{ij} + u_{j(s)} + v_{ij} + e_{ij(s)} \tag{1}$$

where i, j and s indicate individual and sibling cluster, respectively. Each beta represents a single coefficient or a vector of coefficients for each predictor component in the model; X represents age and race, *5-HTTLPR* represents the serotonin transporter promoter genotype, family structure represents the variants in resident parents, SEP refers to parent receipt of PA, support refers to social support, maltreatment refers to childhood maltreatment, and county-level predictor represents PA. The random effect of the family cluster is represented by $u_{j(s)}$, v_{ij} is the random effect of the repeated observations on the same individual, and $e_{ij(s)}$, is the error term. This model allows the random effect of family cluster and the error term to vary by sibling type (Guo & Wang, 2002), denoted by s $(s = mz, dz, fs, hs, co)$. All predictors were set at Wave I values and the outcome variable (depressive symptom score) was assessed across Waves I and II. Interactions among *5-HTTLPR* genotype, childhood maltreatment, and county-level deprivation were explored in models with interaction terms included in which the *ll* genotype, low PA, and no maltreatment were the referent categories and all other covariates were maintained. All models were stratified by gender, and all analyses were conducted using SAS v. 9.2

3. Results

Table 1 presents the descriptive statistics of the sociodemographic variables included in our final model. The average age in both our male (n=512) and female (n=585) samples was

	Males (n=512)		Females (n=585)		Test
	n/mean	%/std	n/mean	%/std	p
Genotype					
SS	112	21.88	109	18.63	0.18
SL	239	46.68	277	47.35	0.82
LL	161	31.45	199	34.02	0.37
Demographics					
Age	16.08	1.66	16.0	1.69	0.43
White	288	56.25	368	62.91	**0.02**
Black	70	13.67	76	12.99	0.74
Hispanic	80	15.63	69	11.79	0.06
Asian	38	7.42	30	5.13	0.12
Other	36	7.03	42	7.18	0.92
Family structure					
Two biological parents	340	66.41	373	63.76	0.36
One biological parents	144	28.13	167	28.55	0.88
Other family structure	28	5.47	45	7.69	0.14
Support and maltreatment					
Social support	4.0	0.54	4.03	0.59	0.88
Exposure to physical or sexual abuse	163	31.84	166	28.38	0.21
Family-level SEP					
Parent receives public assistance	39	7.62	54	9.23	0.34
County-level SEP					
High deprivation	268	52.34	278	47.52	0.11
17-CESD					
Depressive symptom score	9.3	6.04	11.0	7.27	**<0.0001**

Table 1. Sociodemographic characteristics of AddHealth participants included in the present study, stratified by gender.

approximately 16 years (range in males: 12-19; range in females: 12-20). Genotype frequencies for the *5-HTTLPR* locus were in Hardy-Weinberg Equilibrium for both males (χ^2 =0.16, df=1 p=0.69) and females (χ^2 =0.59, df=1 p=0.44). Approximately one-third of adolescents of both genders had been exposed to one or more incidents of physical and/or sexual abuse by an adult caregiver, and approximately half of the male and female samples resided in high deprivation counties. The main predictors of interest (childhood maltreatment, *5-HTTLPR* genotype, and county-level deprivation) did not differ significantly between males and females; however, the average depressive symptom score was significantly higher in female (11.0) vs. male (9.3) adolescents (p<0.001).

A number of predictor variables also showed gender differences in the unadjusted models (Table 2). Notable to this study, however, was the detection in females of a significant

	Male			Female		
	b	p	95% CI		*b*	p	95% CI	
Genotype								
SS	0.08	0.43	-0.12	0.28	**0.25**	**0.04**	**0.02**	**0.49**
SL	-0.13	0.11	-0.29	0.03	**-0.19**	**0.03**	**-0.37**	**-0.02**
LL	0.09	0.30	-0.08	0.27	0.06	0.56	-0.13	0.25
Demographics								
Age in years	0.04	0.15	-0.01	0.08	0.05	0.06	0.00	0.10
White	**-0.31**	**<0.001**	**-0.48**	**-0.14**	**-0.27**	**0.01**	**-0.48**	**-0.07**
Black/African-American	**0.26**	**0.04**	**0.01**	**0.51**	-0.06	0.70	-0.35	0.23
Hispanic/Latino	0.02	0.84	-0.22	0.27	0.13	0.40	-0.18	0.43
Asian	**0.43**	**0.01**	**0.10**	**0.75**	**0.67**	**<0.01**	**0.22**	**1.13**
Other race	0.21	0.23	-0.13	0.55	**0.44**	**0.02**	**0.06**	**0.81**
Family Structure								
Two biological parents	**-0.25**	**0.01**	**-0.43**	**-0.06**	**-0.37**	**<0.001**	**-0.57**	**-0.18**
One-biological parent	**0.24**	**0.01**	**0.05**	**0.44**	**0.32**	**<0.01**	**0.11**	**0.54**
Other family structure	0.10	0.63	-0.29	0.49	0.29	0.13	-0.08	0.66
Support and maltreatment								
Social Support	**-0.67**	**<0.0001**	**-0.80**	**-0.54**	**-0.82**	**<0.0001**	**-0.95**	**-0.69**
Exposure to physical or sexual abuse	0.04	0.64	-0.13	0.20	**0.30**	**<0.01**	**0.11**	**0.49**
Family-level SEP								
Parent receives public assistance	**0.50**	**<0.01**	**0.18**	**0.82**	0.30	0.08	-0.04	0.64
County-level SEP								
High Deprivation	0.16	0.08	-0.02	0.33	0.01	0.93	-0.19	0.21

Table 2. Unadjusted associations predicting standardized depressive symptom score, stratified by gender.

protective effect of the *sl* genotype (b=-0.19, 95% CI: -0.37, -0.02; p=0.03), and a corresponding risk-enhancing effect of the *ss* genotype (b=0.25 95% CI: 0.02, 0.49; p=0.04), with respect to depressive symptom scores. Exposure to maltreatment was also significantly and positively associated with depressive symptom scores in females (b=0.30, 95% CI: 0.11, 0.49; p<0.01); however, for the remaining main predictor of interest, county-level deprivation, no significant association was observed in females (b=0.01, 95% CI: -0.19, 0.21; p=0.93). In contrast, male AddHealth participants showed no significant associations between genotype and depressive symptom scores, or maltreatment and depressive symptom scores (Table 2); however, the association between residing in a high deprivation county and depressive symptom score was marginally significant (b=0.16, 95% CI: -0.02, 0.33; p=0.08).

Table 3 presents the results of our multivariable, multi-level main effects model. Females with the *sl* genotype continued to show significantly decreased depressive symptom scores in this fully adjusted main effects model (b=-0.21, 95% CI: -0.39, -0.03; p=0.02); however, the previously observed positive association between the *ss* genotype and depressive symptom scores in females was attenuated to non-significance (b=-0.03, 95% CI: -0.26, 0.21; p=0.82). The previously observed positive association between maltreatment and depressive

	Male			Female		
	b	p	95% CI	*b*	p	95% CI
Genotype						
SS	-0.01	0.95	-0.21 0.20	-0.03	0.82	-0.26 0.21
SL	-0.05	0.53	-0.22 0.12	**-0.21**	**0.02**	**-0.39 -0.03**
Demographics						
Age in years	0.01	0.63	-0.03 0.05	0.01	0.75	-0.04 0.05
Black/African-American	**0.34**	**0.01**	**0.08 0.59**	-0.02	0.89	-0.29 0.25
Hispanic/Latino	0.11	0.31	-0.11 0.34	0.13	0.33	-0.13 0.40
Asian	**0.51**	**<0.001**	**0.21 0.82**	**0.72**	**<0.001**	**0.33 1.12**
Other race	0.17	0.27	-0.13 0.48	0.20	0.23	-0.12 0.52
Family structure						
One-biological parent	0.09	0.33	-0.09 0.27	**0.31**	**<0.01**	**0.12 0.50**
Other family structure	0.00	0.99	-0.35 0.35	0.27	0.11	-0.06 0.61
Support and maltreatment						
Social Support	**-0.67**	**<0.0001**	**-0.80 -0.54**	**-0.78**	**<0.0001**	**-0.91 -0.65**
Exposure to physical or sexual abuse	-0.06	0.40	-0.21 0.08	0.16	0.07	-0.01 0.33
Family-level SEP						
Parent receives public assistance	**0.45**	**<0.01**	**0.17 0.74**	0.04	0.81	-0.27 0.35
County-level SEP						
High deprivation	0.03	0.77	-0.14 0.19	-0.08	0.38	-0.25 0.10

Table 3. Adjusted main effects model predicted standardized depressive symptom score, stratified by gender.

symptom scores in females was also attenuated in these adjusted main effects models; however, results for this variable remained marginally significant (b=0.16, 95% CI: -0.01, 0.33; p=0.07). As in the unadjusted models, the fully adjusted model revealed no significant associations between genotype and depressive symptom scores, or maltreatment and depressive symptom scores in males (Table 3); and, the previously observed, marginally significant positive association between county-level deprivation and depressive symptom score was markedly attenuated (b=0.03, 95% CI: -0.14, 0.19; p=0.77).

Table 4 presents results from the multi-level, multivariable models with the three-way interaction terms included. Among females, the three-way interaction terms for *5-HTTLPR*

	Male				Female			
	b	p	95% CI		b	p	95% CI	
Genotype								
SS	0.10	0.58	-0.27	0.48	0.07	0.72	-0.34	0.49
SL	0.10	0.49	-0.19	0.39	-0.07	0.61	-0.35	0.20
Demographics								
Age in years	0.01	0.72	-0.04	0.05	0.00	0.93	-0.04	0.05
Black/African-American	0.32	0.02	0.06	0.57	-0.05	0.75	-0.32	0.23
Hispanic/Latino	0.11	0.32	-0.11	0.33	0.13	0.36	-0.14	0.40
Asian	0.52	<0.01	0.21	0.83	0.74	<0.001	0.34	1.15
Other race	0.17	0.29	-0.14	0.47	0.17	0.31	-0.16	0.50
Family structure								
One-biological parent	0.08	0.38	-0.10	0.26	0.32	<0.01	0.13	0.52
Other family structure	-0.02	0.93	-0.37	0.34	0.30	0.08	-0.04	0.64
Support and maltreatment								
Social Support	-0.68	<0.0001	-0.81	-0.54	-0.79	<0.0001	-0.92	-0.65
Exposure to physical or sexual abuse	-0.01	0.95	-0.44	0.41	0.47	0.03	0.04	0.89
Family-level SEP								
Parent receives public assistance	0.45	<0.01	0.16	0.74	-0.01	0.96	-0.32	0.30
County-level SEP								
High deprivation	0.24	0.16	-0.09	0.58	0.17	0.30	-0.16	0.50
Maltreatment* Genotype*County-level SEP								
Maltreatment* S|S * High Deprivation	0.10	0.82	-0.75	0.94	0.97	0.04	0.05	1.89
Maltreatment*S|L* High Deprivation	0.10	0.79	-0.60	0.79	0.86	0.03	0.09	1.63

Table 4. Adjusted interaction model predicted standardized depressive symptom score.

genotype, maltreatment, and county-level deprivation were significant: in the context of both exposure to maltreatment and high deprivation at the county-level, females with the *sl* genotype showed significantly higher depressive symptom scores (b=0.86, 95% CI: 0.09, 1.63; p=0.03), as did females with the *ss* genotype (b=0.97, 95% CI: 0.05, 1.89; p=0.04). In contrast, no significant three-way interaction terms were observed among males.

4. Discussion

The goal of this study was to investigate the joint and interacting effects of genetic variation at the *5-HTTLPR* locus, childhood maltreatment, and macrosocial context in shaping risk for, or resilience to, depressive symptoms in a U.S. adolescent population, controlling for a number of factors previously associated with depression in this population. Results showed that, among females, the *sl* genotype conferred a protective main effect against higher depressive symptom scores; however, interaction models revealed that, among females who were both exposed to childhood maltreatment and resided in high deprivation counties, the *sl* genotype conferred increased risk of higher depressive symptom scores. An additional, risk-enhancing three-way interaction was observed among females carrying the *ss* genotype. In contrast, among males, no significant associations were observed between our predictors of interest and depressive symptom scores in either main effects or interaction models. These findings demonstrate that factors operating at multiple levels—biologic, social, and macrosocial—combine to shape risk for mental illness, and confirm that these factors can differ by gender, particularly in adolescent populations.

Our results confirm and extend previous findings regarding the link between childhood maltreatment and depression. A large body of work has established that exposure to maltreatment during childhood is a potent risk factor for depression (eg (Maniglio, 2010; Powers et al., 2009) and other mental illnesses (Afifi et al., 2008; Molnar et al., 2001; Molnar et al., 2001a; Schilling et al., 2007), with many of these studies identifying gender differences in the effect size associating maltreatment and psychopathology. Nevertheless, the vast majority of these studies has focused on childhood maltreatment as a risk factor for later depression during adulthood. In contrast, there is a paucity of studies examining the relation between childhood maltreatment and adolescent depression. Findings from these studies are mixed, with some studies finding a main effect maltreatment-depression association (e.g. (Åslund et al., 2009; Sesar et al., 2011)) while others fail to find such an association (Brown et al., 1999; Cicchetti, et al., 2007). However, when interaction between genetic variation at the *5-HTTLR* locus and childhood maltreatment is assessed, specific genotypes are implicated in increased risk of depression , particularly among adolescent females (Åslund et al., 2009; Cicchetti et al., 2007), in the subset of individuals who have experience maltreatment. This heterogeneity of effect by genotype suggests that the impact of child maltreatment on adolescent depression is particularly acute among carriers of the *ss* genotype.

Although three-way interactions incorporating genetic, social (i.e. maltreatment) and macrosocial variables have not, to our knowledge, previously been reported, some parallels can be drawn to earlier findings from our own group based on the same cohort. Specifically, earlier work using the AddHealth cohort found that adolescent boys are more susceptible to macro- (i.e, county) level contextual effects on depressive symptoms than their female counterparts, who showed stronger genetic effects on their risk for depression (Uddin et al., 2010). Results of the present study confirm the findings of a main genetic effect on risk of depressive symptoms for adolescent females, and two-way interaction models also showed a marginally significant (p=0.09) interaction whereby adolescent male carriers of the *sl* genotype, showed lower depressive symptom scores when residing in counties with high deprivation (data not shown) consistent with our earlier work (Uddin et al., 2010). More importantly, the present study augments the earlier work by including an important factor known to contribute to subsequent depression, namely childhood maltreatment. Remarkably, the inclusion of this variable in the models presented here effectively negated the protective main effect of the *sl* genotype observed in females in this study and our earlier work. We have previously noted the high levels of genetic variation surrounding the 5-*HTTLPR* locus in different human populations, and have suggested that different alleles and/or genotypes in this region may confer selective advantages in different environments (Uddin et al., 2010), in much the same way as the well-known sickle-cell anemia example. Results of the current study lend support to this hypothesis by demonstrating how the same genotype can, on average, reduce risk of depressive symptoms in females while at the same time increase risk among the subset of females exposed to both childhood maltreatment and adverse county-level social environments.

Findings from this work should be interpreted in light of a number of limitations. The primary limitation of this study is the possibility of information bias. Reports of childhood maltreatment were collected retrospectively and may thus be under reported due to recall difficulties. However, the AddHealth study was specifically designed to collect this potentially sensitive information during adulthood, at a time when most participants would no longer be subject to the care of the potential perpetrator of the maltreatment; this limitation was thus unavoidable. In addition, longitudinal research suggests that adult recall of physical and sexual abuse during childhood may actually underestimate the prevalence of childhood maltreatment (Widom & Kuhns, 1996; Widom et al., 1999). Furthermore, and again because of our reliance on secondary data analysis, we were unable to assess the role of an additional common genetic variation at the 5-*HTTLPR* locus in which a single nucleotide polymorphism renders the *l* allele more functionally similar to the *s* allele (Uddin et al., 2010). Our reliance on the two 5-*HTTLPR* alleles genotyped by AddHealth, however, would likely have biased our results toward the null.

Strengths of our study include the use of a dataset that allowed an assessment of "E" at multiple levels (i.e. adverse experiences and county-level social environment) and that also provided genetic data, allowing us to test three-way interactions defined at multiple levels. An additional strength was the longitudinal design of our investigation, which assessed depressive symptoms across a one-year time frame and excluded individuals who relocated to different counties during this time frame. This approach enhances our ability to make causal inferences regarding the influence of genetic variation, maltreatment, and county level social environment on depressive symptoms in this study population. Furthermore, our study controlled for the family-level analog (parental receipt of public assistance) of our macrosocial predictor of interest, county-level public assistance/deprivation. Our findings are thus less likely to be attributable to confounding by factors more proximal to the individual. Finally, by conducting our analyses stratified by gender, our study was able to detect important differences in the factors influencing depressive symptoms in adolescent females vs. males that may have been otherwise missed. These sex-specific effects render plausible that different triggers, or stressors, may be salient to depression in adolescent males and females and have implications for interventions designed to reduce risk of depressive symptoms following adverse exposures early in life.

5. Conclusion

In conclusion, we have shown that exposure to childhood maltreatment and adverse county-level social environments jointly moderate the effect of genetic variation at the *5-HTTLPR* locus on depressive symptoms in female adolescents. Female adolescents exposed to both childhood maltreatment and county-level deprivation are at significantly increased risk of higher depressive symptom scores if they possess the *sl* or *ss* genotypes at the *5-HTTLPR* locus. Future work should aim to replicate these findings in additional adolescent cohorts, and to understand how factors operating at multiple levels — biologic, social, and macrosocial — interact to shape risk for mental illness in ways that may differ between genders.

6. Acknowledgements

This research uses data from Add Health, a program project directed by Kathleen Mullan Harris and designed by J. Richard Udry, Peter S. Bearman, and Kathleen Mullan Harris at the University of North Carolina at Chapel Hill, and funded by grant P01-HD31921 from the Eunice Kennedy Shriver NICHD with cooperative funding from 23 other federal agencies and foundations. Special acknowledgment is due Ronald R. Rindfuss and Barbara Entwisle for assistance in the original design. Information on how to obtain the Add Health data files is available on the Add Health website (http://www.cpc.unc.edu/addhealth). No direct support was received from grant P01-HD31921 for this analysis. The authors would like to thank Drs. Sandro Galea and Karestan Koenen for helpful comments and discussions regarding this work. This work was supported by NIH grants DA022720, DA022720-S1 and RC1 MH088283-01.

7. References

Afifi, T.O., Enns, M.W., Cox, B.J., Asmundson, G.J., Stein, M.B & Sareen, J. (2008). Population attributable fractions of psychiatric disorders and suicide ideation and attempts associated with adverse childhood experiences. *American Journal of Public Health*, Vol.98, (May 2008), pp. 946-952, ISSN 1541-0048

American Psychiatric Association. (1994). *Diagnostic and statistical manual of mental disorders DSM-IV-TR Fourth Edition (Text Revision)*, ISBN-10: 0890420254 Washington, DC

Åslund, C., Leppert, J., Comasco, E., Nordquist, N., Oreland, L. & Nilsson, K. (2009). Impact of the Interaction Between the 5HTTLPR Polymorphism and Maltreatment on Adolescent Depression. A Population-Based Study. *Behavior genetics*, Vol.39, No.5, (July 2009), pp. 524-531, ISSN 1573-3297

Brown, J., Cohen, P., Johnson, J.G. & Smailes, E.M. (1999). Childhood abuse and neglect: specificity of effects on adolescent and young adult depression and suicidality. *Journal of the American Academy of Child & Adolescent Psychiatry*, Vol.38, No.12, (December 1999), pp. 1490-1496, ISSN 1527-5418

Caspi, A., Sugden, K., Moffitt, T.E., Taylor, A., Craig, I.W., Harrington, H., McClay, J., Mill, J., Martin, J., Braithwaite, A & Poulton, R. (2003). Influence of life stress on depression: moderation by a polymorphism in the 5-HTT gene. *Science*, Vol.301, No. 5631, (July 2003), pp. 386-389, ISSN 0036-8075

Chipman, P., Jorm, A.F., Prior, M., Sanson, A., Smart, D., Tan, X & Easteal, S. (2007). No interaction between the serotonin transporter polymorphism (5-HTTLPR) and childhood adversity or recent stressful life events on symptoms of depression: results from two community surveys. *American Journal of Medical Genetics Part B: Neuropsychiatric Genetics*, Vol.144B, No.4, (June 2007), pp. 561-565, ISSN: 1552-4841

Cicchetti, D., Rogosch, F.A. & Sturge-Apple, M.L. (2007). Interactions of child maltreatment and serotonin transporter and monoamine oxidase A polymorphisms: depressive symptomatology among adolescents from low socioeconomic status backgrounds. *Development and Psychopathology*, Vol.19, No.19, (2007), pp. 1161-1180, ISSN 0954-5794

Druss, B.G., Hwang, I., Petukhova, M., Sampson, N.A., Wang, P.S & Kessler, R.C. (2009). Impairment in role functioning in mental and chronic medical disorders in the United States: results from the National Comorbidity Survey Replication. *Molecular Psychiatry*, Vol.14, (Febuary 2008), pp. 728-737, ISSN 1359-4184

Eley, T.C., Sugden, K., Corsico, A., Gregory, A.M., Sham, P., McGuffin, P., Plomin, R & Craig, I.W. (2004). Gene-environment interaction analysis of serotonin system markers with adolescent depression. *Molecular Psychiatry*, Vol.9, (July 2004), pp. 908-915, ISSN 1359-4184

Greenberg, P.E., Kessler, R.C., Birnbaum, H.G., Leong, S.A., Lowe, S.W., Berglund, P.A & Corey-Lisle, P.K. (2003). The economic burden of depression in the United States: how did it change between 1990 and 2000? *The Journal of clinical psychiatry*, Vol.64, No.12, (December 2003), pp. 1465-1475, ISSN 0160-6689

Guo, G. & Wang, J. (2002). The mixed or multilevel model for behavior genetic analysis. *Behavior genetics*, Vol.32, No.3, (August 2001), pp.37-49, ISSN 1573-3297

Harris, K.M., Halpern, C.T., Smolen, A & Haberstick, B.C. (2006). The National Longitudinal Study of Adolescent Health (Add Health) twin data. *Twin research and human genetics: the official journal of the International Society for Twin Studies*, Vol.9, No.6, (December 2006), pp. 988-997, ISSN 1832-4274

Harris, K.M. (2008). The National Longitudinal Study of Adolescent Health (Add Health), Waves I & II, 1994–1996, Wave III, 2001–2002 [machine-readable data file and documentation], in. Edited by. Chapell Hill, NC, Carolina Population Center, University of North Carolina at Chapel Hill., 2008.

Heils, A., Teufel, A., Petri, S., Stober, G., Riederer, P., Bengel, D & Lesch, K.P. (1996). Allelic variation of human serotonin transporter gene expression. *Journal of Neurochemistry*, Vol.66, No.6, (June 1996), pp. 2621-2624, ISSN 1471-4159

Karg, K., Burmeister, M., Shedden, K & Sen, S. (2011). The serotonin transporter promoter variant (5-HTTLPR), stress, and depression meta-analysis revisited: evidence of genetic moderation. *Archives of General Psychiatry*, Vol.68, (May 2011), pp. 444-454, ISSN 0003-990x

Kaufman, J., Yang, B.Z., Douglas-Palumberi, H., Houshyar, S., Lipschitz, D., Krystal, J.H & Gelernter, J. (2004). Social supports and serotonin transporter gene moderate depression in maltreated children. *Proceedings of the National Academy of Sciences of the United States of America*, Vol.10, No.49, (December 2004), pp. 17316-17321, ISSN 0027-8424

Kessler, R.C., Chiu, W.T., Demler, O., Merikangas, K.R & Walters, E.E. (2005). Prevalence, severity, and comorbidity of 12-month DSM-IV disorders in the National Comorbidity Survey Replication. *Archives of General Psychiatry*, Vol.62, No.6, (June 2005), pp. 617-627, ISSN 0003-990X

Kessler, R.C & Wang, P.S. (2008). The descriptive epidemiology of commonly occurring mental disorders in the United States. *Annual Review of Public Health* Vol.29, (April 2008), pp. 115-129, ISSN 0163-7525

Koenen, K.C., Aiello, A.E., Bakshis, E., Amstadter, A.B., Ruggiero, K.J., Acierno, R., Kilpatrick, D.G., Gelernter, J & Galea, S. (2009). Modification of the association between serotonin transporter genotype and risk of posttraumatic stress disorder in adults by county-level social environment. *American Journal of Epidemiology*, Vol.169, (Febuary 2009), pp. 704-711, ISSN 0002-9262

Koenen, K.C. & Galea, S. (2009). Gene-Environment Interactions and Depression. *JAMA: The Journal of the American Medical Association*, Vol.302, No.5, (August 2011), pp. 1859-1862, ISSN 0098-7484

Koenen, K.C., Uddin, M., Amstadter, A.B & Galea, S. (2010). Incorporating the social environment in genotype environment interaction studies of mental disorders. *International journal of clinical practice*,Vol.64, No.11, (October 2010), pp. 1489–1492, ISSN 1368-5031

Kohout, F.J., Berkman, L.F., Evans, D.A & Cornoni-Huntley, J. (1993). Two shorter forms of the CES-D (Center for Epidemiological Studies Depression) depression symptoms index. *Journal of Aging & Health*, Vol.5, No.2, (May 1993), pp. 179-193, ISSN 0898-2643

Laucht, M., Treutlein, J., Blomeyer, D., Buchmann, A.F., Schmid, B., Becker, K., Zimmermann, U.S., Schmidt, M.H., Esser, G., Rietschel, M & Banaschewski, T. (2009). Interaction between the 5-HTTLPR serotonin transporter polymorphism and environmental adversity for mood and anxiety psychopathology: evidence from a high-risk community sample of young adults. *The international journal of neuropsychopharmacology*, Vol.12, (January 2009), pp. 737-747, ISSN 1461-1457

Lopez-Leon, S., Janssens, A.C., Gonzalez-Zuloeta Ladd, A.M., Del-Favero, J., Claes, S.J., Oostra, B.A & van Duijn, C.M. (2008). Meta-analyses of genetic studies on major depressive disorder. *Molecular psychiatry*, Vol.13, (October 2007), pp. 772-785, ISSN 1476-5578

Lotrich, F.E & Lenze, E. (2009). Gene-Environment Interactions and Depression. *JAMA: The Journal of the American Medical Association*, Vol.302, (2009), pp. 1859a-1862, ISSN 1368-5031

Lupien, S.J., McEwen, B.S., Gunnar, M.R & Heim, C. (2009). Effects of stress throughout the lifespan on the brain, behaviour and cognition. *Nature Reviews Neuroscience*, Vol.10, (June 2009), pp. 434-445, ISSN 1471-0048

Maniglio, R. (2010). Child sexual abuse in the etiology of depression: A systematic review of reviews. *Depression and anxiety*, Vol.27, (2010), pp. 631-642, ISSN 1091-4269

Moffitt, T.E., Caspi, A & Rutter, M. (2005). Strategy for investigating interactiosn between measured genes and measured environments. *Archives of general psychiatry*, Vol.62, (2005), pp. 473-481, ISSN 1538-3636

Molnar, B.E., Berkman, L.F & Buka, S.L. Psychopathology, childhood sexual abuse and other childhood adversities: relative links to subsequent suicidal behaviour in the US. *Psychological Medicine*, Vol.31, (2001), pp. 965-977, ISSN 0033-2917

Molnar, B.E., Buka, S.L & Kessler, R.C. (2001). Child sexual abuse and subsequent psychopathology: results from the National Comorbidity Survey. *American Journal of Public Health*, Vol.91, (2001), pp. 753-760, ISSN 0090-0036

Munafo, M.R., Durrant, C., Lewis, G & Flint, J. (2009). Gene X environment interactions at the serotonin transporter locus. *Biological Psychiatry*, Vol.65, (2009), pp. 211-219, ISSN 0006-3223

Powers, A., Ressler, K.J & Bradley, R.G. (2009). The protective role of friendship on the effects of childhood abuse and depression. *Depression and Anxiety*, Vol.26, (2009), pp. 46-53, ISSN 1091-4269

Radloff, L. (1977). The CES-D scale: A self-report depression scale for research in the general population. *Applied psychological measurement*, Vol.1, (1977), pp. 385-401, ISSN 0146-6216

Risch, N., Herrell, R., Lehner, T., Liang, K.Y., Eaves, L., Hoh, J., Griem, A., Kovacs, M., Ott, J. & Merikangas, K.R. (2009). Interaction between the serotonin transporter gene (5-HTTLPR), stressful life events, and risk of depression: a meta-analysis. *The Journal of the American Medical Association*, Vol.301, (2009), pp. 2462-2471, ISSN 0098-7484

Robert, S.A. (1998). Community-level socioeconomic status effects on adult health. *Journal of health and social behavior*, Vol.39, (1998), pp. 18-37, ISSN 0022-1465

Rodriguez, S., Gaunt, TR & Day, IN. (2009). Hardy-Weinberg equilibrium testing of biological ascertainment for Mendelian randomization studies. *American Journal of Epidemiology*, Vol.169, No.4, (January 2009), pp. 505-514, ISSN 0002-9262

Rutter, M., Thapar, A. & Pickles, A. (2009). Gene-Environment Interactions: Biologically Valid Pathway or Artifact? *Archives of general psychiatry*, Vol.66, (2009), pp. 1287-1289, ISSN 0003-990X

Scheid, J.M., Holzman, C.B., Jones, N., Friderici, K.H., Nummy, K.A., Symonds, L.L., Sikorskii, A., Regier, M.K & Fisher, R. (2007). Depressive symptoms in mid-pregnancy, lifetime stressors and the 5-HTTLPR genotype. *Genes, Brain, and Behavior*, Vol.6, (2007), pp. 453-464, ISSN 1601-1848

Schilling, E.A,. Aseltine, R.H. Jr., & Gore S (2007). Adverse childhood experiences and mental health in young adults: a longitudinal survey. *BMC Public Health*, Vol.7, No.30, (March 2007), ISSN 1471-2458

Schwahn, C. & Grabe, H.J. (2009). Gene-Environment Interactions and Depression. *The Journal of the American Medical Association*, Vol.302, (2009), pp.1859-b-1862, ISSN 0098-7484

Searle, S.R., Casella, G & McCulloch, C.E. (1992). *Variance components: Wiley series in probability and mathematical statistics. Applied probability and statistics.* ISBN 0471621625, Wiley, New York

Sesar, K., Simic, N & Barisic, M. (2011). Multi-type childhood abuse, strategies of coping, and psychological adaptations in young adults. *Croatian medical journal*, Vol.51, (2011), pp. 406-416, ISSN 0353-9504

Shih, R.A., Belmonte, P.L. & Zandi, P.P. (2004). A review of the evidence from family, twin and adoption studies for a genetic contribution to adult psychiatric disorders. *International review of psychiatry*, Vol.16, (2004), pp. 260-283, ISSN 1048-0021

Sjoberg, R.L., Nilsson, K.W., Nordquist, N., Ohrvik, J., Leppert, J., Lindstrom, L. & Oreland, L. (2006). Development of depression: sex and the interaction between environment and a promoter polymorphism of the serotonin transporter gene. *The international journal of neuropsychopharmacology*, Vol.9, (2006), pp. 443-449, ISSN 1461-1457

Surtees, P.G., Wainwright, N.W., Willis-Owen, S.A., Luben, R., Day, N.E & Flint, J. (2006). Social adversity, the serotonin transporter (5-HTTLPR) polymorphism and major depressive disorder. *Biological Psychiatry*, Vol.59, (2006), pp. 224-229, ISSN 0006-3223

Uddin, M., Koenen, K.C., de Los Santos, R., Bakshis, E., Aiello, A.E & Galea, S. (2010). Gender differences in the genetic and environmental determinants of adolescent depression. *Depression Anxiety*, Vol.27, No.7, (July 2010), pp. 658-666, ISSN 1091-4269

Uher, R. & McGuffin, P. (2008). The moderation by the serotonin transporter gene of environmental adversity in the aetiology of mental illness: review and methodological analysis. *Molecular psychiatry*, Vol.13, (2008), pp. 131-146, ISSN 1359-4184

WHO. (2009). *Depression*, Available from:
        <http://www.who.int/mental_health/management/depression/definition/en/>

Widom, C.S. & Kuhns, J.B. (1996). Childhood victimization and subsequent risk for promiscuity, prostitution, and teenage pregnancy: A prospective study. *American Journal of Public Health*, Vol.86, (1996), pp. 1607-1612, ISSN 1541-0048

Widom, C.S., Weiler, B.L & Cottler, L.B. (1999). Childhood victimization and drug abuse: A comparison of prospective and retrospective findings. *Journal of Consulting and Clinical Psychology*, Vol.67, (1999), pp. 867-880, ISSN 0095-8891

11

Mentalizing Skills Deficits in Schizophrenia as a Clue for Drug Choice: Clozapine Versus Other Antipsychotics on Keeping Outpatients Stable

Rosó Duñó[1], Klaus Langohr[2,3], Diego Palao[1] and Adolf Tobeña[4]

[1]Parc Taulí University Hospital, Autonomous University of Barcelona,
[2]Pharmacology Research Unit, Institut Municipal d'Investigació Mèdica, Barcelona
[3]Department of Statistics and Operations Research,
Technical University of Catalonia, Barcelona
[4]Department of Psychiatry and Forensic Medicine, Institute of Neurosciences,
Autonomous University of Barcelona,
Spain

1. Introduction

Despite the proven the efficacy of antipsychotic drugs approximately 10-30% of all schizophrenic patients show poor response or remain resistant to antipsychotic medications, and up to an additional 30% of patients have partial responses to treatment, meaning that they exhibit improvement in psychopathology but continue to have mild to severe symptoms (Barnes, 2011; Miyamoto et al., 2005). The proportion considered to be 'treatment resistant' varies according to the criteria used (Barnes et al., 2003; Barnes, 2011: Conley and Kelly, 2001; Pantelis and Lambert, 2003). A minority (around 10%) of patients receiving conventional or atypical antipsychotics do not achieve remission even after the first episode (Crow et al., 1986; Lambert et al., 2008). More commonly, treatment resistance develops as the illness becomes progressively more unresponsive to medication (Barnes 2011; Wiersma et al., 1998). Kane et al. (1988) defined treatment refractoriness as lack of periods of good functioning for 5 years, no response to two different classes of neuroleptics and presence of moderate to severe symptomatology including positive and negative symptoms, as well as disorganized or violent/aggressive behaviour, thought disorder and suicidal ideation. Predictors associated with an unfavourable response to treatment are cognitive functioning deficits (Rabinowitz et al., 2000), poor premorbid functioning (Crespo-Facorro et al., 2007; Duñó et al., 2008), earlier age of onset (Gogtay et al., 2011), duration of untreated psychosis (Farooq et al., 2009) and male gender (Caspi et al., 2007). It remains uncertain whether treatment resistant schizophrenia should be considered simply as the more severe end of the illness spectrum or as a distinct subtype of schizophrenia for which neurocognitive markers of resistance should be explored (Barnes, 2011).

Social cognition generally refers to mental operations that underlie human transactions, including perceiving and interpreting social stimuli as well as responding to socially relevant inputs, such as dealing with intentions and behaviours of others. Theory of Mind (ToM) or mentalizing, a subdomain of social cognition, is defined as the ability to think about people in terms of their mental states (Green et al., 2008a). The bulk of evidence has shown consistent social cognitive impairments in schizophrenia (Green et al.,2008b), that can be present at early phases (Brüne et al., 2011; Chung et al., 2008; Couture et al., 2008) and persist trough different phases of the illness (Green et al., 2011), and several reviews and meta-analysis have established that patient-control differences on mentalizing skills are large and persistent across the chronic phase of illness (Bora et al., 2009; Brüne 2005).

Clozapine is the only antipsychotic that has been found to show superior efficacy for treatment-resistant patients when compared to conventional and atypical antipsychotic drugs. Clozapine is the most effective antipsychotic for severe refractory schizophrenia (approximately 30-60% of patients who fail to respond to other antipsychotics may respond to clozapine), and moderately refractory illness (Barnes, 2011), Further, there are other important benefits with clozapine, including improvement in cognitive function (Bilder et al., 2002; Machado de Sousa and Hallak, 2002; Purdon et al., 2001), reduction in suicidality (Meltzer et al., 2003) and an anti-hostility action or improvement in persistent aggression and behavioural disturbance (Krakowski et al., 2006; Volavka and Citrome, 2008; Volavka et al., 2004). Despite of the abundance of findings about social cognitive deficits in schizophrenia, only a few reports have related these handicaps to the clinical improvement obtained with antipsychotic treatment. Mizrahi et al. (2007) and Harvey et al. (2006) offered some evidence that the atypical risperidone and olanzapine enhanced performance on particular social cognition abilities (Kee et at., 1998; Littrel et al., 2004). Accordingly, Savina and Beninger (2007) found that olanzapine and clozapine but not typical neuroleptics or risperidone may either improve ToM ability or protect against its decline, probably by restoring or improving neural activation at the mPFC. Another study in the same line carried out by Lund et al. (2002) cohered with these results. Contrary to that, Sergi et al. (2007) and Penn et al. (2009) found no differences among medications or within each medication group over time, on these measures. In remitted schizophrenics anomalies in social cognition were worse in the more severe patients (Sprong et al., 2007) and some of the abovementioned studies reported reductions of social cognitive dysfunctions with a specific antipsychotic drug. In this context, the present study attempted to determine which pharmacological treatment (conventional, atypical antipsychotics or clozapine) exhibited superior efficacy to improve ToM skills and whether the deficits on ToM might be linked with resistance to antipsychotic treatment in stable schizophrenic patients. Given that abnormalities in mentalizing are particularly severe in patients with poor premorbid adjustment (Duñó et al., 2008), and that poor premorbid adjustment is considered a factor of refractoriness to treatment, we expected to find a link between the degree of ToM deficit and an increased risk of antipsychotic drug resistance.

2. Method

Fifty-eight schizophrenic patients fulfilling diagnostic and statistical manual (DSM) IV criteria were recruited in a consecutive fashion during the years 2001–2005. Subjects who did not give their consent to participate and those with a visual or auditory disability limiting test application, neurological disease, or another chronic/acute condition that could interfere with cognitive performance were not recruited. Patients with additional DSM-IV diagnosis on Axis I/II were also not recruited. Participants showing an IQ below 70 (Blyler et al., 2000) were excluded from the study. All subjects were on clinical remission at 5 months after discharge from the Day Hospital of the Psychiatry Unit, Parc Taulí University

Hospital (Sabadell-Barcelona, Spain). Clozapine treatment was prescribed only to patients who met the criteria for antipsychotic treatment resistance (Kane et al., 1988).

The schizophrenic group was compared to a control group of forty-eight patients with no psychiatric diagnosis who had been admitted to the Orthopedics and Surgery Department of the same hospital. Control subjects were recruited at the same time as the group with schizophrenia and were matched by sex, age and educational level. The exclusion criteria for this group included a history of psychiatric disorders, the presence of psychopathology and distress at the time of the evaluation according to the three global indices of the Symptom Checklist-90-Revised scale (SCL-90-R) (Positive Symptom Total, Global Severity Index, Positive Symptom Distress Index) (Martinez-Azumendi et al., 2001) medical prescription of psychoactive drugs and an IQ score below 70 (Blyler et al., 2000). Sociodemographic factors of this group are described in Table 1.

2.1 Assessment

Patient's symptom severity was assessed with the positive and negative syndrome scale (PANSS) (Kay et al., 1987). Premorbid adjustment with the Premorbid Adjustment Scale (PAS) (Cannon-spoor et al., 1982; Silverstein et al., 2002). Four false belief ToM tasks were applied: two first-order tasks, "the cigarettes" (Happé, 1994) and "Sally and Anne" (Baron-Cohen, 1989) and two second-order tasks, "the burglar" (Happé and Frith, 1994) and "the ice-cream van" (Baron-Cohen et al., 1985). Stories were read aloud by the examiner and subjects had to listen and answer two questions. The first one (a ToM question) had to be answered on the basis of the mental state of one of the characters and concerned that character's false belief within the situation. The second one (control question) reflected the subject's comprehension of the story. These tasks were rated according to the following:

- correct ToM (task score = 1): correct answers in both ToM and control questions;
- ToM deficit (task score = 0): failure in ToM question and correct answer in control question;
- comprehension error: correct answer in ToM question and failure in control question or failure in both (data in this category omitted from the analysis).

Patients were excluded from the study if they showed comprehension errors in more than two ToM tasks. If the comprehension error was in a second-order ToM task, none of the second-order ToM tasks were considered for analysis, while first-order ones were. The same criteria were applied when comprehension errors appeared in first-order ToM tasks. Subsequently, three categorical subgroups of ToM performance were established for both first- and second-order tasks by adding up scores as follows: 0=two tasks with scores of 0 (severe ToM deficit); 1=one task scoring 1 and the other scoring 0 (low ToM performance); 2=scoring of 1 in both tasks (good ToM performance). Neurocognitive measures were grouped into several domains, from basic to high-level processing according to Nuechterlien et al. (2004) criteria: Speed processing (Trail Making Test A (TMT-A) (Reitan, 1993), Working Memory (Digit Span Backward) (Wechsler, 1999), Executive functions (Stroop Color-Word (Golden, 1994), Trail Making Test B [TMT-B] (Reitan, 1993), Block Design (Wechsler, 1999).

Antipsychotic treatment included 3 groups of drugs: conventional, atypical (olanzapine, risperidone aripiprazol) and clozapine. Drug doses for each group were converted to haloperidol equivalents (mg/day). Patients were assessed on these all measures at 5 months after discharge from hospital, except PANSS scale, which was further administrated at start and end of hospitalization.

Long-term Follow-up: 6-10 years later these patients were contacted again through telephone calls. All were retraced except 3 who were dead, 4 who had changed address and 2 who were hospitalized. From the remaining, 21 patients refused to collaborate and 24 accepted and were re-examined. Symptom severity was assessed with the positive and negative syndrome scale (PANSS) (Kay et al., 1987) and ToM tasks were assessed applying the same tasks and methodology as stated above.

2.2 Statistical analysis

Socio-demographic data as well as neuropsychology and social cognition measures were compared in patients and controls by means of either the X^2-test (for categorical variables) or t-tests. Relations among antipsychotic treatment and haloperidol equivalents doses with PANSS scale were studied through descriptive analysis. Comparative analysis between social cognition and dosage of haloperidol equivalents were carried out through U Mann-Whitney tests. Relations between first- and second-order ToM tasks scores and antipsychotic treatment were studied by the X^2-tests. Ordinal regression models were employed to analyze the association between the results of first-order and second-order ToM tasks with socio-demographic variables, premorbid adjustment, neuropsychological scores and antipsychotic treatment as possible explanatory variables of treatment resistance. Starting with regression models including gender and PAS for social isolation, further explanatory variables were included if they significantly improved the model fit and yielded maximum R-square values. Several links for ordinal regression models were considered and those that yielded maximum R-square values were chosen. Finally, it was proved that the models for first- and second-order ToM tasks held the assumption of parallel lines (Chen and Meharry, 2004). Statistical analysis was performed with the statistical software packages SPSS, version PASW 18 version 18.0.0 and R, v. 2.11.1, in particular using the contributed package "exact RankTests" (Hothorn and Hornik, 2011). P-values below 0.05 were considered statistically significant. For the long term follow-up measures only a descriptive analysis was carried out.

3. Results

Sociodemographic and clinical data of schizophrenic patients and controls are shown in Table 1, as well as, neuropsychological and social cognition measures in Table 2. Clear differences between patients and controls appeared in independence, paternity and occupational status. Premorbid adjustment in the patients was poor, worsening from childhood into late adolescence. Patients scored significantly lower in Trail Making Test A, Stroop word-colour and Trail Making Test B. Table 3 displays changes over time in PANSS scale in relation to antipsychotic drugs and dosage haloperidol equivalents at discharge and follow-up study. Total PANSS scores improved over time in all groups. Patients on clozapine had higher scores at each PANSS subscales at baseline and lesser scores at the end of assessment. At the long-term follow-up these scores in general decreased slightly, being more pronounced for atypical and clozapine. First- and second-order ToM tasks performance relations to mean dosage of haloperidol equivalents are shown in Table 4. Dosage haloperidol equivalents were inferior in category 2 on both measures.

	Schizophrenia group (N=58)	Control group (N=48)	p-value
Males	41 (70.7%)	36 (75.0%)	
Age	31.4 (8.1)	33.9 (8.6)	
Years of education =< 8 years	42 (72.4%)	37 (77.1%)	
Living with own family	15 (25.9%)	35 (72.9%)	χ^2=23.336; p<0.001
Children	8 (13.8%)	26 (54.2%)	χ^2=19.650; p<0.001
Employed	12 (20.7%)	41 (85.4%)	χ^2=44.014; p<0.001
Age of illness onset	21.6 (4.9)		
Psychiatric diagnosis (DSM-IV)			
Paranoid schizophrenia	39 (67.2%)		
Non-paranoid schizophrenia	8 (13.7%)		
Schizofreniform disorder	6 (10.3%)		
Schizoaffective disorder	5 (8.6%)		
Global activity (DSM-IV)	61.6 (11.7)		
SCL-90-R[1]			
Positive Symptom Total		24.9 (11.2)	
Global Severity Index		0.27 (0.12)	
Positive Symptom Distress Index		1.19 (0.20)	
PAS			
Childhood	0.27 (0.2)		
Early adolescence	0.39 (0.2)		
Late adolescence	0.44 (0.2)		
Years of illness evolution	9.6 (7.7)		
Drugs			
Mean dose haloperidol equivalents (mg/day)	8.7 (7.3)		
Conventional antipsychotic	14 (24.1%)		
Atypical antipsychotic	35 (60.3%)		
Mixed antipsychotic	6 (10.3%)		
Clozapine[2]	17 (29.3%)		
None[3]	3 (5.2%)		
Anticholinergic	8 (13.8%)		
Antidepressant	15 (25.9%)		

Results are presented as mean (standard deviation) in case of continuous variables and as frequency (%) in case of categorical variables. Gender, age, and educational level were matching variables; hence, no statistical tests for comparison are applied.
[1] Mean normative values: Positive Symptom Total, 25.32 (SD: 14.3); Global Severity Index, 0.51 (0.36); Positive Symptom Distress Index, 1.75 (0.48).
[2] Patients on clozapine from the total 35 on atypical antipsychotics.
[3] At evaluation, 5 months after discharge.
DSM-IV-Diagnostic and Statistical Manual Disorders, Fourth Edition;
SCL-90-R-Symptom Checlist-90-Revised; PANSS=Positive and Negative Syndrome Scale.

Table 1. Sociodemographic and clinical characteristics of study cohort

Figure 1a and 1b display relations between antipsychotic drugs and performance of first-order ToM tasks at discharge and follow-up respectively: 78.6% of patients performed correctly at discharge, with a slight non-significant advantage for atypical drugs, whereas 83% performed right, with a moderate advantage for clozapine at follow-up. Figure 2a and 2b display antipsychotic drugs and performance of second-order ToM tasks at discharge and follow-up: 63.9% of patients performed correctly at discharge, with a slight non-significant advantage for atypical drugs, whereas 79.2% performed right, with moderate advantage for clozapine at follow-up study. Tables 5a and 5b show the variables included in the ordinal regression models for first- and second-order ToM tasks, respectively. The negative sign of the regression coefficients corresponding to premorbid adjustment (PAS social isolation) in both models indicates a negative relationship between that variable and the outcome. That is, ordinal regression analysis revealed a main association between deficits in first-order and second-order ToM tasks both with poor social premorbid adjustment (social isolation). In first-order ToM tasks, deficits were also related to poor performance on Trail Making Test B. The test showed the highest significant association between second-order ToM tasks with block design, males and clozapine treatment. R-square values amounted to 0,300 and 0.657, respectively. No association was found between first-order ToM tasks with variables of treatment resistance, whereas second-order ToM tasks deficits were linked to factors of unfavourable response to treatment.

	Schizophrenia group (N=58)	Control group (N=48)	p-value
Neuropsychological measures			
General cognition abilities			
Intelligence Quotient	96.8 (19.2)	104.1(19.5)	t=-1.918: p=0.060
Speed of processing			
Trail Making Test A	43.1 (16.8)	30.9(10.1)	**t=4.333; p=0.000**
Working Memory			
Digit span backward	5.5 (1.1.9)	5.3(1.7)	t=0.708 p=0.481
Executive function			
Stroop word color	36.1 (11.2)	42.3 (10.7)	**t=-2833; p=0.006**
Trail Making Test B	106.9 (51.9)	84.8 (27.3)	**t= 2.829; p=0.01**
Block design	40.6 (11.9)	44.1 (11.6)	t=-1504; p=0.136
Social cognition measures			
ToM category			
First order			
0	11.8%	0%	
1	11.8%	0%	**χ²=12602; p=0.002**
2	76.5%	100%	
Second order			
0	11.5%	4.%	
1	26.9%	10.6%	**χ²=6917; p=0.031**
2	61.5%	85.1%	

Results are presented as mean (standard deviation) in case of continuous variables and as frequency (%) in case of categorical variables

Table 2. Neuropsychology and social cognition measures of study cohort

PANSS	Conventional	Atypical	Clozapine
POSITIVE **Main measures**			
Hospitalization starts	20.9(4.9)	15.2(7.2)	22.8 (6.6)
Hospitalization ends	13.8(3.9)	10.5(4.7)	13.1 (4.1)
5 month after discharge	12.0(3.9)	10.2(3.7)	13.7 (4.3)
Follow-up	12.8(3.9)	10.6(3.1)	10.6(4.9)
NEGATIVE **Main measures**			
Hospitalization starts	21.9(9.5)	28.7(10.4)	27.4 (13.5)
Hospitalization ends	13.8(4.0)	10.5(4.7)	13.1 (4.1)
5 month after discharge	18.5(7.4)	18.8(10.8)	14.1 (10.5)
Follow-up	19.0(12.3)	11.7(6.9)	13.4(6.1)
GENERAL **Main measures**			
Hospitalization starts	43.2(9.5)	46.5(10.5)	48.9(8.3)
Hospitalization ends	33.7 (5.7)	34.6(12.8)	31.8(8.9)
5 month after discharge	34.1 (8.0)	31.6(9.7)	30.4(10.1)
Follow-up	27.2(9.5)	26.0(12.0)	25.9(8.3)
TOTAL **Main measures**			
Hospitalization starts	88.0(19.2)	90.4(19.3)	97.7(23.9)
Hospitalization ends	66.9 (11.9)	62.9(22.2)	66.5(13.2)
5 month after discharge	65.1 (15.1)	61.1(18.8)	58.1(22.7)
Follow-up	59.0(24.5)	48.3(18.5)	49.9(13.3)
DOSE HALOPERIDOL **equivalents (mg/day)**			
Main measures	13.2 (8.4)	4.3 (2.4)	10.3 (6.6)
Long term Follow-up	17.6 (5.4)	8.3 (7.3)	13.2 (7.5)

Results presented as mean (standard deviation). For Main measures N=58: Conventional N=19; Atypical
N=21; Clozapine N=16; A Follow-up N= 24: Conventional N=5; Atypical N=7; Clozapine N=12

Table 3. PANSS changes over time in relation to antipsychotic medication and dose of
haloperidol equivalents (mg/day) in schizophrenics patients

ToM Tasks	Discharge N=58	Follow-up N=24
First-Order ToM Tasks		
Category 0 + Category 1	(N=12) 11.9 (8.0)	(N=4) 14.3 (8.3)
Category 2	(N=46) 7.3 (6.7)	(N=20) 13.2 (8.1)
p value	U=190.500 p=0.009*	
Second-order ToM Tasks		
Category 0+ Category 1	(N=20) 10.4 (7.1)	(N=5) 17.8 (5.1)
Category 2	(N=38) 7.5 (7.4)	(N=19) 13.3 (8.4)
p value	U=276.000 p=0.052	

Results are presented as mean (standard deviation) of mean dosage of haloperidol equivalents. Analysis of distribution between ToM tasks categories with mean dosage of haloperidol at discharge were carried out with the Mann-Whitney test; *p<0.05 level of significance

Table 4. Relations between first- and second-order ToM tasks performance and mean dosage of haloperidol equivalents at discharge and follow-up of the schizophrenia group

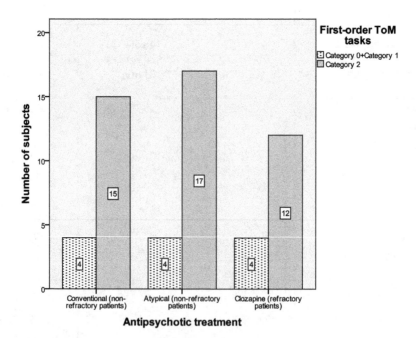

*Conventional (non-refractory patients): mixed antipsychotic group is included within this group. Percentage of good performance at ToM tasks were: conventional 26.8%, atypical 30.4% and clozapine 21.4%; (X^2=0.194; p=0.908).

(a)

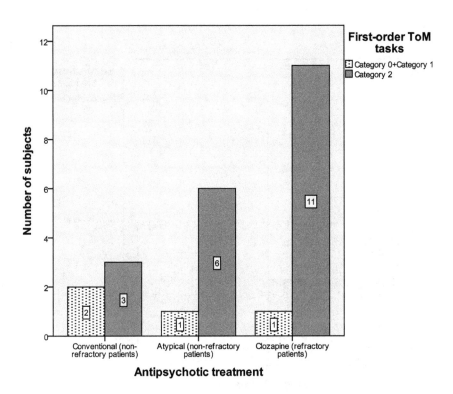

*Conventional (non-refractory patients): mixed antipsychotic group is included within this group.
Percentage of good performance at ToM tasks were: conventional 12.5%, atypical 25.0% and clozapine
45.8%.

(b)

Fig. 1. (a) Antipsychotic treatment type and first-order ToM tasks at discharge study
(b) Antipsychotic treatment type and first-order ToM tasks at the long term follow-up in a
subsample of the schizophrenia patients

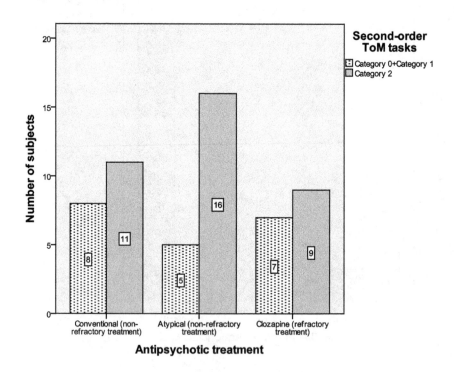

*Conventional (non-refractory patients): mixed antipsychotic group is included within this group.
Percentage of good performance ToM tasks were: conventional 19.1%, atypical 28.6% and clozapine
16.1% ; (X^2=2.084; p=0.353)

(a)

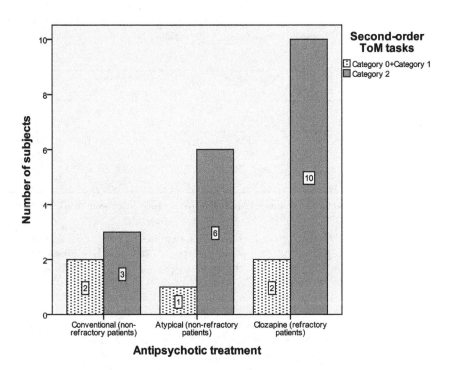

*Conventional (non-refractory patients): mixed antipsychotic group is included within this group.
Percentage of good performance ToM tasks were: conventional 12.5%, atypical 25.0% and clozapine
41.7%.

(b)

Fig. 2. (a) Antipsychotic treatment type and second-order ToM tasks at discharge study
(b) Antipsychotic treatment type and second-order ToM tasks at the long term follow-up in
a subsample of the schizophrenia patients

	Regression coefficient	95% Confidence interval	p-value
Threshold [ToM1 = 0]	-3.225	(-4.700; -1.750)	<0.001
Threshold [ToM1 = 0]	-2.667	(-4.057; -1.278)	<0.001
PAS: Social isolation	-1.990	(-3.754; -0.227)	0.027
Trail B	-0.009	(-0.016; -0.001)	0.026
Males	-0.385	(-1.357; 0.586)	0.586

The link function applied was the probit link. Pseudos R-square values amounted to: 0.224 (Cox and Snell); 0.300 (Nagelkerke); and 0.184 (McFadden).

Table 5a. Regression coefficients of an ordinal model to explore the relative weight of first order ToM tasks at predicting treatment resistance factors including premorbid adjustment (social isolation), trail B and gender as explanatory variables

	Regression coefficient	95% Confidence interval	p-value
Threshold [ToM2 = 0]	-5.975	(-12.251; 0.300)	0.062
Threshold [ToM2 = 0]	-0.317	(-4.673; 4.040)	0.887
PAS: Social isolation	-14.003	(-26.340; -1.666)	0.026
Blocks design	0.291	(0.033; 0.549)	0.027
Clozapine	-3.379	(-6.734; -0.025)	0.048
Males	-5.580	(-10.775; -0.385)	0.035

The link function applied was the Cauchy link. Pseudos R-square values amounted to: 0.551 (Cox and Snell); 0.657 (Nagelkerke); and 0.440 (McFadden).

Table 5b. Regression coefficients of an ordinal model to explore the relative weight of second-order ToM tasks at predicting treatment resistance factors including premorbid adjustment (social isolation), blocks design, clozapine and gender as explanatory variables

4. Discussion

This study identified distinctive responses on ToM performance with different antipsychotic medications in stable schizophrenics: initially patients responded relatively better with atypical antipsychotics in contrast to clozapine and conventional agents. Nevertheless, over time clozapine provided some hints of better restoration of mentalizing abilities than other antipsychotics agents. Also, the findings confirmed predictors of unfavourable response to antipsychotic treatment in patients with poor mentalizing deficits. These predictors include male gender, social isolation (poor premorbid adjustment), low performance in block design and receiving clozapine treatment at start higher severity. That constellation of factors characterized a well-studied subgroup of patients having a poor prognosis. Cohering with previous findings, the present sample of stabilized schizophrenia outpatients showed difficulties across diverse interpersonal functions in contrast to healthy controls: they were mainly less independent, with no children, and either unemployed or disabled. Decreased premorbid adjustment across age epochs in which full-blown schizophrenia symptoms appear has also been found in other studies (Strous et al., 2004; Vourdas et al., 2003). Schizophrenic patients performed worse than control group on both first and second order

ToM tasks, without differences in intelligence quotient measures. Regarding the links between ToM performance and antipsychotic medication, the results showed drug's positive effects on mentalizing abilities with a tendency to increase over the years in the restricted subsample re-examined at follow-up meaning perhaps that the deficits in social cognitive abilities were relatively restored over the long-term. After discharge the patients who had been prescribed atypical antipsychotic drugs displayed a modest superiority on mentalizing skills in contrast with those receiving conventional antipsychotic or clozapine. Almost a decade later, in the follow-up, clozapine showed a modest trend of better efficacy, despite that at least a fraction of those patients were highly resistant to treatment and showed deep second-order mentalizing handicaps when first studied at the start of the study.This trend may cohered with Savina and Berninger (2007) findings, showing that clozapine (and olanzapine) improves ToM abilities due to the enhancement of mPFC function, although they measured that over the short-term. Dosage of antipsychotic was lower in patients with good performance on mentalizing skills, indicating less illness severity.

The accumulating evidence suggests that improvement in cognitive function might be expected to follow reduction of psychotic symptoms, with differences between antipsychotics at improving cognitive performance, being rather modest and never normalizing cognitive function (Barnes, 2011; Lieberman et al., 2005). Also, the literature suggests a parallel path for both atypical antipsychotics in non-resistant patients and clozapine in resistant ones at improving psychosis and cognition deficits (O'Carroll, 2000; Keefe and Fenton, 2007). It is worth noting that clozapine treatment remains as one of the most effective for schizophrenia and consensus treatment guidelines from a wide range of prominent expert panels specify that (APA, 2004; Goodwin et al., 2009; NICE, 2010), recommending its use after the failure of 2 adequate trials with other antipsychotics, including an atypical one, to get adequate response or in patients with persistent suicidal gestures or ideation. So it would be desirable to introduce clozapine in appropriate time and dosages (Joober and Boksa, 2010), to improve social cognitive abilities as well as to enhance pro-social function (Toua et al., 2010; Möller et al., 2011).

Concerning disease state at baseline, before treatment commencement, it is important to highlight that second-order ToM tasks deficits disclosed well-characterized factors related with poor prognosis: male gender, (Caspi et al., 2007), poor premorbid functioning (Duñó et al., 2008; Strous et al., 2004) and executive functioning deficits, specifically planning and coordination dysfunction (Béchard-Evans et al., 2010; Koelkebeck et al., 2010; Rabinowitz et al., 2000), together with particular drug regimes (clozapine) required to achieve a quick clinical stabilization (Barnes, 2011). Severe deficits in social cognition have been repeatedly shown along these factors (Duñó et al., 2008; Montreuil et al., 2010; Schenkel et al., 2005; Uhlhaas and Silverstein 2005). It is interesting to note that mentalizing deficits had not been previously described as a predictor factor of poor response to treatment. Therefore it is important to note that refractory responses to drug treatment ought to be expected in patients with poor mentalizing skills especially if they are accompanied with these factors of poor outcome.

This study had obvious limitations. The ToM tasks employed, although widely used in the literature, have not been fully validated. The study characterized a substantial homogeneous sample, but at the long term follow-up study half of the sample did not accept to collaborate again thus restricting the weight of those results. In conclusion, our findings reflect beneficial effects of antipsychotic agents at restoring ToM ability, especially clozapine, in a sample of stabilized schizophrenics. Also we found second-order ToM tasks deficits as a predictor factor of poor response to antipsychotic treatment together with others well described in the literature: male gender, poor premorbid adjustment, executive dysfunctions (coordination-planning) and clozapine at baseline (higher clinical severity).

5. References

American Psychiatric Association. Practice guideline for the treatment of patients with schizophrenia, second edition. Am J Psychiatry 2004; 161:1-56.

Barnes TR; Schizophrenia Consensus Group of British Association for Psychopharmacology. Evidence-based guidelines for the pharmacological treatment of schizophrenia: recommendations from the British Association for Psychopharmacology. J Psychopharmacol 2011; 25: 567-620.

Barnes TR, Buckley P, Schulz SC. Treatment-resistant schizophrenia. In: Hirsch SR and Weinberger D (eds) Schizophrenia. Oxford: Blackwell Publishing; 2003.

Baron-Cohen S. The autistic child's theory of mind: a case of specific developmental delay. J Child Psychol Psychiatry 1989; 30: 285-297.

Baron-Cohen S, Leslie AM, Frith U. Does the autistic child have a "theory of mind"? Cognition 1985; 21: 37-46

Béchard-Evans L, Iyer S, Lepage M, Joober R, Malla A. Investigating cognitive deficits and symptomatology across pre-morbid adjustment patterns in first-episode psychosis. Psychol Med 2010; 40: 749-59.

Bilder RM, Goldman RS, Volavka J, Czobor P, Hoptman M, Sheitman B, Lindenmayer JP, Citrome L, McEvoy J, Kunz M, Chakos M, Cooper TB, Horowitz TL, Lieberman JA. Neurocognitive effects of clozapine, olanzapine, risperidone, and haloperidol in patients with chronic schizophrenia or schizoaffective disorder. Am J Psychiatry 2002; 159: 1018-28.

Bora E, Yucel M, Pantelis C. Theory of mind impairment in schizophrenia: meta-analysis. Schizophr Res 2009; 109: 1-9.

Blyler CR, Gold JM, Iannone VN, Buchanan RW. Short form of the WAIS-III for use with patients with schizophrenia. Schizophrenia Res 2000; 46: 209–15.

Brüne M. "Theory of mind" in schizophrenia: a review of the literature. Schizophr Bull 2005; 31:21-42.

Brüne M, Abdel-Hamid M, Lehmkämper C, Sonntag C. Mental state attribution, neurocognitive functioning, and psychopathology: what predicts poor social competence in schizophrenia best?. Schizophr Res 2007; 92: 151-9.

Brüne M, Ozgürdal S, Ansorge N, von Reventlow HG, Peters S, Nicolas V, Tegenthoff M, Juckel G, Lissek S. An fMRI study of "theory of mind" in at-risk states of psychosis: comparison with manifest schizophrenia and healthy controls. Neuroimage 2011; 55: 329-37.

Cannon-Spoor HE, Potkin G, Wyatt RJ. Premorbid Adjustment Scale (PAS). Schizophrenia Bull 1982; 8: 480–4.

Caspi A, Reichenberg A, Weiser M, Rabinowitz J, Shmushkevich M, Lubin G, Nahon D, Vishne T, Davidson M. Premorbid behavioral and intellectual functioning in

schizophrenia patients with poor response to treatment with antipsychotic drugs.
    Schizophr Res 2007; 94: 45-9.
Chen CK, Meharry JH Jr. Using ordinal regression model to analyze student satisfaction
    questionnaires. IR Applications 2004; 26: 1-13.
Chung YS, Kang DH, Shin NY, Yoo SY, Kwon JS. Deficit of theory of mind in individuals at
    ultra-high-risk for schizophrenia. Schizophr Res 2008; 99: 111-8.
Conley RR and Kelly DL. Management of treatment resistance in schizophrenia. Biol
    Psychiatry 2001; 50: 898–911.
Couture SM, Penn DL, Addington J, Woods SW, Perkins DO. Assessment of social
    judgments and complex mental states in the early phases of psychosis. Schizophr
    Res 2008; 100: 237-41.
Crespo-Facorro B, Pelayo-Terán JM, Pérez-Iglesias R, Ramírez-Bonilla M, Martínez-García
    O, Pardo-García G, Vázquez-Barquero JL. Predictors of acute treatment response in
    patients with a first episode of non-affective psychosis: sociodemographics,
    premorbid and clinical variables. J Psychiatr Res 2007;41: 659-66.
Crow TJ, MacMillan JF, Johnson AL and Johnstone EC The Northwick Park study of first
    episodes of schizophrenia II: a randomized controlled trial of prophylactic
    neuroleptic treatment. Br J Psychiatry 1986; 148: 120–27.
Duñó R, Pousa E, Miguélez M, Palao D, Langohr K, Tobeña A. Poor premorbid adjustment
    and dysfunctional executive abilies predict theory of mind deficits in stabilized
    schizophrenia outpatients. Clin Schizophr Relat Psychoses 2008; 2: 205-216.
Farooq S, Large M, Nielssen O, Waheed W. The relationship between the duration of
    untreated psychosis and outcome in low-and-middle income countries: a
    systematic review and meta analysis. Schizophr Res 2009; 109: 15-23.
Gogtay N, Vyas NS, Testa R, Wood SJ, Pantelis C. Age of onset of schizophrenia:
    perspectives from structural neuroimaging studies. Schizophr Bull 2011; 37: 504-13.
Golden CJ. Stroop — test de colores y palabras. Madrid: TEA Editores; 1994.
Goodwin G, Fleischhacker W, Arango C, Baumann P, Davidson M, de Hert M, Falkai P,
    Kapur S, Leucht S, Licht R, Naber D, O'Keane V, Papakostas G, Vieta E, Zohar J
    Advantages and disadvantages of combination treatment with antipsychotics
    ECNP Consensus Meeting, March 2008, Nice. Eur Neuropsychopharmacol 2009;
    19:520-32.
Green MF, Penn DL, Bentall R, Carpenter WT, Gaebel W, Gur RC, Kring AM, Park S,
    Silverstein SM, Heinssen R. Social cognition in schizophrenia: an NIMH workshop
    on definitions, assessment, and research opportunities. Schizophr Bull 2008a; 34:
    1211-20.
Green MF, Leitman DI. Social cognition in schizophrenia. Schizophr Bull 2008b; 34: 670-2.
Green MF, Bearden CE, Cannon TD, Fiske AP, Hellemann GS, Horan WP, Kee K, Kern RS,
    Lee J, Sergi MJ, Subotnik KL, Sugar CA, Ventura J, Yee CM, Nuechterlein KH.
    Social Cognition in Schizophrenia, Part 1: Performance Across Phase of Illness
    Schizophr Bull 2011. doi:10.1093/schbul/sbq171
Happé F. An advanced test of theory of mind: understanding of story characters' thoughts
    and feelings by able autistics, mentally handicapped, and normal children and
    adults. J Autism Dev Disord 1994; 24: 129-154.
Happé F, Frith U. Theory of mind in autism. In: Schopler E, Mesiboy G, editors. Learning
    and cognition in autism. New York: Plenum Press; 1994.

Harvey PD, Patterson TL, Potter LS, Zhong K, Brecher M. Improvement in social competence with short-term atypical antipsychotic treatment: a randomized, double-blind comparison of quetiapine versus risperidone for social competence, social cognition, and neuropsychological functioning. Am J Psychiatry 2006; 163:1918-25.

Hothorn T, Hornik K. exactRankTests: exactRankTests: Exact Distributions for Rank and Permutation Tests. R package version 0.8-20. http://CRAN.R-project.org/package=exactRankTests; 2011.

Joober R, Boksa P. Clozapine: a distinct, poorly understood and under-used molecule. J Psychiatry Neurosci 2010; 35:147-9.

Kane JM, Honigfeld G, Singer J, Meltzer H. Clozapine in treatment-resistant schizophrenics. Psychopharmacol Bull 1988; 24:62-7

Kay SR, Fiszbein A, Opler LA. The positive and negative syndrome scale (PANSS) for schizophrenia. Schizophr Bull 1987; 13: 261-76.

Kee KS, Kern RS, Marshall BD Jr, Green MF. Risperidone versus haloperidol for perception of emotion in treatment-resistant schizophrenia: preliminary findings. Schizophr Res 1998; 31: 159-65.

Keefe RS, Fenton WS. How should DSM-V criteria for schizophrenia include cognitive impairment?. Schizophr Bull 2007;33: 912-20.

Koelkebeck K, Pedersen A, Suslow T, Kueppers KA, Arolt V, Ohrmann P. Theory of Mind in first-episode schizophrenia patients: correlations with cognition and personality traits. Schizophr Res 2010; 119: 115-23.

Krakowski MI, Czobor P, Citrome L, Bark N and Cooper TB. Atypical antipsychotic agents in the treatment of violent patients with schizophrenia and schizoaffective disorder. Arch Gen Psychiatry 2006; 63: 622–629.

Lambert M, Naber D, Schacht A, Wagner T, Hundemer HP, Karow A, Huber CG, Suarez D, Haro JM, Novick D, Dittmann RW, Schimmelmann BG. Rates and predictors of remission and recovery during 3 years in 392 never-treated patients with schizophrenia. Acta Psychiatr Scand 2008; 118:220-9.

Lieberman JA, Stroup TS, McEvoy JP, Swartz MS, Rosenheck RA, Perkins DO, Keefe RS, Davis SM, Davis CE, Lebowitz BD, Severe J, Hsiao JK; Clinical Antipsychotic Trials of Intervention Effectiveness (CATIE) Investigators. Effectiveness of antipsychotic drugs in patients with chronic schizophrenia. N Engl J Med 2005;353:1209-23.

Littrell KH, Petty RG, Hilligoss NM, Kirshner CD, Johnson CG. Improvement in social cognition in patients with schizophrenia associated with treatment with olanzapine. Schizophr Res 2004; 66: 201-2.

Lund A, Kroken R, Thomsen T, Hugdahl K, Smievoll AI, Barndon R, Iversen J, Landrø NI, Sundet K, Rund BR, Ersland L, Lundervold A, Asbjørnsen. A"Normalization" of brain activation in schizophrenia. An fMRI study. Schizophr Res 2002; 58: 333-5.

Machado de Sousa JP, Hallak JE Neurocognitive functioning and facial affect recognition in treatment-resistant schizophrenia treated with clozapine. Schizophr Res 2008; 106:371-2.

Martínez-Azumendi O, Fernández-Gómez C, Beitia-Fernández M.[Factorial variance of the SCL-90-R in a Spanish out-patient psychiatric sample]. Actas Esp Psiquiatr 2001; 29: 95-102.

Mentalizing Skills Deficits in Schizophrenia as a Clue for Drug Choice: Clozapine Versus Other Antipsychotics on
Keeping Outpatients Stable

237

Meltzer HY, Alphs L, Green AI, Altamura AC, Anand R, Bertoldi A, Bourgeois M, Chouinard G, Islam MZ, Kane J, Krishnan R, Lindenmayer JP, Potkin S; International Suicide Prevention Trial Study Group. Clozapine treatment for suicidality in schizophrenia: International Suicide Prevention Trial (InterSePT). Arch Gen Psychiatry 2003; 60:82-91.

Mizrahi R, Korostil M, Starkstein SE, Zipursky RB, Kapur S. The effect of antipsychotic treatment on Theory of Mind. Psychol Med 2007; 37:595-601.

Miyamoto S, Duncan GE, Marx CE, Lieberman JA. Treatments for schizophrenia: a critical review of pharmacology and mechanisms of action of antipsychotic drugs. Mol Psychiatry 2005; 10:79-104.

Möller M, Du Preez JL, Emsley R, Harvey BH. Isolation rearing-induced deficits in sensorimotor gating and social interaction in rats are related to cortico-striatal oxidative stress, and reversed by sub-chronic clozapine administration. Eur Neuropsychopharmacol 2011; 21:471-83.

Montreuil T, Bodnar M, Bertrand MC, Malla AK, Joober R, Lepage M. Social cognitive markers of short-term clinical outcome in first-episode psychosis. Clin Schizophr Relat Psychoses 2010; 4:105-14.

National Institute for Health and Clinical Excellence (NICE). NICE Clinical Guideline 82: Schizophrenia: core interventions in the treatment and management of schizophrenia in adults in primary and secondary care (update). London (UK): NICE; 2009. Available: www.nice.org.uk/CG082 (accessed 2010 Mar. 26).

Neuchterlein KH, Barch DM, Gold JM, Golberg TE, Green MF, HeatonRK. Identification of separable cognitive factors in schizophrenia. Schizophr Res 2004; 72:29-39.

O'Carroll R. Cognitive impairment in schizophrenia. Adv Psychiatr Treatment 2000; 6: 161-168.

Pantelis C and Lambert TJ Managing patients with "treatment-resistant" schizophrenia. Med J Aust 2003; 178 (Suppl): S62-S66.

Penn DL, Keefe RS, Davis SM, Meyer PS, Perkins DO, Losardo D, Lieberman JA. The effects of antipsychotic medications on emotion perception in patients with chronic schizophrenia in the CATIE trial. Schizophr Res. 2009; 115: 17-23.

Purdon SE, Labelle A and Boulay L. Neuropsychological change in schizophrenia after 6 weeks of clozapine. Schizophr Res 2001; 48: 57-67.

Rabinowitz J, Reichenberg A, Weiser M, Mark M, Kaplan Z, Davidson M. Cognitive and personality functioning during the decade prior to first hospitalization and early course of psychotic illness. Br J Psychiatry 2000; 177: 26-32.

Reitan RM. Validity of the trail making test as an indicator of organic brain damage. Percept Mot Skills 1993; 8: 271-76.

Savina I, Beninger RJ. Schizophrenic patients treated with clozapine or olanzapine perform better on theory of mind tasks than those treated with risperidone or typical antipsychotic medications. Schizophr Res 2007; 94: 128-38.

Schenkel LS, Spaulding WD, Silverstein SM. Poor premorbid social functioning and theory of mind deficit in schizophrenia: evidence of reduced context processing?. J Psychiatr Res 2005; 39: 499-508.

Sergi MJ, Rassovsky Y, Widmark C, Reist C, Erhart S, Braff DL, Marder SR, Green MF. Social cognition in schizophrenia: relationships with neurocognition and negative symptoms. Schizophr Res 2007; 90:316-24.

Silverstein ML, Mavrolefteros G, Close D. Premorbid adjustment and neuropsychological performance in schizophrenia. Schizophrenia Bull 2002; 28: 157–165.

Sprong M, Schothorst P, Vos E, Hox J, van Engeland H. Theory of mind schizophrenia: meta-analysis. Br J Psychiatry 2007; 191:5-13.

Strous RD, Alvir JM, Robinson D, Gal G, Sheitman B, Chakos M, Lieberman JA. Premorbid functioning in schizophrenia: relation to baseline symptoms, treatment response, and medication side effects. Schizophr Bull 2004; 30:265-78.

Toua C, Brand L, Möller M, Emsley RA, Harvey BH. The effects of sub-chronic clozapine and haloperidol administration on isolation rearing induced changes in frontal cortical N-methyl-D-aspartate and D1 receptor binding in rats. Neuroscience 2010; 165:492-9.

Uhlhaas PJ, Silverstein SM. Perceptual organization in schizophrenia spectrum disorders: empirical research and theoretical implications. Psychol Bull 2005; 131: 618-32.

Volavka J and Citrome L. Heterogeneity of violence in schizophrenia and implications for long-term treatment. Int J Clin Pract 2008; 62: 1237–45.

Volavka J, Czobor P, Nolan K, Sheitman B, Lindenmayer JP, Citrome L, McEvoy JP, Cooper TB, Lieberman JA. Overt aggression and psychotic symptoms in patients with schizophrenia treated with clozapine, olanzapine, risperidone, or haloperidol. J Clin Psychopharmacol 2004; 24:225-8.

Vourdas A, Pipe R, Corrigall R, Frangou S. Increased developmental deviance and premorbid dysfunction in early onset schizophrenia. Schizophr Res 2003; 62: 13-22.

Wechsler D. Escala de inteligencia Wechsler para adultos. WAIS III. Madrid: TEA Editores; 1999.

Wiersma D, Nienhuis FJ, Slooff CJ and Giel R. Natural course of schizophrenic disorders: a 15-year follow-up of a Dutch incidence cohort. Schiz Bull 1998; 24: 75–85.

12

An Update on Psychotic Depression

John Matthews
Harvard Medical School
USA

1. Introduction

There has been a debate since the 1980's whether delusional depression or psychotic depression is a distinct psychiatric disorder. (Glassman & Roose, 1981) Currently, DSM-IV-TR classifies psychotic symptoms in patients with major depressive disorder as a severity specifier. However, researchers in the area of major depressive disorder, with psychotic features (PMD) believe that PMD is a distinct disorder based on not only the phenomenological presentation, but family studies, course of illness, biological findings, and treatment as well. This lack of recognition of PMD as being a distinct disorder has contributed to the limited amount of research funding for this disorder in spite of a prevalence in the general population of 0.4-0.6%. (Johnson et al., 1991; Ohayon and Schatzberg, 2002) This chapter will provide an update on studies that support PMD as being a distinct psychiatric disorder.

2. Phenomenology of PMD

The DSM-IV-TR definition of PMD is major depressive disorder plus delusions or hallucinations. Early studies report that delusions occur in one half to two-thirds of adults and hallucinations occur alone in 3-25%. However, in our more recent studies, delusions co-occur with hallucinations in as many as 67% of patients with PMD. (Matthews 2002, 2008) The most common delusions include: persecution, suspiciousness, paranoia, sin, guilt, ideas of reference, and somatic. (Frangos et al, 1983) Fifty percent or more experience more than one kind of delusion. (Dubovsky, 1992) Keller (2006) reported that patients with PMD score higher on unusual thought content, psychomotor retardation, and guilt then NPMD. Interestingly, a formal thought disorder occurs in only 20% of patients with PMD, thus, psychotically depressed patients who present with a formal thought disorder are more likely to have a diagnosis of either bipolar disorder or schizophrenia. The most common hallucinations are auditory and visual and they occur with equal frequency. (Schatzberg and Rothshild, 1992) Tactile and olfactory hallucinations may occur but usually with other types of hallucinations. In one study, olfactory hallucinations occurred in 40% of PMD patients. (Matthews et al., 2002) Dissociative symptoms in the absence of abuse may occur with greater frequency in PMD than NPMD. The psychotic symptoms of PMD may present as mood congruent or mood incongruent. In a study of 40 PMD inpatients , 26 (65%) had mood congruent (MC) and 14 (35%) had mood incongruent (MI) psychotic symptoms; 71% of patients with MC experienced at least 1 MI symptom and 50% of patients with MI experienced at least 1 MC psychotic symptom. (Burch et al., 1994) In a 10-year study by Maj et al. (2007), 10% of 452 PMD patients had both MC and MI psychotic symptoms. Having MC or MI or both does not predict response to treatment or prognosis. (Rothschild, 2009)

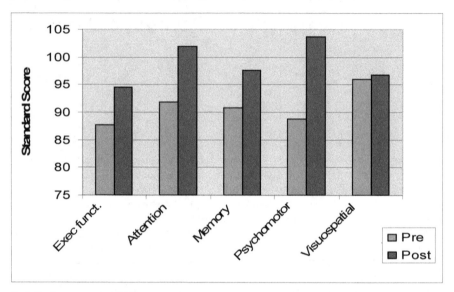

Fig. 1. (Matthews et al., 2010)

As with schizophrenia and bipolar disorder, patients with major depressive disorder exhibit cognitive deficits as a part of their clinical presentation. However, patients with PMD show greater performance deficits on specific neuropsychological tasks than patients with major depressive disorder, without psychotic features (NPMD). (Gomez et al., 2006) In addition, patients with PMD demonstrate more difficulty processing, manipulating and encoding new information than patients with NPMD (Gomez et al., 2006) In a meta-analysis of five studies, Fleming et al. (2004) showed that patients with PMD scored significantly lower on neuropsychological measures of executive function, verbal memory, and psychomotor speed than patients with NPMD.

We also found that found that patients with PMD scored significantly lower on executive function, verbal memory, and psychomotor speed than patients with NPMD. (Figure 1) (Matthews, et al., 2010)The mean scores on these three measures for PMD were greater than one standard deviation below the mean for the general population. The total score on the BPRS predicted the lower scores on executive function, verbal memory, and psychomotor speed, whereas, the HAM-D-17 did not. We also found that these cognitive deficits significantly improved with remission of PMD; thus, the cognitive deficits were state dependent (Table 1).

In order to control for the possible impact of medications on cognitive function, Hill et al., (2004) studied first episode PMD, Schizoaffective, Schizophrenia versus NPMD and healthy controls. There were significant differences between PMD and NPMD on several neuropsychological tasks; however, PMD was more similar to, but less severe, than performances by first break schizophrenics. (Figure 2) Hill hypothesized that the cognitive deficits found in PMD and schizophrenia may involve similar brains systems.

- Executive function
  - Pre -Treatment 87.76 (±18.89)
  - Post -Treatment 94.52 (±15.58) *
- Memory
  - Pre-Treatment 90.85 (±10.87)
  - Post- Treatment 97.57 (±14.36)
- Psychomotor
  - Pre-Treatment 88.82 (±30.51)*
  - Post-Treatment 103.77 (±25.39) *

* p < .01

Table 1. (Matthews, et al., 2010)

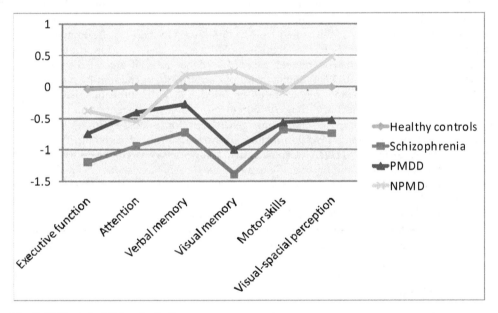

Fig. 2. (Hill et al., 2004; adapted)

3. Differential diagnoses

The diagnosis of PMD is often missed. Rothschild et al., (2008) found that in the NIMH Study of Pharmacotherapy of Psychotic Depression (STOP-PD), which was located at 4 academic medical centers, only 65% (85/130) of clinicians made an accurate diagnosis. Missed diagnoses on inpatient units were significantly less than in the emergency room; 18% (13/74) versus 39% (22/56) ($\chi 2=7.64$, p<.01) respectively. Distinctions between PMD and schizoaffective disorder or bipolar disorder are most problematic. In schizoaffective disorder, psychotic symptoms are not confined to mood disturbance, whereas, in PMD, psychotic symptoms co-occur with symptoms of depression. However, Maj et al., (2007) found that 10% of PMD with mood incongruent psychosis met criteria for schizoaffective disorder, depressed type. Studies have shown that a subset of patients with PMD eventually experience a manic or hypomanic episode. This is particularly true for early onset PMD. Between 40-75% of adolescents with PMD convert to bipolar disorder (Askiskal et al., 1983; Strober and Carlson, 1982). Maj et al., (2007) found a switch rate of 10.1% for PMD versus a switch rate of 5% for NPMD in an adult population (n=452) over a 10-year period.

4. Family studies/genetics

There is limited data to support PMD as being a genetic disorder. In the case of NPMD, twin studies have demonstrated that there is a genetic factor that is passed on from one generation to the next. In a review of twin studies in NPMD, Sullivan and Kendler (2001) estimated heritability to be 37%, with a significant component of individual environmental risk. Brown et al., (1994) found that only 20% of patients with PMD could identify a significant stressor in the 6 month period prior to a new episode onset compared to 72% in patients with NPMD. These results might reflect differences in the procurement of homogeneous populations or the genetic loading or both. Rothschild (2009) summarized the family studies of first degree relatives comparing PMD and NPMD and found that the first degree relatives of PMD had higher rates of PMD, higher rates of bipolar disorder by a factor of 6 (Weissman et al., 1984), higher rates of cyclothymia in children by a factor of 3 (Weissman et al., 1988), and higher rates of NPMD if PMD probands had a post-dexamethsone serum cortisol of >15 ug/dl (Bond et al., 1986). A number of candidate genes have been have been proposed including genes for: dopamine-β-hydroxylase (DBH); dopamine D4 receptor gene; glycogen synthase kinase-3 gene; and serotonin transporter gene (5-HT1A; 5-HT2C; 5-HT 2A receptor gene). The gene for the DBH activity has been most promising based on the findings that five of six studies have shown decreased DBH activity in PMD. (Rothschild, 2009) Schatzberg et al., (1985) have hypothesized that a decrease in DBH enzyme activity may be important as to why depressed patients may become psychotic; reduced DBH activity results in a decrease in conversion of dopamine to norepinephrine thus increasing the availability of dopamine. The gene encoding DBH is located on chromosome 9q34; the adenosine allele predicts psychosis. (Craig et al., 1998; Wood et al., 2002)

5. Comorbidity

There is very little literature on the co-morbid psychiatric disorders in PMD. In a clinical trial of the combination of olanzapine plus fluoxetine, Matthews et al., (Figure3) found that anxiety disorders were among the most common; especially panic disorder.

6. Biology of PMD

Although there have been a few EEG and imaging studies using CT and MRI scans in depression, the most consistent findings have been with the dysregulation of the hypothalamic-pituitary-adrenal axis (HPA-axis). Table 2 summarizes the findings.

Researchers have know since the 1970's that cortisol is elevated in patients with NPMD (Carroll et al. 1981; Brown et al., 1985); however, the dysregulation of the HPA-axis is even more pronounced in PMD. Twenty-four hour urinary free cortisol is significantly higher in PMD than in NPMD and patients with PMD also have higher rates of dexamethasone

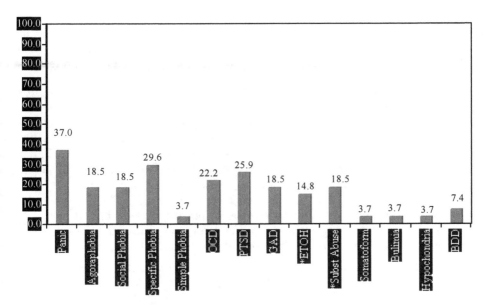

Fig. 3. (Matthews et al., 2002)

- • ↑ cortisol in urine, blood, and CSF
- • ↑ cortisol response to ACTH
- • ↑ size of both pituitary and adrenal glands
- • ↑ secretion of CRH
- • ↑ CRH in CSF
- • ↑ CRH messenger RNA in PVN
- • ↑ ACTH response to CRH challenge

Table 2. Evidence for HPA-axis Hyperactivity

stimulation test (DST) non-suppression than patients with NPMD. (Nelson and Davis, 1997; Schatzberg et al., 1992) The presence of psychotic symptoms accounts for most of the variance and severity of depression does not account for the differences. (Schatzberg et al., 1992) In a meta-analysis of 14 studies (12/14 inpatient), the DST non-suppression rates were 64% for PMD (n=276) and 41% for NPMD (n=708) (p<0.001) with a sensitivity of 64% and specificity of 59% using a post-dexamethasone cortisol serum level cut off of ≥5 ug/dL. (Nelson & Davis, 1997) These differences between PMD and NPMD DST non-suppression appear to be due to the presence of psychosis since Nelson and Davis, in another meta-analysis of 19 studies of NPMD, showed that there were no significant differences in DST non-suppression rates of inpatients with or without melancholic features; the rates were 38% versus 33% respectively (p=0.74) The DST non-suppression rate for non-melancholic outpatients (n=138) was 12%. Using a cut off for DST non-suppression of ≥15 ug/dL, Schatzberg et al., (1983) improved on the specificity (93%) but, not on the sensitivity (50%) of DST. Rothschild et al., (1982) demonstrated that the DST distinguished PMD from schizophrenia; the DST non-suppression rate for PMD was 57% and 0% for psychotic schizophrenics. The dysregulation of the HPA-axis is a state rather than a trait phenomenon. There is normalization of the HPA-axis with treatment (Carroll et al., 1981). Using the combined DST and corticotropic releasing hormone (CRH) infusion test, Kunugi et al. (2006) reported significant decreases in ACTH (p=.007) and cortisol (p=.002) levels with response to treatment in patients with PMD.

The mechanism for the hyperactivity of the HPA-axis is based on studies that suggest glucocorticoid-mediated feedback impairment at the level of the pituitary and hypothalamus. (de Kloet et al.,1998; Young et al., 1991) Specifically, glucocorticoid receptors are located in the cytoplasm of cells and consist of two types, GR I and GR II. The GR I receptors are the high affinity receptors for endogenous glucocorticoids and are responsible for the diurinal regulation of cortisol; whereas, the GR II receptors are the low affinity glucocorticoid receptors and are important when cortisol levels are high, such as in stress or depression. It is hypothesized that, in depression, there is an impairment in the translocation of the glucocorticoid receptor from the cytoplasm into the nucleus; once activated by cortisol, the glucocorticoid receptor translocates in to the nucleus to complete the feedback by binding to DNA. (Figure 4; adapted) (Parionte and Miller, 2001; adapted) Interestingly,

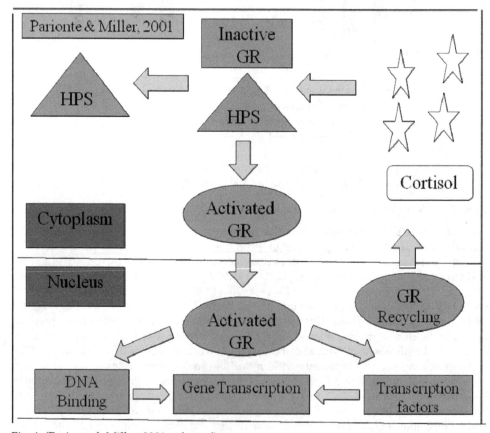

Fig. 4. (Parionte & Miller, 2001; adapted)

preclinical studies have shown that serotonin re-uptake blockers (SSRIs) and tricyclic antidepressants (TCAs) facilitate the translocation of the activated glucocorticoid receptors from the cytoplasm to the nucleus. Parionte and Miller (2001) suggest that this mechanism may provide one possible explanation for how treatment with antidepressants results in normalization of the HPA-axis hyperactivity in patients with depression.

While there was research focusing on HPA-axis dysregulation, there was another line of research evaluating dopamine (DA) activity in PMD versus NPMD. Previous studies have shown that CSF levels of a metabolite of DA, homvanillic acid (HVA), are low in patients with NPMD. (Sher et al., 2006; Reddy et al., 1992) However, Rothschild et al., (1987) showed that DA plasma levels are elevated in PMD, but not in NPMD. Others have shown that HVA is elevated in blood and CSF in PMD, but not in NPMD. (Sweeney et al., 1978; Aberg-Wistedt et al., 1985) The relationship between the findings of HPA-axis dysregulation and elevated DA in PMD was realized by Langlais et al., (1984; 1985) and others (Wolkowiz et al., 1986; Rothschild et al., 1984, 1987; Banki et al., 1983) who showed that glucocorticoids can increase DA in rat brain and human plasma and increase HVA in rat brain and human CSF. Based on these findings, Schatzberg and Rothschild hypothesized that psychotic symptoms in depression were secondary to the effects of hypercortisolemia on DA systems. (Schatzberg & Rothschild, 1992; Schatzberg et al.,1985) Maguire et al., (1987) showed a positive correlation between plasma free HVA and post dexamethasone log plasma cortisol levels ($r=0.59$; $p=0.02$).

7. Treatment straegies for PMD

The observations that DA activity is elevated in PMD have provided the rationale for the findings that antipsychotic medications significantly improve response rates when combined with antidepressant medications. Spiker et al., (1985) carried out one of the first randomized, double-blind prospective studies. Patients were randomized to amitriptyline monotherapy, perphenazine monotherapy, or combined amitriptyline plus perphenazine over a 5 week period; the response rates were 41% (7/17), 19% (3/16), and 78% (14/18) respectively. These results established the standard of practice of using combined antidepressant and antipsychotic medications for the treatment of PMD from that point forward. With the introduction of SSRIs, SNRIs, atypical antidepressants and atypical antipsychotic medications, there have been new treatment strategies using SSRI or SNRI monotherapy, atypical antipsychotic monotherapy, or atypical antipsychotic medications combined with an SSRI, or SNRI. In a series of 6-week treatment studies of PMD using SSRI or SNRI monotherapy, Gatti et al., (1996) and Zanardi et al., (1996;2000) showed high remission rates with fluvoxamine (84%), sertraline (72%), and venlafaxine (50%). In addition, Zanardi et al., (1997), in a 30 month, maintenance, open study of fluvoxamine remitters, found a relapse rate of only 20%. However, these studies lacked a control group and a validated instrument for the identification of psychosis.(Rothschild & Phillips, 1999) In addition, there has been no replication of these results. In an 8-week open study comparing the efficacy of sertraline monotherapy in PMD (n=25) versus NPMD (n=25)), Simpson et al., (2003) found remission rates of 16% and 64% in patients with PMD and NPMD respectively (p=.001).

The atypical antipsychotics block both 5-HT2 and DA receptors, which, theoretically, make them potential candidates for treating both depression and psychosis. There was a series of case reports and small open studies in the 1990's suggesting that atypical antipsychotic monotherapy was effective in treatment resistant PMD. (Ranyan and Meltzer, 1996; Dassa et al., 1993; Lane and Chang 1998; Hillert et al., 199) To test the efficacy of atypical antipsychotic monotherapy, Muller-Siecheneder et al., (1998) compared the efficacy of risperidone monotheray (n=16) versus the combination of haloperidol and amitriptyline (n=18) in the treatment of PMD. Both arms of the study showed improvement in depression and psychosis, but combined treatment was significantly better than monotherapy on scores for depression, BRMES, (p=.002) and psychosis, BPRS, (p=.016) More recent studies also support the value of combined atypical antipsychotic and antidepressant medications over atypical antipsychotic monotherapy. Rothschild et al., (2004) reported on two identical parallel trials where PMD patients were randomized to combined olanzapine/fluoxetine (OFC), olanzapine monotherapy (OLAN), or placebo (PLB); the HAM-D-24 response rates were 63.6%, 34.9%, and 28% respectively in Trial 1. Olanzapine/fluoxetine response rates were significantly higher than OLAN monotherapy (p=.027) and PLB (=.004). There were no significant differences among the three arms in Trial 2. (Figure 5)

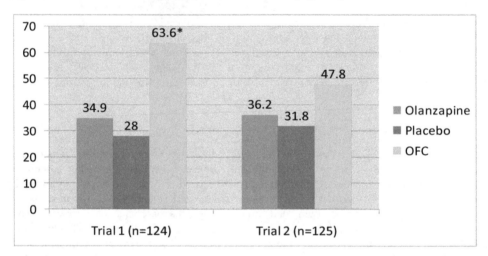

Fig. 5. (Rothschild et al., 2004; adapted) 8-Week Randomized Trial Olanzapine vs. OFC vs. PI (HAM-D-24 Response Rates - Trial: 1 OFC vs. Olan *p=.027; OFC vs. Pl p=.004)

The only other randomized clinical trial comparing combined atypical antipsychotic/antidepressant with atypical antipsychotic monotherapy was the STOP-PD study, A National Institutes of Mental Health funded, multi-center study, reported by Meyers et al., (2009). (Figure 6)

In the STOP-PD study, patients were randomized to olanzapine plus sertraline (OLAN/SERT) (n=129) or olanzapine plus placebo (OLAN/PLB) (n=130) and treatment was continued for 12 weeks. The OLAN/SERT group remission rate separated from the remission rate for the OLAN/PLB group at week-8; the remission rate for OLAN/SERT continued to be significantly better than the remission rate for the OLAN/PLB group through week-12 (Hochberg α level of .05 from χ2 analysis). Remission rates at last assessments were 41.9% and 23.9% for the OLAN/SERT and OLAN/PLB groups respectively. There is only one randomized controlled study comparing combined atypical antipsychotic and antidepressant medications with antidepressant monotherapy. Wijkstra et al., (2010a), in a 7-week trial, randomized patients to combined quetiapine plus venlafaxine

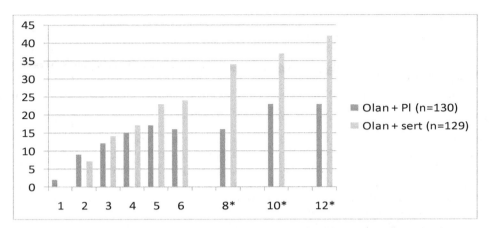

Fig. 6. (Meyer et al., 2009; adapted) STOP-PD: Remission for Olan + Sertraline vs. Olan + Placebo (* Hochberg α level of .05 from χ2 analysis)

(QUET/VEN) (n=42), venlafaxine monotherapy (VEN) (n=39), or impramine monotherapy (IMI) (n=41). There were no significant differences among the three groups with regards to remission rates. However, there was a significant difference with regards to HAM-D-17 response rates (response rate=50% reduction in HAM-D-17 from baseline and HAM-D-17 score at endpoint of ≤14) between QUET/VEN versus VEN (RD=32.5{95%CI:11.8; 53.2) at week-7. Based on these four randomized controlled studies, combined treatment with an atypical antipsychotic medication with an antidepressant is recommended. There have been no randomized controlled studies with the partial dopamine agonist, aripiprazole. In an open study, Matthews et al., (2009) published the first study combining aripiprazole with the SSRI, escitalopram. (Figure 7) Patients on this combination treatment showed remission rates of 42% by week-4 and 50% by week-7. Matthews et al., (2009) suggested that this rapid response may be due to the possibility that the SSRI, escitalopram, augmented the antipsychotic effect of aripiprazole through the established relationship of raphe nucleus serotonin inhibitory activity on ventral tegmental area dopamine cells and the possible augmentation of escitalopram by aripiprazole through 5HT2A blocking.

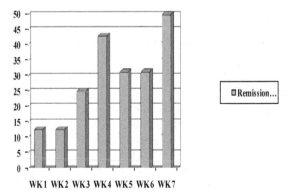

Fig. 7. (Matthews et al., 2009; adapted) PMD Remission Times: Aripiprazole/Escitalopram

Studies by Rothschild et al., (1999) and Kaiya et al., (1990) suggest that atypical antipsychotics are superior to typical antipsychotic medications for the treatment of PMD based on efficacy and time to response. Based on current findings, the ideal treatment for PMD might be the combination of an atypical antipsychotic with either an SSRI or SNRI; however, there needs to be a head-to-head trial comparing an SSRI or SNRI with a norepinephrine uptake blocker in combination with an atypical antipsychotic medication in order to validate this hypothesis. (Matthews, et al., 2009)

Recent research has used a novel approach for the treatment of PMD by targeting the HPA-axis hyperactivity associated with PMD. (Thakore & Dinan, 1995) There have been two strategies, inhibition of cortisol synthesis and blockade of the GR II receptors with antagonists. In a 4-week randomized, double blind, placebo controlled study of 20 medication –free NPMD patients, eight of whom had elevated cortisol levels, Wolkowitz et al., (1999) randomized patients to ketoconazole (400-800 mg/d) or placebo for 4 weeks. Ketoconazole was associated with improvements in depression ratings only in those patients with elevated cortisols. Forty-eight percent of ketoconazole treated hypercortisolemic patients showed a significant drop in HAM-D-21 compared to 6.6% of the placebo group (p<.03). In preclinical studies, mifepristone has been shown to be an antagonist at the GR II receptor. (de Kloet et al., 1998) This finding has lead to a series of studies assessing the efficacy and safety of mifepristone (RU486) in the treatment of PMD. Early studies by Belanoff et al., (2001, 2002) and Simpson et al., (2003) (Figure 8) demonstrated improvement in both depression and psychosis in a dose dependent manner.

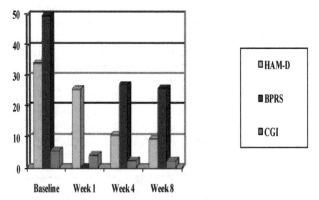

Fig. 8. (Simpson et al., 2005 adapted)   Mifepristone: N=20; 6-week course; open-label; LOCF

However, more recent studies point to psychosis as the primary target of response. (DeBattista et al., 2006) Blasey et al., (2009), in a multi-site study (n=29), 56 day, placebo controlled study, demonstrated a rapid reduction in the Brief Psychiatric Rating Scale-Positive Symptoms Subscale (BPRS-PSS) in only 7 days with mifepristone compared to placebo; response rates were defined as a 50% reduction in BPRS-PSS from baseline at both days 7 and 56. BPRS-PSS response rate was determined by mifepristone plasma level. (Figure 9)

Patients with mifepristone plasma levels ≥1800 ng/ml were more likely to respond than patients on placebo; however, there were differences in responses between the original 20 research sites versus the 9 added research sites (Intent-to-treat: OR=2.4, p=.03; Initial sites: OR=4.1, p=.002).

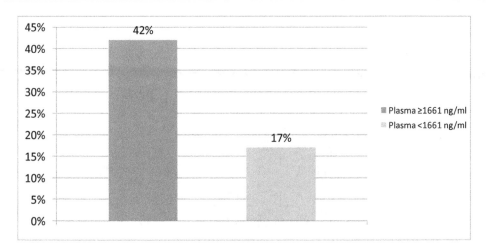

Fig. 9. (Blasey et al., 2009; adapted) Mifepristone: BPRS-PSS Response Rate at Days 7 and 56 (50% ↓ from Baseline; p=.018) (n=207)

Electroconvulsive therapy has been shown to be very effective in treating both neurovegetative symptoms of depression and psychosis. In an early review by Solan et al., (1988) they concluded that ECT response rates in PMD were not significantly different than the response rates in NPMD. However, two more recent studies have shown that the presence of psychosis is a predictor of ECT response in major depressive disorder. Petrides et al., (2001) found that completer remission rates for PMD (n=77) versus NPMD (n=176) were 95% and 83% respectively. Figure 10)

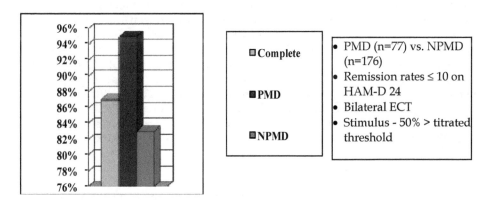

Fig. 10. (Petrides et al., 2001,adapted) ECT Remission Rates in Psychotic vs. Nonpsychotic MDD

In an European study, Birkenhager et al., (2003) found response rates of 92% and 55% in delusional depression versus non delusional depression respectively; remission rates were 57% and 24% respectively. (Figure 11)

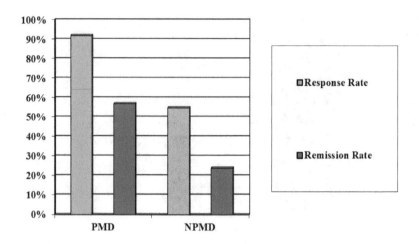

Fig. 11. (Birkenhager et al., 2003; adapted) ECT Response in Delusional vs. Non-delusional Depressed Inpatients

There is no evidence that psychotherapy alone is effective in the treatment of PMD as is the case for mild to moderate NPMD outpatients. (Rush et al., 1977) Gaudiano and Herbert (2006) combined Acceptance and Commitment Therapy (ACTto enhanced treatment as usual (ETAU) (n=19) versus ETAU (n=21) in an inpatient populations of PMD. Acceptance and Commitment Therapy focuses on acceptance of one's distress rather than ruminating about contributing factors from the past and/or worries about future negative predictions, both of which are out of one's absolute control. Acceptance allows one to observe one's distress as an opportunity to learn and thus improve problem solving. Acceptance also enables one to proceed with achieving value-based goals; thus, with acceptance, value-based goals can be achieved in spite of one's distress. Gaudiano and Herbert taught patients to accept their psychotic symptoms without judgment and to proceed with achieving their value-based goals. For their primary outcome measure, they found that 44% of ACT+ETAU versus 0% of ETAU had a ≥ 2 standard deviation improvement at discharge from baseline on total BPRS ($\chi 2=5.14$, p<.05). In addition, there were no significant differences in change scores from baseline to discharge between the two groups on the BPRS-PSS subscale, but the percent change scores on the BPRS mood subscale from baseline to discharge for ACT+ETAU versus ETAU were 70% and 30% respectively ($\chi 2=3.60$, p=.058).

8. Longitudinal course of PMD

Patients with PMD have a more severe course to their illness compared to patients with NPMD. At one year follow-up, patients with PMD were more likely to be in an episode, had significantly higher numbers of episodes, and psychiatric hospitalizations. (Robinson and Spiker, 1985) Data from the Epidemiology Catchment Area (ECA) study found that patients with PMD, compared with NPMD, have significantly greater impairment in functioning as measured by percent on public assistance (17.5% of PMD; 7.2%of NPMD) and on disability (15.9% of PMD; 6.7% of NPMD). (Johnson et al., 1991) As with schizophrenia and bipolar disorder, PMD is associated with higher rates of morbidity and mortality from medical conditions. Vythilingam et al., (2003) found that the mortality rate was two-fold higher for PMD versus NPMD and that 88% of the deaths were due to medical disorders.

In a 10-year prospective study, Coryell, et al., (1996) found that patients with PMD spent more weeks in full major depressive disorder than patients with NPMD. (Figure 12)

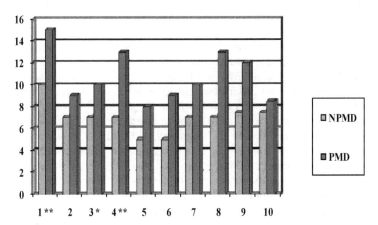

Fig. 12. (Coryell et al., 1996; adapted) Number of Weeks in Full Major Depression (10 YEARS) (*p < .05; **p < .01)

They also found that the recovery period was significantly prolonged with PMD versus NPMD. The percents of patients who had not recovered from their index episodes of PMD versus NPMD were 36.4% versus 28.2% at year-1 (p<.05), 19.7% versus 7.8% at year- 5 (p<.001), and 14.3% versus 4.6% at year-10 (p<.001) respectively. However, when compared to schizophrenia, Tsaung and Coryell, (1992) showed that recovery rates from index psychotic episodes were significantly better for PMD versus schizophrenia: 54% versus 4% at year-1, 75% versus 18% at year- 5; and 75% versus 21% at year-8 respectively (Wilcoxon $\chi 2$=15.4, df=1, p<0.0001). Wijkstra et al., (2010b) showed that remission rates continue to improve by 27.5% over a 4-month continuation of the same medications that resulted in meeting criteria for response at week-7. Thus, for patients who have responded partially, but have not achieved remission, continuation of treatment for another few months may provide added benefit.

As noted above, PMD is a highly relapsing disorder. Aaronson et al., (1988) reported on a 3-year retrospective study of 52 PMD inpatients who had achieved remission by discharge. Forty-five of the 52 patients (86%) relapsed over the 3-year period following discharge. There were 98 episodes of relapse among the 45 patients who relapsed. Eight-two (82.5%) of the 98 episodes occurred within the first year after discharge from inpatient treatment. Seventy-one (86%) of the first year relapses occurred with patients on no antipsychotic medications or tapering doses of antipsychotic medications. Twenty-nine (41%) of the 71 relapses associated with antipsychotic medications changes occurred despite stable doses of antidepressants. The relapse rate for patients on stable doses of antidepressant and antipsychotic medications during year-1 was 13.4%. In addition, 42% of the first year relapses occurred in the first 3-month period of discontinuation or decrease in dose of antipsychotic medications. Aronson et al., (1988) concluded that combined treatment with antipsychotic and antidepressant medications beyond the first year of recovery is recommended. Coryell, et al., (1996) reported on the percent of PMD patients on antidepressant and antipsychotic medications at the time of first relapse after achieving remission. They found 48 % were on antidepressant but only 20% were on antipsychotic medications.

There have been few accessible guidelines available for clinicians to use in deciding maintenance treatment of PMD. In a survey of 304 practicing clinicians, who were attending a psychopharmacology course sponsored by the Department of Psychiatry at Massachusetts General Hospital in 2001, Matthews, (2001) queried clinicians as to whether they continued their PMD patients on antidepressant and antipsychotic medications beyond 12 months after they achieved remission. Fifty-six percent of the clinicians indicated that they continued antidepressant medications beyond 12 months, whereas, only 16% reported that they continued antipsychotic medications beyond 12 months. Rothschild and Duval, (2003) provided potential guidelines for clinical decision making regarding maintenance treatment for PMD. They reported on 40 patients diagnosed with PMD who had achieved remission after 5 weeks of acute treatment with the combination of perphenazine plus fluoxetine. These patients were continued on the combination treatment for an additional 4 months; at the end of the 4-month continuation phase, they were tapered off perphenazine and continued on fluoxetine monotherapy for an additional 8 months of maintenance treatment. There were no relapses during the 4-month continuation phase; however, 8 (27%) of the 30 patients who continued into the maintenance phase relapsed. Rothschild and Duval reported that the predictors of relapse included a longer index episode, a history of more frequent episodes, an earlier age of onset of PMD, and less than 30 years of age at index episode. In the recent STOP-PD study, Andreescu et al., (2007) reported on the adequacy of pharmacological treatment on the first 100 patients at study entry. The rates of adequate or high doses of antidepressants, antipsychotics, and combined antidepressant/antipsychotic medications were 48%, 6%, and 5% respectively.

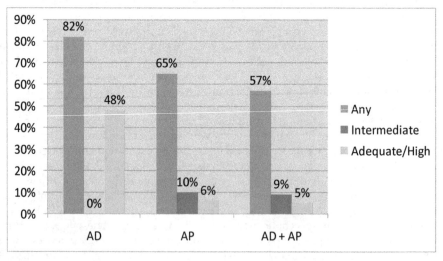

Fig. 13. (Andreescu et al., 2007; adapted) STOP-PD: Adequate Pharmacological Treatment on Study Entry (n=100)

(Figure 13) Interestingly, these finding are comparable with results reported by Mulsant et al. (1997), who found that only 4% (2/53) of PMD patients referred for ECT received an adequate medication trial, whereas 52% (70/134) of NPMD patients received an adequate medication trial. In addition, 47% (25/53) of PMD received either no antipsychotic medication or the duration treatment with an antipsychotic medication was for less than three weeks. Only 15% received antipsychotic doses greater than 200 mg daily of chlorpromazine equivalents. Thus, it appears that prescribing practices for PMD had not changed significantly for the 10- year period from 1997 to 2007. (Figure 14) Unfortunately, there have been very few acute and long-term clinical trials for the treatment of PMD compared with NPMD, bipolar disorder, or schizophrenia; thus, there is minimal data available to serve as a guideline for practicing clinicians.

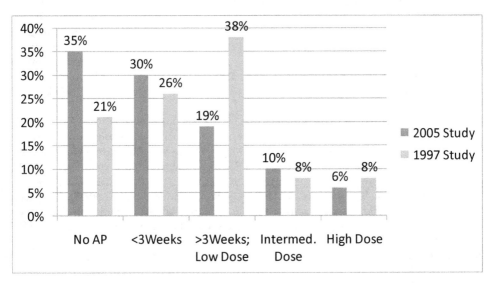

Fig. 14. (Andreescu et al., 2007; adapted) STOP-PD: % Receiving Adequate Antipsychotics at Study Entry in 2005 vs. 1997

9. Conclusions

Combined antidepressant and antipsychotic treatment continues to be the standard for acute and maintenance treatment of PMD. Selective Serotonin Reuptake Inhibitor monotherapy may be effective in treating PMD during the acute, continuation, and maintenance phases; however, there advantage may be in helping to augment atypical antipsychotic medications in treating psychotic symptoms, but further studies are required. Atypical antipsychotics in combination with SSRIs may increase the response rate and decrease the time to response. SSRIs may augment atypical antipsychotics by inhibiting DA cells and atypical antipsychotics may augment SSRIs by blocking 5HT 2A receptors; however, studies are needed to support these hypotheses. Preliminary data suggests mifepristone, a glucocorticoid receptor antagonist, treats psychotic symptoms in PMD rapidly and the response has durability beyond discontinuation of the drug after only 7 days of treatment. Psychotic features in major depressive disorder predict response to ECT.

Psychotic major depression is a highly relapsing illness with a long recovery period, therefore, long-term prophylactic treatment with combined antidepressant and an antipsychotic medications is recommended.

10. References

Aberg-Wistedt, A., Wistedt, B., Bertilsson, L., Higher (1985). Higher CSF Levels of HVA and 5-HIAA in Delusional Compared to Nondelusional Depression (letter). Arch Gen Psychiatry, Vol. 42 (1985), pp. 925-926, ISSN 0003-990X.

Akiskal, H.S., Walker, P., Puzantian, V.R., et al (1983). Bipolar Outcome in the Course of Depressive Illness: Phenomenological, Familial, and Pharmacologic Predictors. *Journal of Affective Disorders*, Vol. 5 (1983), pp. 115-128, ISSN 0165-0327.

American Psychiatric Association. (1994). *Diagnostic and Statistical Manual of Mental Disorders* (4th edition), American Psychiatric Association, ISBN 0890420645, Washington, DC.

Andreescu, C., Mulsant, B.H., Peasley-Micklus, C., et al (2007). The Study of Pharmacotherapy of Psychotic Depression (STOP-PD) Collaborative Study Group: Persisting Low Use of Antipsychotics in the Treatment of Major Depressive Disorder with Psychotic Features. Journal of Clinical Psychiatry, Vol. 68 (2007), pp. 194-200.

Andreescu, C., Mulsant, B.H., Peasley-Miklus, C., Rothschild, A.J., Flint, A.J., Heo, M., Caswell, M., Whyte, E.M. & Meyers, B.S. (2007). Persisting Low Use of Antipsychotics in the Treatment of Major Depressive Disorder with Psychotic Features. *Journal of Clinical Psychiatry*, Vol.68, No.2, (February 2007), pp. 194-200, ISSN 0160-6689

Aronson, T.A., Shukla, S., Gujavarty, K., Hoff, A., DiBuono, M. & Khan, E. (1988). Relapse in Delusional Depression: a Retrospective Study of the Course of Treatment. *Comprehensive Psychiatry*, Vol.29, No.1, (January-February 1988), pp. 12-21, ISSN 0010-440X

Banki, C.M., Arato, M., Papp, Z. (1983). Cerebrospinal Fluid Biochemical Examinations: Do They Reflect Clinical or Biological Differences? Biological Psychiatry, Vol. 18 (1983), pp. 1033-1044, ISSN 0006-3223.

Belanoff, J.K., Flores, B.H., Kalezhan, M., Sund, B. & Schatzberg, A.F. (2001). Rapid Reversal of Psychotic Depression Using Mifepristone. *Journal of Clinical Psychopharmacology*, Vol.21, No.5, (October 2001), pp. 516-521, ISSN 0271-0749

Belanoff, J.K., Rothschild, A.J., Cassidy, F., DeBattista, C., Baulieu, E.E., Schold, C. & Schatzbert, A.F. (2002). An Open Label Trial of C-1074 (Mifepristone) for Psychotic Major Depression. Biological Psychiatry, Vol.52, No.5, (September 2002), pp. 386-392, ISSN 0006-3223

Birkenhager, A.K., Pluijms, E.M. & Lucius, S.A.P. (2003). ECT Response in Delusional versus Non-Delusional Depressed Inpatients. *Journal of Affective Disorders*, Vol.74, No.2, (April 2003), pp. 191-195, ISSN 0165-0327

Blasey, C.M., DeBattista, C., Roe, R., Block, T. & Belanoff, J.K. (2009). A Multisite Trial of Mifepristone for the Treatment of Psychotic Depression: A Site-by-Treatment Interaction. *Contemporary Clinical Trials*, Vol.30, No.4, (July 2009), pp. 284-288, ISSN 1551-7144

Bond, T.C., Rothschild, A.J., Lerbinger, J., et al (1986). Delusional Depression, Family, History, and DST Response: A Pilot Study. Biological Psychiatry, Vol. 21 (1986), pp. 1239-1246, ISSN 0006-3223.

Brown, W.A., Keitner, G., Qualls, C.B., Haier, R. (1985). The Dexamethasone Suppression Test and Pituitary-adrenocortical Function. Arch Gen Psychiatry, Vol. 42, No. 2 (February 1985), pp. 121-3, ISSN 0003-990X.

Brown, G.W., Harris, T.O., Hepworth, C (1994). Life Events and Endogenous Depression: A Puzzle Re-examined. Arch Gen Psychiatry, Vol. 51, No. 7 (Jul 1994), pp. 525-34, 0003-990X.

Burch, E., Anton, R., Carson, W. (1994). Mood Congruent and Incongruent Psychotic Depressions: Are They the Same? Journal of Affective Disorders, Vol. 31 (1994), pp. 275-280, ISSN 0165-0327.

Carroll, B.J., Feinburg, M., Greden, J.F., Tarika, J., Albala, A.A., Haskett, R.F., James, N.M., Kronfol, Z., Lohr, N., Steiner, M., de Vigne, J.P., Young, E. (1981). A Specific Laboratory Test for the Diagnosis of Melancholia: Standardization, Validation, and Clinical Utility. Arch Gen Psychiatry, Vol. 38, No. 1 (January 1981), pp. 15-22.

Coryell, W., Leon, A., Winokur, G., Endicott, J., Keller, M., Akiskal, H. & Slomon, D. (1996). Importance of Psychotic Features to Long-Term Course in Major Depressive Disorder. American Journal of Psychiatry, Vol.153, No.4, (April 1996), pp. 483-489, ISSN 0002-953X

Craig, S.P., Buckle, V.J., Lamouroux, A., et al (1998). Dopamine Beta-Hydroxylase: Two Polymorphisms in Linkage Disequilibrium at the Structural Gene DBH Associate with Biochemical Phenotypic Variation. Human Genetics, Vol. 102 (1998), pp. 533-540, ISSN 0301-0171.

Dassa, D., Kaladjian, A., Azorin, J.M. & Giudicelli, S. (1993). Clozapine in the Treatment of Psychotic Refractory Depression. British Journal of Psychiatry, Vol.163, (December 1993), pp. 822-824, ISSN 0007-1250

DeBattista, D., Belanoff, J., Glass, S., Khan, A., Horne, R.L., Blasey, C., Carpenter, L.L. & Alva, G. (2006). Mifepristone versus Placebo in the Treatment of Psychosis in Patients with Psychotic Major Depression. Biological Psychiatry, Vol.60, No.12, (December 2006), pp. 1343-1349, ISSN 0006-3223

De Kloet, E.R., Vreugdenhil, E., Oitzl, M.S., Joels, M. (1998). Brain Corticosteroid Receptor Balance in Health and Disease. Endocrine Reviews, Vol. 19, No. 3 (1998), pp. 269-301, ISSN 0163-769X.

Dubovsky, S.L. & Thomas, M. (1992). Psychotic Depression: Advances in Conceptualization and Treatment. Hospital and Community Psychiatry, Vol.43, No.12, (December 1992), pp. 1189-1198, ISSN 0022-1597

Fleming, S.K., Blasey, C., Schatzberg, A.F. (2004). Neuropsychological Correlates of Psychotic Features in Major Depressive Disorders: a Review and Meta-Analysis. Journal of Psychiatric Research, Vol. 38 (2004), pp. 27-35, ISSN 0022-3956.

Frangos, E., Athanassenas, G., Tsitourides, P., Psilolignos, P. & Katsanou, N. (1983). Psychotic Depressive Disorder: A Separate Entity? Journal of Affective Disorders, Vol.5, No.3, (August 1983), pp. 259-265, ISSN 0165-0327

Gatti, F., Bellini, L., Gasperini, M., Perez, J.P., Zanardi, R. & Smeraldi, E. (1996). Fluvozamine Alone in the Treatment of Delusional Depression. American Journal of Psychiatry, Vol.153, No.3, (March 1996), pp. 414-416, ISSN 0002-953X

Glassman, A.H. & Roose, S.P. (1981). Delusional Depression: A Distinct Clinical Entity? *Archives of General Psychiatry*, Vol.38, No.4, (April 1981), pp. 424-427, ISSN 0003-990X

Gomez, R.G., Fleming, S.H., Keller, J., Flores, B., Kenna, H., DeBattista, C., Solvason, B., Schatzberg, A.F. (2006). The Neuropsychological Profile of Psychotic Major Depression and Its Relation to Cortisol. Biological Psychiatry, Vol. 60, No. 5 (February 2006), pp. 472-8, ISSN 0006-3223.

Guadiano, B.A. & Herbert, J.D. (2006). Acute Treatment of Inpatients with Psychotic Symptoms Using Acceptance and Commitment Therapy: Pilot Results. *Behaviour Research and Therapy*, Vol.44, No.3, (March 2006), pp. 415-437, ISSN 0005-7967

Hamilton, M. (1960). A Rating Scale for Depression. *Journal of Neurology, Neurosurgery, & Psychiatry*, Vol.23, No.1, (February 1960), pp. 56-62, ISSN 00223050

Hill, S.K., Keshavan, M.S., Thase, M.E., et al (2004). Neuropsychological Dysfunction in Antipsychotic-Naïve First-Episode Unipolar Psychotic Depression. *American Journal of Psychiatry*, Vol. 161 (2004), pp. 996-1003, ISSN 0002-953X.

Hillert, A., Maier, W., Wetzel, H. & Benkert, O. (1992). Risperidone in the Treatment of Disorders with a Combined Psychotic and Depressive Syndrome – A Functional Approach. *Pharmacopsychiatry*, Vol.25, No.5, (September 1992), pp. 213-217, ISSN 0176-3679

Johnson, J., Horwath, E., Weissman, M.M. (1991). The Validity of Major Depression with Psychotic Features Based on a Community Sample. Arch Gen Psychiatry, Vol. 48 (1991), pp. 1075-1081, ISSN 0003-990X.

Kaiya, H. & Takeda, N. (1990). Sulpiride in the Treatment of Delusional Depression. *Journal of Clinical Psychopharmacology*, Vol.10, No.2, (April 1990), pp. 147, ISSN 0271-0749

Keller, J., Gomez, R., Kenna, H., Poesner, J., DeBattista, C., Flores, B., Schatzberg, A. (2006). Detecting Psychotic Major Depression Using Psychiatric Rating Scales. Journal of Psychiatric Research, Vol. 40, Issue 1 (February 2006), pp. 22-29, ISSN 0022-3956.

Kunugi, H., Ida, I., Owashi, T., Kimura, M., Inoue, Y., Nakagawa, S., Yabana, T., Urushibara, T., Kanai, R., Aihara, M., Yuuki, N., Otsubo, T., Oshima, A., Kudo, K., Inoue, T., Kitaichi, Y., Shirakawa, O., Isogawa, K., Nagayama, H., Kamijima, K., Nanko, S., Kanba, S., Higuchi, T., Mikuni, M (2006). Assessment of the Dexamethasone/CRH Test as a State-Dependent Marker for Hypothalamic-Pituitary-Adrenal (HPA) Axis Abnormalities in Major Depressive Episode: A Multicenter Study. *Neuropsychopharmacology*, Vol. 31 (2006), pp. 212-220, ISSN 0893-133X.

Lane, H.Y. & Chang, W.H. (1998). Risperidone Monotherapy for Psychotic Depression Unresponsive to Other Treatments. *Journal of Clinical Psychiatry*, Vol.59, No.11, (November 1998), pp. 624, ISSN 0160-6689

Langlais P.J., Rothschild A.J., Schatzberg A.F., Cole J.O., Bird E.D. (1984). Dexamethasone Elevates Dopamine in Human Plasma and Rat Brain. *Psychopharmacol Bull.*, Vol. 20, No. 3 (Summer 1984), pp. 365-70, ISSN 0048-5764.

Maj, M., Pirozzi, R., Magliano, L., Fiorillo, A. & Bartoli, L. (2007). Phenomenology and Prognostic Significance of Delusions in Major Depressive Disorder: A 10-Year Prospective Follow-Up Study. *Journal of Clinical Psychiatry*, Vol.68, No.9, (September 2007), pp. 1411-1417, ISSN 0160-6689

Matthews, J.D., Bottonari, K.A., Polania, L.M., Mischoulon, D., Dording, C.M., Irving, R., Fava, M. (2002). An Open Study of Olanzapine and Fluoxetine for Psychotic Major

Depressive Disorder: Interim Analyses. *Journal of Clinical Psychiatry*, Vol. 63, No. 12 (December 2002), pp. 1164-70, ISSN 0160-6689.

Matthews, J.D., Siefert, C., Dording, C., Denninger, J.W., Park, L., van Nieuwenhuizen, A.O., Sklarsky, K., Hilliker, S., Homberger, C., Rooney, K., Fava, M. (2009). An Open Study of Aripiprazole and Escitalopram for Psychotic Major Depressive Disorder. *Journal of Clinical Psychopharmacology*, Vol. 29, No. 1 (February 2009), pp. 73-6, ISSN 0271-0749.

Matthews, J.D. (2010). Improvements in Cognitive Functioning During Inpatient Hospitalization for Unipolar and Bipolar Depression with and Without Psychotic Features. Poster Presentation, American Psychiatric Association Annual Meeting, New Orleans, LA, 2010.

Matthews, J.D. (2001). Psychotic Major Depression: Prescribing Practices – 304 Clinicians Surveyed. Unpublished Data (2001).

Meyers, B.S., Flint, A.J., Rothschild, A.J., Mulsant, B.H., Whyte, E.M., Peasley-Miklus, C., Papademetriou, E., Leon, A.C. & Heo, M. (2009). A Double-Blind Randomized Controlled Trial of Olanzapine Plus Sertraline versus Olanzapine Plus Placebo for Psychotic Depression. *Archives of General Psychiatry*, Vol.66, No.8, (August 2009), pp. 838-847, ISSN 0003-990X

Muller-Siecheneder, F., Muller, M.J., Hillert, A., Szegedi, A., Wetzel, H. & Benkert, O. (1998). Risperidone versus Haloperidol and Amitriptyline in the Treatment of Patients with a Combined Psychotic and Depressive Syndrome. *Journal of Clinical Psychopharmacology*, Vol.18, No.2, (April 1998), pp. 111-120, ISSN 0271-0749

Mulsant, B.H., Hasket, R.F., Prudic, J., Thase, M.E., Malone, K.M., Mann, J.J., Pettinatie, H.M. & Sackeim, H.A. (1997). Low Use of Neuroleptic Drugs in the Treatment of Psychotic Major Depression. *American Journal of Psychiatry*, Vol.154, No.4. (April 1997), pp. 559-561, ISSN 0002-953X

Nelson, J.C. & Davis, J.M. (1997). DST Studies in Psychotic Depression: A Meta-Analysis. *American Journal of Psychiatry*, Vol.154, No.11, (November 1997), pp. 1497-1503, ISSN 0002-953X

Ohayon, M.M. & Schatzberg, A.F. (2002). Prevalence of Depressive Episodes with Psychotic Features in the General Population. *American Journal of Psychiatry*, Vol.159, No.11, (November 2002), pp.1855-1861, ISSN 0002-953X

Pariante, C.M. & Miller, A.H. (2001). Glucocorticoid Receptors in Major Depression: Relevance to Pathophysiology and Treatment. *Biological Psychiatry*, Vol.49, No.5, (March 2001), pp. 391-404, ISSN 0006-3223

Petrides, G., Fink, M., Husain, M.M., Knapp, R.G., Rush, A.J., Mueller, M., Rummans, T.A., O'Connor, K.M., Rasmussen, K.G., Berstein, H.J., Biggs, M., Bailine, S.H. & Keller, C.H. (2001). ECT Remission Rates in Psychotic versus Nonpsychotic Depressed patients: A Report from CORE. *Journal of ECT*, Vol.4, No.4, (December 2001), pp. 244-253, ISSN 1095-0680

Ranyan, R. & Meltzer, H.Y. (1996). Acute and Long-Term Effectiveness of Clozapine in Treatment-Resistant Psychotic Depression. *Biological Psychiatry*, Vol.40, No.4, (August 1996), pp. 253-258, ISSN 0006-3223

Reddy, P.L., Khanna, S., Subhash, M.N., Channabasavanna, S.M., Sridhara Rama Rao, B.S (1992). CSF Amine Metabolites in Depression. *Biological Psychiatry*, Vol. 31, (1992), pp. 112-118, ISSN 0006-3223.

Robinson, D.G., Spiker, D.G. (1985). Delusional Depression: A One Year Follow-Up. *Journal of Affective Disorders*, Vol. 9 (1985), pp. 79-83, ISSN 0165-0327.

Rothschild, A., Langlais, P., Schatzberg, A., Walsh, F., Cole, J., Bird, E. (1984). Dexamethasone Increases Plasma Free Dopamine in Man. *Journal of Psychiatric Research*, Vol. 18, No. 3 (1984), pp. 217-223, ISSN 0022-3956.

Rothschild, A.J., Bates, K.S., Boehringer, K.L. & Syed, A. (1999). Olanzapine Response in Psychotic Depression. *Journal of Clinical Psychiatry*, Vol.60, No.2, (February 1999), pp. 116-118, ISSN 0160-6689

Rothschild, A.J. & Phillips, K.A. (1999). Selective Serotonin Reuptake Inhibitors and Delusional Depression. *American Journal of Psychiatry*, Vol.156, No.6, (June 1999), pp. 977-978, ISSN 0002-953X

Rothschild, A.J. & Duval, S.E. (2003). How Long Should Patients with Psychotic Depression Stay on the Antipsychotic Medication? *Journal of Clinical Psychiatry*, Vol.64, No.4, (April 2003), pp. 390-396, ISSN 0160-6689

Rothschild, A.J., Schatzberg, A.F., Langlais, P.J., Lerbinger, J.E., Miller, M.M., Cole, J.O (1987). Psychotic and Nonpsychotic Depressions: I. Comparison of Plasma Catecholamines and Cortisol Measures. *Psychiatry Res*, Vol. 20, No. 2, (Feb 1987), pp. 143-53, ISSN 0165-1781.

Rothschild, A.J., Schatzberg, A.F., Rosenbaum, A.H., et al (1982). The Dexamethasone Suppression Test as a Discriminator Among Subtypes of Psychotic Patients. British Journal of Psychiatry, Vol. 141 (1982), pp. 471-474, ISSN 0007-1250.

Rothschild, A.J., Williamson, D.J., Tohen, M.F., Schatzberg, A., Andersen, S.W., Van Campen, L.E., Sanger, T.M. & Tollefson, G.D. (2004). A Double-Blind, Randomized Study of Olanzapine and Olanzapine/Fluoxetine Combination for Major Depression with Psychotic Features. *Journal of Clinical Psychopharmacology*, Vol.24, No.4, (August 2004), pp. 365-373, ISSN 0271-0749

Rothschild, A.J., Winer, J., Flint, A.J., Mulsant, B.H., Whyte, E.M., Heo, M., Fratoni, S., Gabriele, M., Kasapinovic, S. & Meyers, B.S. (2008). Missed Diagnosis of Psychotic Depression at 4 Academic Medical Centers. *Journal of Clinical Psychiatry*, Vol.69, No.8, (August 2008), pp. 1293-1296, ISSN 0160-6689

Rothschild, AJ (2009). Clinical Manual for Diagnosis and Treatment of Psychotic Depression, American Psychiatric Association ISBN 978-1-58562-292-4, Washington, DC.

Rush, A.J., Beck, A.T., Kovacs, M., Hollon, S. (1977). Comparative Efficacy of Cognitive Therapy and Pharmacotherapy in the Treatment of Depressed Outpatients. *Cognitive Therapy Research*, Vol. 1 (1997), pp. 17-37, ISSN 0147-5916.

Schatzberg, A. & Rothschild, A.J. (1992). Psychotic (Delusional) Major Depression: Should it be Included as a Distinct Syndrome in DSM-IV? *American Journal of Psychiatry*, Vol.149, No.6, (June 1992), pp. 733-745, ISSN 0002-953X

Schatzberg, A.F., Rothschild, A.J., Langlais, P.J., et al (1985). A Corticosteroid/Dopamine Hypothesis for Psychotic Depression and Related States. Journal Psychiatric Research, Vol. 19 (1985), pp. 57-64, ISSN 0022-3956.

Schatzberg, A.F., Rothschild, A.J., Stahl, J.B., Bond, T.C., Rosenbaum, A.H., Lofgen, S.B., MacLaughlin, R.A., Sullivan, M.A., Cole, J.O. (1983). The Dexamethasone Suppression Test: Identification of Subtypes of Depression. American Journal of Psychiatry, Vol. 140, No. 1 (January 1983), pp. 88-91.

Sher, L., Mann, J.J., Traskman-Bendz, L., Winchel, R., Huang, Y., Fertuck, E., Stanley, B. Lower Cerebrospinal Fluid Homovanillic Acid Levels in Depressed Suicide Attempters. *Journal of Affective Disorders*, Vol. 90, Iss. 1 (January 2006), pp. 83-89, ISSN 0165-0327.

Simpson, G.M., Sheshai, A., Rady, A., Kingsbury, S.J. & Fayek, M. (2003). Sertraline as Monotherapy in the Treatment of Psychotic and Nonpsychotic Depression. *Journal of Clinical Psychiatry*, Vol.64, No.8, (August 2003), pp. 959-965, ISSN 0160-6689

Solan, W.J., Khan, A., Avery, D.H. & Cohen, S. (1988). Psychotic and Nonpsychotic Depression: Comparison of Response to ECT. *Journal of Clinical Psychiatry*, Vol.49, No.3, (March 1988), pp. 97-99, ISSN 0160-6689

Spiker, D.G., Cofsky, W.J., Dealy, R.S., Griffin, S.J., Hanin, I., Neil, J.F., Perel, J.M., Rossi, A.J. & Soloff, P.H. (1985). The Pharmacological Treatment of Delusional Depression. *American Journal of Psychiatry*, Vol.142, No.4, (April 1985), pp. 430-436, ISSN 0002-953X

Strober, M., Carlson, G. (1982). Bipolar Illness in Adolescents with Major Depression: Clinical, Genetic, and Psychopharmacologic Predictors in a Three to Four Year Prospective Follow-Up Investigation. *Arch Gen Psychiatry*, Vol. 39 (1982), pp. 549-555, ISSN 0003-990X.

Sullivan, P., Kendler, K. (2001). Genetic Case-control Studies in Neuropsychiatry. *Arch Gen Psychiatry*, Vol. 58 (2001), pp. 1015-1024, ISSN 0003-990X.

Thakore, J.H. & Dinan, T.G. (1995). Cortisol Synthesis Inhibition: A New Treatment Strategy for the Clinical and Endocrine Manifestations of Depression. *Biological Psychiatry*, Vol.37, No.6, (March 1995), pp. 364-368, ISSN 0006-3223

Tsuang, D. & Coryell, W. (1993). An 8-Year Follow-Up of Patients with DSM-III-R Psychotic Depression, Schizoaffective Disorder, and Schizophrenia. *American Journal of Psychiatry*, Vol.150, No.8, (August 1993), pp. 1182-1188, ISSN 0002-953X

Vythilingam, M., Chen, J., Bremner, J.D., Mazure, C.M., Maciejewski, P., Nelson, J.C. (2003). Psychotic Depression and Mortality. *American Journal of Psychiatry*, Vol. 160, No. 3 (March 2003), pp. 574-576, ISSN 0002-953X.

Weissman, M.M., Prusoff, B.A., Merikangas, K.R. (1984). Is Delusional Depression Related to Bipolar Disorder? American Journal of Psychiatry, Vol. 141 (1984), pp. 892-893, ISSN 0002-953X.

Weissman, M.M., Warner, V., Prusoff, J.K., et al (1988). Delusional Depression and Bipolar Sepctrum: Evidence for a Possible Association From a Family Study of Children. *Neuropsychopharmacology*, Vol. 1 (1988), pp. 257-264.

Wijkstra, J., Burger, H., van den Broek, W.W., Birkenhager, T.K., Janzing, J.G.E., Boks, M.P.M., Bruijn, J.A., van der Loos M.L.M., Breteler, L.M.T., Ramaekers, G.M.G.I., Verkes, R.J. & Nolen, W.A. (2010a). Treatment of Unipolar Psychotic Depression: A Randomized, Double-Blind Study Comparing Imipramine, Venlafaxine, and Venlafaxine Plus Quetiapine. *Acta Psychiatrica Scandinavica*, Vol.121, No.3, (March 2010), pp. 190-200, ISSN 0001-690X

Wijkstra, J., Burger, H., van den Broek, W.W., Birkenhager, T.K., Janzing, J.G.E., Boks, M.P.M., Bruijn, J.A., van der Loos M.L.M., Breteler, L.M.T., Verkes, R.J. & Nolen, W.A. (2010b). Long-Term Response to Successful Actue Pharmacological Treatment of Psychotic Depression. *Journal of Affective Disorders*, Vol.123, No.1-3, (June 2010), pp. 238-242, ISSN 0165-0327

Wolkowitz, O.M., Doran, A.R., Breier, A., Roy, A., Jimerson, D., Sutton, M., Golden, R., Paul, S., Pickar, D (1987). The Effects of Dexamethasone on Plasma Homovanillic Acid and 3-Methoxy-4-hydroxyphenylglycol. *Arch Gen Psychiatry*, Vol. 44 (Sept 1987), pp. 782-1017, ISSN 0003-990X.

Wolkowitz, O.M., Reus, V.I., Chan, T., Manfredi, F., Raum, W., Johnson, R. & Canick, J. (1999). Antiglucocorticoid Treatment of Depression: Double-Blind Ketoconazole. *Biological Psychiatry*, Vol.45, No.8, (April 1999), pp. 1070-1074, ISSN 0006-3223

Wood, J.G., Joyce, P.R., Miller, A.L., et al (2002). A Polymorphism in the Dopamine Beta-Hydroxyglase Gene is Associated with "Paranoid Ideation" in Patients with Major Depression. *Biological Psychiatry*, Vol. 51 (2002), pp. 365-376, ISSN 0002-3223.

Young, E.A., Haskett, R.F., Murphy-Weinberg, V., Watson, S.J. & Akil, H. (1991). Loss of Glucocorticoid Fast Feedback in Depression. *Archives of General Psychiatry*, Vol.48, No.8, (August 1991), pp. 693-699, ISSN 0003-990X

Zanardi, R., Franchini, L., Gasperini, M., Perez, J. & Smeraldi, E. (1996). Double-Blind Controlled Trial of Sertraline versus Paroxetine in the Treatment of Delusional Depression. *American Journal of Psychiatry*, Vol.153, No.12, (December 1996), pp. 1631-1633, ISSN 0002-953X

Zanardi, R., Franchini, L., Gasperini, M., Smeraldi, E. & Perez, J. (1997). Long-Term Treatment of Psychotic (Delusional) Depression with Fluvoxamine: And Open Pilot Study. *International Clinical Psychopharmacology*, Vol.12, No.4, (July 1997), pp. 195-197, ISSN 0268-1315

Zanardi, R., Franchini, L., Serretti, A., Perez, J. & Smeraldi, E. (2000). Venlafaxine versus Fluvoxamine in the Treatment of Delusional Depression: A Pilot Double-Blind Controlled Study. *Journal of Clinical Psychiatry*, Vol.61, No.1, (January 2000), pp. 26-29, ISSN 0160-6689

Permissions

The contributors of this book come from diverse backgrounds, making this book a truly international effort. This book will bring forth new frontiers with its revolutionizing research information and detailed analysis of the nascent developments around the world.

We would like to thank Prof. Dr. Luciano L'Abate, for lending his expertise to make the book truly unique. He has played a crucial role in the development of this book. Without his invaluable contribution this book wouldn't have been possible. He has made vital efforts to compile up to date information on the varied aspects of this subject to make this book a valuable addition to the collection of many professionals and students.

This book was conceptualized with the vision of imparting up-to-date information and advanced data in this field. To ensure the same, a matchless editorial board was set up. Every individual on the board went through rigorous rounds of assessment to prove their worth. After which they invested a large part of their time researching and compiling the most relevant data for our readers. Conferences and sessions were held from time to time between the editorial board and the contributing authors to present the data in the most comprehensible form. The editorial team has worked tirelessly to provide valuable and valid information to help people across the globe.

Every chapter published in this book has been scrutinized by our experts. Their significance has been extensively debated. The topics covered herein carry significant findings which will fuel the growth of the discipline. They may even be implemented as practical applications or may be referred to as a beginning point for another development. Chapters in this book were first published by InTech; hereby published with permission under the Creative Commons Attribution License or equivalent.

The editorial board has been involved in producing this book since its inception. They have spent rigorous hours researching and exploring the diverse topics which have resulted in the successful publishing of this book. They have passed on their knowledge of decades through this book. To expedite this challenging task, the publisher supported the team at every step. A small team of assistant editors was also appointed to further simplify the editing procedure and attain best results for the readers.

Our editorial team has been hand-picked from every corner of the world. Their multi-ethnicity adds dynamic inputs to the discussions which result in innovative outcomes. These outcomes are then further discussed with the researchers and contributors who give their valuable feedback and opinion regarding the same. The feedback is then collaborated with the researches and they are edited in a comprehensive manner to aid the understanding of the subject.

Apart from the editorial board, the designing team has also invested a significant amount of their time in understanding the subject and creating the most relevant covers. They scrutinized every image to scout for the most suitable representation of the subject and create an appropriate cover for the book.

The publishing team has been involved in this book since its early stages. They were actively engaged in every process, be it collecting the data, connecting with the contributors or procuring relevant information. The team has been an ardent support to the editorial, designing and production team. Their endless efforts to recruit the best for this project, has resulted in the accomplishment of this book. They are a veteran in the field of academics and their pool of knowledge is as vast as their experience in printing. Their expertise and guidance has proved useful at every step. Their uncompromising quality standards have made this book an exceptional effort. Their encouragement from time to time has been an inspiration for everyone.

The publisher and the editorial board hope that this book will prove to be a valuable piece of knowledge for researchers, students, practitioners and scholars across the globe.

List of Contributors

Vesna Švab
University Ljubljana, Slovenia

Adrian Furnham and Kate Telford
Research Department of Clinical, Educational and Health Psychology, University College London, UK

John E. Berg
Oslo and Akershus University College, Oslo, Norway

Aline Drapeau
Département de psychiatrie – Université de Montréal, Canada
Centre de recherche Fernand-Seguin – Hôpital Louis. H. Lafontaine, Canada
Département de médecine sociale et préventive – Université de Montréal, Canada

Alain Marchand
École de relations industrielles – Université de Montréal, Canada
Institut de recherche en santé publique – Université de Montréal, Canada

Dominic Beaulieu-Prévost
Département de sexologie – Université du Québec à Montréal, Canada

Arabinda Narayan Chowdhury
Northamptonshire Healthcare NHS Foundation Trust, Stuart Road Resource Centre, Corby Northants NN17 1RJ, UK

Javier Contreras
University of Costa Rica, Costa Rica

Śpila Bożena and Urbańska Anna
Department of Psychiatry Medical University of Lublin, Poland

Tsuyoshi Hattori, Shingo Miyata and Akira Ito
Taiichi Katayama and Masaya Tohyama, Osaka University, Japan

M. Dalvi
William Harvey Hospital, Ashford Kent, Kent &Medway NHS& Social Care Partnership Trust, Kent, UK

Monica Uddin
Center for Molecular Medicine and Genetics and Department of Psychiatry and Behavioral Neurosciences, Wayne State University, Detroit, MI, USA

Erin Bakshis and Regina de los Santos
Department of Epidemiology, University of Michigan School of Public Health, Ann Arbor, MI, USA Rosó

Rosó Duñó and Diego Palao
Parc Taulí University Hospital, Autonomous University of Barcelona, Spain

Klaus Langohr
Pharmacology Research Unit, Institut Municipal d'Investigació Mèdica, Barcelona, Spain
Department of Statistics and Operations Research, Technical University of Catalonia, Barcelona, Spain

Adolf Tobeña
Department of Psychiatry and Forensic Medicine, Institute of Neurosciences, Autonomous University of Barcelona, Spain

John Matthews
Harvard Medical School, USA